Neurobehavioral Aspects of Cerebrovascular Disease

Neurobehavioral Aspects of Cerebrovascular Disease

Edited by

ROBERT A. BORNSTEIN, Ph.D.

Associate Professor, Department of Psychiatry
Director, Neuropsychology Laboratory
Ohio State University, Columbus, Ohio

and

GREGORY G. BROWN, Ph.D.

Director, Cognitive Neuroscience Laboratory
Neuropsychology Division, Psychiatry Department
Henry Ford Hospital, Detroit, Michigan

New York Oxford
OXFORD UNIVERSITY PRESS
1991

Oxford University Press

Oxford New York Toronto
Delhi Bombay Calcutta Madras Karachi
Petaling Jaya Singapore Hong Kong Tokyo
Nairobi Dar es Salaam Cape Town
Melbourne Auckland

and associated companies in
Berlin Ibadan

Published by Oxford University Press, Inc.,
200 Madison Avenue, New York, New York 10016

Oxford is a registered trademark of Oxford University Press

Library of Congress Cataloging-in-Publication Data
Neurobehavioral aspects of cerebrovascular disease
edited by Robert A. Bornstein and Gregory G. Brown.
p. cm. Includes bibliographic references. Includes index.
ISBN 0-19-505431-8
1. Cerebrovascular disease—Diagnosis.
2. Neuropsychological tests.
I. Bornstein, Robert A. II. Brown, Gregory G.
[DNLM: 1. Brain—physiopathology.
2. Cerebrovascular Disorders—complications.
3. Cerebrovascular Disorders—psychology.
4. Neuropsychology.
WL 355 N494] RC388.5.N46 1991
616.8′1—dc20 DNLM/DLC
for Library of Congress
90-7381

9 8 7 6 5 4 3 2 1

Printed in the United States of America
on acid-free paper

To

Sandy B.
and
Sandy B.

Preface

The history of the study of brain behavior relationships is intimately linked with cerebral vascular disease. Contemporary concepts of localization of function derive in large part from work with patients who had focal cerebral vascular lesions. Broca, Wernicke, and others were the forerunners of twentieth century investigators of localized brain functions. In addition to anatomic localization, studies of patients with vascular lesions were instrumental in developing models of overall brain organization. More recently, studies of patients with focal vascular lesions have had an important role in the development of models of neurobehavioral functions. For example, reports by Goodglass, Geschwind, and others from the Boston VA Medical Center have helped define the neurological and anatomic correlates of language. Heilman and his colleagues at the University of Florida have used findings from patients with focal lesions to elucidate models of the apraxias and neglect syndromes. Many of the patients in these studies had cerebral vascular disease.

In addition to studying specific aspects of higher cognitive function, investigators have increasingly directed their attention to the neurobehavioral consequences of particular diseases. There is now a large body of literature documenting the behavioral correlates of such conditions as Alzheimer's disease, epilepsy, Huntington's disease, Parkinson's disease, and closed head injury. Consistent with the prominence of cerebral vascular disease in the history of the study of brain behavior relationships, it is noteworthy that one of the first volumes devoted to the behavioral aspects of a particular disease dealt with cerebral vascular disorders (Benton, 1970). It is now more than 20 years since that book was published, and the numerous technical and theoretical advances since then warrant a re-exploration of the neurobehavioral aspects of cerebral vascular disease.

Perhaps the most dramatic change to have occurred in the past 20 years has been the development of techniques for imaging brain structure and function. Computed axial tomography (CAT), magnetic resonance imaging (MRI), Xenon inhalation cerebral blood flow (CBF), positron emission tomography (PET), and single photon emission computed tomography (SPECT) have all been introduced since 1970. These and other emerging technologies will play an increasingly important role in the next decade in studies of the pathophysiology of cerebral vascular disease.

The first part of this book, therefore, describes some of the newer methods for studying brain structure and function, and reviews their contributions to an understanding of the consequences of stroke. The second part deals with the diverse behavioral effects of cerebral vascular disease. This section includes discussions of the cognitive and emotional sequelae of both ischemic and hemorrhagic stroke, as well as the relationship between stroke risk factors and cognitive deficit. The role of patients with focal lesions in building models of cognitive function is also covered. The third part concerns treatment and rehabilitation of stroke patients. The management and remediation of cognitive and language deficits, the mechanisms underlying recovery of function, and the potential impact of surgical interventions are discussed.

We would like to take this opportunity to express our appreciation to the contributors to this volume. In addition, we acknowledge the efforts and patience of our secretaries Janet Knauss, Jean Close, and Shirley Craley who prepared the numerous drafts of the book. We are particularly grateful for the support and editorial assistance provided by Jeffrey House at Oxford University Press. The preparation of this volume was supported in part by grants from the National Institute of Mental Health (MH42209 and MH45649, R.A.B.) and grants from the National Institute of Health (NS23393, G.G.B.).

Columbus, Ohio R. A. B.
Detroit, Michigan G. G. B.
December, 1990

Contents

II CLINICAL NEUROPSYCHOLOGY OF STROKE

III RECOVERY AND TREATMENT

Contributors

ANNE D. BAIRD
Staff Neuropsychologist
Neuropsychology Division
Psychiatry Department
Henry Ford Hospital
Detroit, Mich.

ARTHUR L. BENTON
Emeritus Professor of Psychology and Neurology
University of Iowa
Iowa City, Iowa

KAREN I. BOLLA
Assistant Professor of Neurology
Department of Neurology
The Johns Hopkins University School of Medicine
Baltimore, Md.

ROBERT A. BORNSTEIN
Associate Professor
Department of Psychiatry
Director, Neuropsychology Laboratory
Ohio State University
Columbus, Ohio

GREGORY G. BROWN
Director, Cognitive Neuroscience Laboratory
Neuropsychology Division
Psychiatry Department
Henry Ford Hospital
Detroit, Mich.

JEFFREY L. CUMMINGS
Director, Neurobehavior Unit
West Los Angeles Veterans Affairs Medical Center (Brentwood Division)
Associate Professor of Neurology Psychiatry, & Biobehavioral Sciences
UCLA School of Medicine
Los Angeles, Calif.

MICHAEL S. GAZZANIGA
Andrew W. Thompson Professor of Psychiatry (Neurosciences)
Program in Cognitive Neuroscience
Department of Psychiatry
Dartmouth Medical School
Hanover, N.H.

VLADIMIR HACHINSKI
Richard and Beryl Ivey Professor and Chairman
Department of Clinical Neurological Sciences
The University of Western Ontario
University Hospital
London, Ontario
Canada

JIM HOM
Director, Neuropsychology Laboratory
Department of Psychiatry
University of Texas Southwestern Medical School
Dallas, Tex.

MARK P. KELLY
Head Injury Unit
Montebello Hospital
Baltimore, Md.

DAVID KNOPMAN
Associate Professor of Neurology
Department of Neurology
University of Minnesota Hospitals
Minneapolis, Minn.

STEVEN R. LEVINE
Staff Neurologist
Department of Neurology
Center for Stroke Research
Henry Ford Hospital
Detroit, Mich.

MICHAEL E. MAHLER
Associate Director, Neurobehavior Unit
West Los Angeles Veterans Affairs Medical Center (Brentwood Division)
Assistant Professor of Neurology
UCLA School of Medicine
Los Angeles, Calif.

GHAUS MALIK
Staff Neurosurgeon
Department of Neurological Surgery
Henry Ford Hospital
Detroit, Mich.

MANFRED J. MEIER
Professor and Director
Neuropsychology Laboratory
Departments of Neurosurgery & Psychiatry
University of Minnesota Medical School
Minneapolis, Minn.

E. JEFFREY METTER
National Institute on Aging
Gerontology Research Center
Baltimore, Md.

PATRICIA A. REUTER-LORENZ
Assistant Professor
Program in Cognitive Neuroscience
Department of Psychiatry
Dartmouth Medical School
Hanover, N.H.

ROBERT G. ROBINSON
Professor and Chairman
Department of Psychiatry
University of Iowa
Iowa City, Iowa

ALAN RUBENS
Professor and Head
Department of Neurology
University of Arizona
Arizona Health Sciences Center
Tucson, Ariz.

MARTHA TAYLOR SARNO
Speech & Language Pathology Department
Rusk Institute of Rehabilitation Medicine
New York University Medical Center
New York, N.Y.

OLA SELNES
Associate Professor of Neurology
The Johns Hopkins University School of Medicine
Baltimore, Md.

BRETT E. SKOLNICK
Director, Cerebral Blood Flow Laboratory
Department of Neurology
Graduate Hospital
Philadelphia, Pa.

KEVIN SPICER
Research Fellow
Cognitive Neuroscience Laboratory
Neuropsychology Division
Psychiatry Department
Henry Ford Hospital
Detroit, Mich.

SERGIO E. STARKSTEIN
Director of Behavioral Neurology
Institute of Neurological Investigation
Buenos Aires, Argentina

SILVIA E. STRAUMAN
Research Fellow
Department of Psychiatry
Hennepin County Medical Center
Minneapolis, Minn.

DAVID E. TUPPER
Director of Clinical Services
New Medico Rehabilitation and Skilled Nursing Center of Troy
Troy, N.Y.

K.M.A. WELCH
Chairman, Department of Neurology
Director, Center for Stroke Research
Henry Ford Hospital
Detroit, Mich.

SAMUEL WIEBE-VELAZQUEZ
Department of Clinical Neurological Sciences
The University of Western Ontario
University Hospital
London, Ontario
Canada

Neurobehavioral Aspects of Cerebrovascular Disease

1

Cerebrovascular Disease in the History of Clinical Neuropsychology

ARTHUR L. BENTON

> From the theoretical point of view, it is important to stress that it is the patient with the ischemic infarct who is the most important source of knowledge concerning the clinical syndromes of the aphasias and their localizations. Thrombotic cerebrovascular disease is by far the most important cause of aphasia in the adult. These patients can be studied over long periods of stability. At postmortem examination the lesions found are often well defined and can be mapped precisely together with the resultant secondary degenerations.
> Geschwind (1970, p. 30)

Few would dispute the soundness of Geschwind's assertion, and indeed it holds for other specific cognitive disabilities as well as the aphasic disorders. Nor is it any longer necessary to wait for the results of an autopsy study to identify the locus and extent of a focal brain lesion.

A detailed account of how developments in cerebrovascular anatomy and physiology, neurodiagnostic techniques, and clinical observation interacted with each other to effect progress in the understanding of brain-behavior relations would require a treatment of monographic length. The more modest aim of this chapter is to provide some indications of this progress by citing representative examples of observations and discoveries that reflect developments over the centuries. These examples should make it clear that the observed behavioral effects of cerebrovascular disease have played a significant role in fostering the growth of knowledge and thought about brain-behavior relations, particularly with respect to the issue of cerebral localization of function.

FROM HIPPOCRATES TO MORGAGNI

Apoplexy must have been known since time immemorial. In line with their concepts of humoral pathology, Greek physicians variously ascribed this disorder to excessively dry, cool, or phlegmatic states of the brain, to the flow of black bile to the veins, or to excessive filling of the veins (Creutz, 1934; Clarke, 1963). Galen implicated excessive phlegm as the cause. "Apoplexy and epilepsy arise from the accumulation of phlegmatic humors in the ventricles of the brain" (Siegel, 1968, p. 306). Although there were at times vague references to the circulatory system over the course of the following centuries, the association between stroke and cerebrovascular disease was tenuous until the appearance of Johann Jakob Wepfer's *ObservationesAnatomicae* in 1658 (Donley, 1909; Major, 1945, pp. 429–443; Hoessly, 1965; Gawel, 1982).

Wepfer's contribution was truly epoch-making. An accomplished anatomist, he demolished the Galenic concept of the *rete mirabile* and instead showed that the internal carotid arteries penetrated the dura and entered the brain where it divided into its branches. He was the first to demonstrate through postmortem study that stroke was caused by intracranial hemorrhage, both intracerebral and subdural. He differentiated between hemorrhage and occlusion and indicated that each could produce stroke. He presented a description of the circle of Willis that, however, was somewhat less complete than the description of Thomas Willis (1664). More importantly, Willis was the first to point out the functional significance of these anastamoses, or "material conjoinings," in providing protective compensation for the effects of occlusion of a single vessel (Meyer & Hierons, 1962; Gawel, 1982).

Giovanni Battista Morgagni's (1769) great compilation of clinicopathologic correlations included many descriptions of cases of apoplexy. One of his major concerns was to emphasize the relation between paralysis on one side of the body and disease in the opposite cerebral hemisphere, i.e., to affirm the soundness of the doctrine of contralateral innervation. He also described speechlessness in combination with stroke-produced unilateral paralysis; and, in fact, analysis of his brief case reports discloses a definite trend toward a preferential association between speechlessness and *right* hemiplegia (Benton, 1984).

EARLY OBSERVATIONS

From the beginning it was obvious that apoplexy could produce gross mental changes such as confusion, obtundity, and speechlessness as well as motor and sensory disabilities. Wepfer himself suggested that the occurrence of mental changes was contingent on the part of the brain that was affected.

Cerebrovascular disease furnished the setting for the first analyses of specific behavioral disabilities that appeared during the seventeenth century, when it was noted that stroke could produce distinctive aphasic syndromes of medical and psychological interest. Johann Schmidt in 1673 described pure alexia without agraphia as a permanent residual of a stroke-produced aphasia. Peter Rommel in 1683 described a "rare aphonia" resulting from stroke in which a patient with practically complete loss of expressive speech nevertheless retained the capacity for rote recitation of prayers. Later, in 1745, Olof Dalin called attention to still another distinctive clinical picture, i.e., complete loss of expressive speech with retention of the ability to sing (Benton & Joynt, 1960).

Stroke also provided the opportunity for the first unequivocal description of pure anomic aphasia by Gerard Van Swieten in 1742–6. "I have seen many patients whose cerebral functions were quite sound after recovery from apoplexy, except for this one deficit: In designating objects, they could not find the correct names for them" (Benton and Joynt, 1960). In passing, it may be noted that Van Swieten was the first clinician to add embolic occlusion to the causes of stroke (McHenry, 1969).

The earliest descriptions of aphasic disorder that would be considered comprehensive and detailed by modern standards appeared during the second half of the nineteenth century. Johann A.P. Gesner (1770) wrote a chapter about 7000 words in length in which he analyzed the behavior of a patient who manifested a florid jargon aphasia after a stroke (Benton, 1965). Crichton (1798) described a striking case of stroke-produced paraphasia and invoked association theory to explain the patient's disability.

These early descriptions of diverse types and patterns of language disability enriched knowledge of aphasic symptomatology, but they contributed almost nothing to an understanding of brain-behavior relations. By the end of the eighteenth century the course of the major cerebral arteries had been described, at least in a sketchy way; but in all probability the findings were not widely known and were of major interest only to anatomists. The cerebral hemispheres were generally seen as a homogeneous structure to which different authors assigned different functions and only a few parts of which had been assigned names. Functional abnormality was ascribed to dryness, rigidity, or congestion of the brain substance. On the behavioral side, apart from the detailed descriptions of aphasic disability that have been cited, there was little behavioral analysis beyond the traditional division of mind into perception, reasoning, and memory. Thus there was little possibility of establishing meaningful correlations between behavior and the status of the brain.

NINETEENTH CENTURY

The first half of the nineteenth century was a period of significant advance along all fronts. Gall's (Gall and Spurzheim, 1809/1967) conception of the brain as a collection of organs, each of which subserved a specific mental faculty or disposition, as well as his emphasis on the cerebral hemispheres, generated a rancorous controversy and made localization of function in the brain a topic of major concern. The investigations of Rolando, Burdach, Cruveilhier, Leuret, and other anatomists established the basis for modern descriptions of the cerebral hemispheres and their convulutions. At the same time, histologic study of nerve fibers and their functional properties effectively displaced humoral doctrine and established the concept of neural transmission (Clark and O'Malley, 1968; Meyer, 1971).

The dispute over cerebral localization took two forms. There was first the broad issue of whether there was specialization of function in the brain. The influential physiologist Flourens insisted that the cerebral hemispheres operated as a unit, that each region subserved the same functions, and that the severity of behavioral impairment after brain insult was related to the quantity of tissue destroyed and not to its locus (Soury, 1899, pp. 518–527; Clark and O'Malley, 1968, pp. 483–488). His concept of a hemispheric *action commune* (later Lashley's laws of equipotentiality and mass action) was accepted by many clinicians who regarded Gall's system as absurd and who, in any case, were not able to find consistent relations between specific types of disability and lesions in specific areas of the brain. However, Flourens' position (derived from ablation studies on pigeons and chickens!) was contested by other clinicians, more on logical grounds than on established correlations between observed defects and identified lesion sites. For example, the physicians of the Salpetrière and the Pitié pointed to the discrete deficits produced by stroke—e.g., monoplegia of an arm or of a leg, hemiplegia with or without sensory impairment, sensory impairment without paralysis—as evidence that specific cerebral centers governing these functions must exist. Postmortem examination did indeed disclose limited areas of hemorrhage or infarction in these patients. Nevertheless, it was not possible to achieve agreement about the precise location of the presumed centers.

Broca's Discovery

The second aspect of the dispute centered around the specific placement of centers for speech and the "memory of words" in the frontal lobes by Gall and his ardent champion, Bouillaud (1825). The acrimonious debate was resolved only during the 1860s when Paul Broca brought forth convincing autopsy evidence of an association between nonfluent aphasic disorder and frontal lobe disease. Of his first two patients, reported in 1861 (Broca, 1861a,b,c), the first (probably) and the second (certainly) had suffered from strokes. The first patient (Leborgne) had an extensive lesion in the posterior region of the left frontal lobe implicating the third and second gyri as well as generalized softening throughout the hemisphere. Broca interpreted the findings as supportive of the Gall-Bouillaud thesis that the center for speech was in the frontal lobes. However, he noted that the primary lesion was in the third frontal gyrus, and he raised the question of whether a more precise localization might be possible. When his second patient (Lelong) proved to have a deep well demarcated lesion in the third and second frontal gyri of the left hemisphere, Broca could not help but be forcibly impressed by the fact that the same area was implicated in both cases.

By early 1863 Broca had collected eight cases of "aphemia" resulting from lesions of probable vascular etiology in the third frontal gyrus of the left hemisphere. At the same time about a dozen confirmatory cases of varying etiology—stroke, abscess, tumor, trauma—had been reported by others. Subsequently, he himself described a number of cases of traumatic aphasia, all referable to injury of the third frontal gyrus of the left hemisphere (Broca, 1864a,b). He therefore identified this area (in either hemisphere) as the cerebral center for articulated speech. He was also convinced that the crucial lesion was in the left frontal gyrus but at the time hesitated to advance a conclusion that was so much at variance with preconceptions about the essential equivalence of the two hemispheres. However, by 1865 steadily accumulating observations on the consequences of unilateral strokes emboldened him to announce that "we speak with the left hemisphere" (Broca, 1865, p. 384).

Prosopagnosia and Achromatopsia

A stroke probably involving bilateral occlusion of the posterior cerebral artery provided the setting for the first description of a patient with prosopagnosia and its frequent accompaniment, achromatopsia. In 1867 Antonio Quaglino and Giambattista Borelli (ophthalmologists in Pavia and Turin, respectively) reported the case of a 54-year-old man who was seen 1 year after his stroke. He had a left visual field defect, but central visual acuity was excellent; he read without difficulty and had no motor deficits. His chief complaints were that he no longer recognized the faces of familiar persons and that objects in the environment looked pale and devoid of color. Quaglino and Borelli argued that their case supported the basic thesis of localization of function in the brain.

Some 20 years later prosopagnosia and achromatopsia, either singly or in combination, were again described and now correlated with focal brain disease. For example, Wilbrand's (1892) prosopagnosic patient showed bilateral inferior occipitotemporal infarction on postmortem examination, as did Heidenhain's (1927) patient. This lesional localization (almost always bilateral but occasionally right-sided) has been repeatedly confirmed in vascular and neoplastic cases (Meadows, 1974b; Damasio et al., 1982; Benton, 1985). Similarly, both complete achromatopsia and hemiachromatopsia were reported and related to focal brain disease. In 1888 Verrey described right hemiachromatopsia in a stroke patient resulting from a hemorrhagic cyst in the left inferior occipital lobe. Mackay and Dunlop (1899) described a patient with a complete achromatopsia who had bilateral inferior occipital lobe infarctions. This strikingly specific lesional localization has also been repeatedly confirmed (Meadows, 1974a; Damasio et al., 1980).

Dejerine and Pure Alexia

As has been noted, during the seventeenth century Schmidt called attention to the rather striking phenomenon of loss of reading ability with preservation of the capacity to write as a sequela of stroke. Many descriptions of the condition, which was by then called "pure wordblindness" and which was often attributed on theoretical grounds to destruction or dysfunction of a "reading center" in the angular gyrus, appeared during the 1870s and 1880s. No clinicopathologic correlations were made, however, until 1892, when Dejerine published his famous postmortem study of a case of pure alexia following a stroke. His patient, an educated man and accomplished musician, suddenly lost the ability to read musical scores as well as conventional written material. Yet he could write, perform music from memory, and showed no difficulty in the expression or understanding of oral speech. He had a right visual field defect—in all probability a hemiachromatopsia, not a hemianopia (Damasio, 1983).

Autopsy study disclosed infarctions in the territory of the left posterior cerebral artery, specifically, the mesial occipital area and the splenium of the corpus callosum. Dejerine inferred that the lesions had the effect of preventing the transmission of visual information to the language centers of the left hemisphere, thus making reading impossible while leaving the interpretation of nonverbal visual stimuli intact. His concept of pure wordblindness as a disconnection symptom, and not the result of destruction of a "reading center," was validated by later investigators who showed that variations in the clinical picture (e.g., with or without right visual field defect) could be related to varying locations of the infarcts produced by occlusion of the left posterior cerebral artery (Geschwind, 1965; Geschwind and Fusillo, 1966; Benson and Geschwind, 1969; Greenblatt, 1973; Ajax et al., 1977; Vincent et al., 1977).

TWENTIETH CENTURY

Detailed knowledge of the distribution of the cerebral arteries, their anastomoses, functional interrelations and variations, and the cortical and subcortical areas served by their branches was achieved through a long series of studies beginning with those of Duret (1874) and Heubner (1874) and followed by, among others, those of Beevor (1908), Shellshear (1920); Foix and Levy (1927) and Pfeiffer (1928). Given this firm anatomic basis, clinicians were encouraged to attempt to identify the characteristic symptomatic manifestations of specific vascular abnormalities, in effect establishing a vascular system of cerebral localization.

Charles Foix was the pioneer worker in this endeavor. In a remarkable series of papers based on thorough anatomic study of the cerebrovascular system, he and his coworkers described the symptomatic features associated with occlusion of the vessels at various points along their course as well as of occlusion of individual branches. For example, Foix and Hillemand (1925) presented a detailed description of the "syndromes" of the anterior cerebral artery, a topic that was later taken up by Critchley (1930). A more or less specific combination of symptoms resulted from alterations in specific branches of the artery, e.g., monoplegia, particularly of the leg, from involvement of the predominantly cortical-subcortical distribution. Of particular interest is their observation that defective vascular supply to the corpus callosum, mainly through occlusion of the pericallosal artery, produced unilateral ideomotor apraxia of the left hand. When explaining the disability, Foix and Hilleman accepted the model of Liepmann and Maas (1907), postulating a break in the connection between a "command center" in the left supramarginal territory and the right motor area. In his equally detailed exposition, Critchley (1930) also called attention to left ideomotor apraxia as a consequence of callosal infarction; in addition, he emphasized that some degree of general mental impairment is invariably present. He noted that transitory expressive speech disorder may occur with left-sided lesions.

Subsequently Foix (1926; Foix and Levy, 1927) dealt with the pathologic anatomy of the aphasic disorders and the syndromes of the middle cerebral artery and its branches. He introduced the first topic with the statement that:

> Aphasia is above all dependent upon cerebral softening. Not that one cannot encounter aphasic syndromes caused by tumors, hemorrhages and abscesses, but the great majority of cases, more than nine out of ten, depend upon cerebral softening. . . . Hence this study is devoted largely to cerebral softening, first the pathologic anatomy of Wernicke aphasia, then Broca aphasia and finally the so-called pure forms. [Foix, 1926, p. 787]

Under the heading of Wernicke aphasia, various forms of fluent aphasic disorder were discussed, e.g., *grand aphasie de Wernicke;* fluent aphasia with particularly severe impairment in reading (referable to involvement of the angular gyrus); amnesic aphasia (which he regarded as a forme fruste of Wernicke aphasia). He identified the posterior temporal artery with its distribution to the hinder parts of the first and second temporal gyri as the principal artery of aphasia. *Grande aphasie de Wernicke,* i.e., the combination of fluent aphasia with ideational apraxia and right hemianopia, is referable to involvement of the posterior parietal and occipitoparietal arteries in addition to that of the posterior temporal. Occlusion of the posterior parietal and occipitotemporal arteries produces a fluent aphasia of moderate degree with severe alexia.

Similarly, under the heading of Broca aphasia, Foix discussed various forms of nonfluent speech disorder, ranging from apraxia of speech to global aphasia, and their correlations with the site, extent, and depth of cerebral softenings. Among other observations, he noted that the alexia shown by some Broca patients appeared to be associated with occlusion of the precentral artery. The report of Foix and Levy (1927) regarding the syndromes produced by lesions of the middle cerebral artery and its branches also dealt in large part with the aphasic disorders but in a complementary way, i.e., proceeding from the pathology to the symptom.

The topic was again addressed by Davison and colleagues (1934) in a systematic study based on a sample of 48 patients with a single vascular lesion selected from a pool of about 200 cases. Their findings generally confirmed earlier observations (e.g., Critchley on the occurrence of general mental impairment in disease of the anterior cerebral artery) and in many instances indicated that localized vascular abnormality produces distinctive clinical pictures. Their conclusion was that "cerebral localization on the basis of vascular supply, although difficult and necessitating caution in interpretation, can still be definitely established. We were able, on the basis of our study of 48 cases, to demonstrate definite syndromes accompanying occlusion of the anterior and middle cerebral arteries or their branches" (Davison et al., 1934, p. 465).

Critchley (1930), and indeed earlier observers, had noted that transient disturbances of speech could be produced by infarction of the left anterior cerebral artery. One form of disturbance was identified by Rubens (1975) in two patients as transcortical motor aphasia, i.e., the symptom complex of impoverished conversational speech, preserved capacity for repetition, echolalia, and relative preservation of understanding of speech. One of his patients had persisting apraxia and tactile anomia in the left hand pointing to involvement of the corpus callosum. The thrust of Rubens' contribution was to emphasize the importance of the left mesial and superior premotor region in the mediation of speech and language, a finding in accord with observations on surgical, epileptic, and traumatically injured patients. Later reports discussed the anatomic and clinical significance of transcortical motor aphasia as a component of the syndrome of the anterior cerebral artery (Damasio and Kassel, 1978; Alexander and Schmitt, 1980).

Disease of the anterior cerebral artery has also been related to the complex syndrome of akinetic mutism and a variety of behavioral deviations, including attentional disturbances, memory defects, and personality changes in the affected patients. Detailed study of these patients has given rise to a deeper understanding of the functional properties of different sectors of the frontal lobes (Damasio and Van Hoesen, 1983; Damasio, 1985; Stuss and Benson, 1986).

EPILOGUE

This chapter has presented some examples of how cerebrovascular disease brought to light certain specific defects in mentation and behavior and how in due time it was possible to relate these defects to specific abnormalities of the cerebral circulation. Strokes producing infarcts in a limited cerebral territory provided the opportunity for a variety of observations, such as those of Schmidt on pure alexia, Van Swieten on anomia, and Quaglino and Borelli on prosopagnosia and achromatopsia. Although it was not possible to identify the pathologic basis for the defects, these observations not only enriched clinical knowledge but also carried implications for localization theory. Broca's revolutionary correlation of nonfluent aphasic disorder with left frontal lobe disease ushered in an era of clinicopathologic study designed to elucidate brain-behavior relations. With progress in knowledge of the cerebrovascular system, attention was focused on the distinctive syndromes associated with abnormalities at various loci of the system.

Trauma, surgical intervention, tumor, and degenerative disease can also produce the same symptoms and symptom complexes as those resulting from stroke, either by a direct effect on the parenchyma or through injury to a blood vessel. Some examples that may be cited are pure alexia after surgical resection (Levin and Rose, 1979), prosopagnosia associated with tumor or surgical resection (Hécaen and Angelergues, 1962; Meadows, 1974b), and traumatic transcortical motor aphasia (Kleist, 1934; Rubens, 1976). Although these cases are less common than those of vascular etiology, they can provide information as useful as that derived from vascular cases. Moreover, individual variation as well as overlapping in the distributions of the vascular supply of the brain may complicate diagnostic inference (H. Damasio, 1983). Nevertheless, as Geschwind noted and the contributions in this volume illustrate, the ischemic infarct is the most valuable experiment of nature available for the clinical study of brain-behavior associations.

REFERENCES

Ajax, E.T., Schenkenberg, T., and Kostaljanetz, M. (1977). Alexia without agraphia and inferior splenium. *Neurology,* **27,** 685–688.

Alexander, M., and Schmitt, M.A. (1980). The aphasia syndrome of stroke in the left anterior cerebral artery territory. *Arch. Neurol.,* **37,** 97–100.

Beevor, C.E. (1908). On the distribution of the different arteries supplying the human brain. *Philos. Transact. R. Soc.,* **B200,** 1–55.

Benson, D.F., and Geschwind, N. (1969). The alexias. In: P.J. Vinken and G.W. Bruyn, eds., *Handbook of Clinical Neurology,* Vol. 4. Amsterdam: North Holland.

Benton, A.L. (1965). Johann A.P. Gesner on aphasia. *Med. Hist.,* **9,** 54–60.

Benton, A.L. (1984). Hemispheric dominance before Broca. *Neuropsychologia,* **22,** 807–811.

Benton, A.L. (1985). Visuoperceptual, visuospatial and visuoconstructive disorders. In: K.S. Heilman and E. Valenstein, eds., *Clinical Neuropsychology,* pp. 151–185. New York: Oxford University Press.

Benton, A.L., and Joynt, R.J. (1960). Early descriptions of aphasia. *Arch. Neurol.,* **3,** 205–222.

Bouillaud, J.-B. (1825). Recherches cliniques propres à démontrer que la perte de la parole correspond à la lésion des lobules antérieurs du cerveau. *Arch. Gén. Méd.,* **8,** 25–45.

Broca, P. (1861a). Nouvelle observation d'aphémie produite de la moitié postérieure des deuxième et troisième circonvolutions frontales gauches. *Bull. Soc. Anat.,* **36,** 398–407.

Broca, P. (1861b). Perte de la parole, ramollissement chronique et destruction partielle du lobe antérieur gauche. *Bull. Soc. Anthropol.,* **2,** 235–238.

Broca, P. (1861c). Remarques sur le siège de la faculté du langage articulé, suives d'une observation d'aphémie. *Bull. Soc. Anat.,* **36,** 330–357.

Broca, P. (1864a). Deux cas d'aphémie traumatique produite par des lésions de la troisième circonvolution frontale gauche. *Bull. Soc. Chir.,* **5,** 51–54.

Broca, P. (1864b). Sur le siège du langage articulé; aphémie traumatique; lésion de la troisième circonvolution frontale. *Bull. Soc. Anthropol.,* **5,** 362–365.

Broca, P. (1865). Sur le siège de la faculté du langage articulé. *Bull. Soc. Anthropol.,* **6,** 377–393.

Clarke, E. (1963). Apoplexy in the Hippocratic writings. *Bull. Hist. Med.,* **37,** 301–314.

Clarke, E., and O'Malley, C.D. (1968). *The Human Brain and Spinal Cord.* Berkeley: University of California Press.

Creutz, W. (1934). Die Neurologie des 1.-7. Jahrhunderts n. Chr. Leipzig: Thieme.

Critchley, M. (1930). The anterior cerebral artery, and its clinical syndromes. *Brain,* **55,** 120–165.

Critchton, A. (1798). *An Inquiry into the Nature and Origin of Mental Derangement.* London: T. Cadell Jr. & W. Davies.

Damasio, A. (1983). Pure alexia. *Trends Neurosci.,* **6,** 93–96.

Damasio, A.R. (1985). The frontal lobes. In: K.S. Heilman and E. Valenstein, eds., *Clinical Neuropsychology,* pp. 339–402. New York: Oxford University Press.

Damasio, A., Damasio, H., and Van Hoesen, G.W. (1982). Prosopagnosia: anatomic basis and behavioral mechanisms. *Neurology,* **32,** 331–341.

Damasio, A.R., and Kassel, N.F. (1978). Transcortical motor aphasia in relation to lesions of the supplementary motor area. *Neurology,* **28,** 396.

Damasio, A.R., and Van Hoesen, G.W. (1983). Emotional disturbances associated with lesions of the limbic frontal lobe. In: K.M. Heilman and P. Satz, eds., *Neuropsychology of Human Emotion,* pp. 85–110. New York: Guilford Press.

Damasio, A., Yamada, T., Damasio, H., Corbett, J., and McKee, J. (1980). Central achromatopsia: behavioral, anatomic and physiologic aspects. *Neurology,* **30,** 1064–1071.

Damasio, H. (1983). A computed tomographic guide to identification of cerebral vascular territories. *Arch. Neurol.,* **40,** 138–142.

Davidson, C., Goodhart, S.P., and Needles, W. (1934). Cerebral localization in cerebrovascular disease. *Res. Publ. Assoc. Res. Nerv. Ment. Dis.,* **13,** 435–465.

Dejerine, J. (1892). Contribution à la l'étude anatomopathologique et clinique des différentes varietés de cécité verbale. *Mem. Soc. Biol.,* **4,** 61–90.

Donley, J.E. (1909). John James Wepfer, a renaissance student of apoplexy. *Bull. Johns Hopkins Hosp.,* **20,** 1–8.

Duret, H. (1874). Recherches anatomiques sur la circulation de l'encéphale. *Arch. Physiol. Norm. Pathol.,* **1,** 60–91, 316–353, 664–693, 919–957.

Foix, C. (1926). Sur l'anatomie pathologique de l'aphasie. *Ann. Anat. Pathol.,* **3,** 787–814.

Foix, C., and Hillemand, P. (1925). Les syndromes de l'artére cérébrale antérieure. *Encephale,* **20,** 209–232.

Foix, C., and Levy, M. (1927). Les ramollissements sylviens. *Rev. Neurol. (Paris),* **2,** 1–51.

Gall, F.J., and Spurzheim, G. (1809). *Recherches sur le Systeme Nerveux en Général, et Sur Celui du Cerveau en Particulier.* Paris: F. Schoell (reprint, Amsterdam: Bonset, 1967).

Gawel, M. (1982). The development of concepts concerning cerebral circulation. In: F.C. Rose, ed., *Historical Aspects of the Neural Sciences,* pp. 171–178. New York: Raven Press.

Geschwind, N. (1965). Disconnection syndromes in animals and man. *Brain,* **88,** 237–295, 585–644.

Geschwind, N. (1970). Language disturbances in cerebrovascular disease. In: A.L. Benton, ed., *Behavioral Change in Cerebrovascular Disease,* pp. 29–36. New York: Harper & Row.

Geschwind, N., and Fusillo, M. (1966). Color naming defects in association with alexia. *Arch. Neurol.,* **15,** 137–146.

Gesner, J.A.P. (1770). *Samlung von Beobachtungen aus der Arzneigelahrtheit und Naturkunde.* Nördlingen: C.G. Beck.

Greenblatt, S. (1973). Alexia without agraphia or hemianopia; anatomical analysis of an autopsied case. *Brain,* **96,** 307–318.

Hécaen, H., and Angelergues, R., (1962). Agnosia for faces (prosopagnosia). *Arch. Neurol.,* **7,** 92–100.

Heidenhain, A. (1927). Beitrag zur Kenntnis der Seelenblindheit. *Monatsschr. Psychiatr. Neurol.,* **66,** 61–116.

Heubner, H.B.O. (1874). *Die luetische Erkrankung der Hirnarterien.* Leipzig: Vogel.

Hoessley, G.F. (1965). Intracranial hemorrhage in the seventeenth century. *J. Neurosurg.* **24,** 493–496.

Kleist, K. (1934). *Gehirnpathologie.* Leipzig: Barth.

Levin, H.S., and Rose, J.E. (1979). Alexia without agraphia in a musician after transcallosal removal of a left ventricular meningioma. *Neurosurgery,* **4,** 168–174.

Liepmann, H., and Maas, O. (1907). Fall von linkseitiger Agraphie und Apraxie bei rechtseitiger Lahmung. *J. Psychol. Neurol.,* **10,** 214–227.

Mackay, G. and Dunlop, J.C. (1899). The cerebral lesions in a case of complete acquired colour-blindness. *Scott. Med. Surg. J.,* **5,** 503–512.

Major, R.H. (1945). *Classic Descriptions of Disease,* 3rd ed. Springfield, IL: Charles C Thomas.

McHenry, L.C. (1969). *Garrison's History of Neurology.* Springfield, IL: Charles C Thomas.

Meadows, J.C. (1974a). Disturbed perception of colours associated with localized cerebral lesions. *Brain,* **97,** 615–632.

Meadows, J.C. (1974b). The anatomical basis of prosopagnosia. *J. Neurol. Neurosurg. Psychiatry,* **37,** 489–501.

Meyer, A. (1971). *Historical Aspects of Cerebral Anatomy.* London: Oxford University Press.

Meyer, A., and Hierons, R. (1962). Observations on the history of the "circle of Willis." *Med. Hist.* **6,** 119–130.

Morgagni, G.B. (1769). *The Seats and Causes of Disease, Investigated by Anatomy,* translated by B. Alexander. London: A. Millar & T. Cadell.

Pfeiffer, R.A. (1928). *Die Angioarchitektonik der Grosshirnrinde.* Berlin: Springer.

Quaglino, A., and Borelli, G. (1867). Emiplegia sinistra con amaurosi; guaragione; perdita totale della percezione dei colori and della memoria della configurazione degli oggetti. *G. Oftalmol. Ital.,* **10,** 106–117.

Rubens, A.B. (1975). Aphasia with infarction in the territory of the anterior cerebral artery. *Cortex,* **11,** 239–250.

Rubens, A.B. (1976). Transcortical motor aphasia. In: H. Whitaker and H.A. Whitaker, eds., *Studies in neurolinguistics,* Vol. 1, pp. 293–303. New York: Academic Press.

Shellshear, J.L. (1920). The basal arteries of the forebrain and their functional significance. *J. Anat.,* **15,** 27–35.

Siegel, R.E. (1968). *Galen's System of Physiology and Medicine.* Basel: Karger.

Soury, J. (1899). *Le Système Nerveux Central.* Paris: Carre & Naud.

Stuss, D.T. and Benson, D.F. (1986). *The Frontal Lobes.* New York: Raven Press.

Verry, D. (1888). Hémiachromatopsie droite absolute. *Arch. Ophthalmol.,* **8,** 289–300.

Vincent, F.M., Sadowsky, C.H., Saunders, R.L., and Reeves, A.G. (1977). Alexia without agraphia, hemianopia or color naming defect: a disconnection syndrome. *Neurology*, **27**, 689–691.

Wilbrand, H. (1892). Ein Fall von Seelenblindheit und Hemianopsie mit Sectionsbefund. *Dtsch. Z. Nervenheilk.*, **2**, 361–387.

Willis, T. (1664). *Cerebri Anatome*. London: J. Flesher.

I

Basic Ischemic, Biochemical, and Metabolic Mechanisms of Stroke

2

Focal Brain Ischemia and Stroke: Pathophysiology and Acid-Base Status

K.M.A. WELCH AND STEVEN R. LEVINE

Stroke most often results from occlusion of a single intracranial artery that causes incomplete ischemia. Despite the general knowledge that an ischemic level of blood flow damages nerve cells, there is little consensus about the specific biochemical mechanisms that ultimately cause the damage. Whatever they may be, the processes leading to cell death are triggered by the failure of nerve cells to produce the biochemical energy cells needed to function (Welch and Barkley, 1986).

This chapter presents a basic discussion of the pathophysiology of ischemic stroke and reviews the evidence that changes in brain hydrogen ion concentrations (pH) may moderate the energy failure and structural breakdown of cells during brain ischemia. The chapter is divided into four parts. The first part is a primer on cell energy metabolism and the synthesis and breakdown of phospholipids. It may be skipped by those familiar with the concepts and terminology of phosphate metabolism. The second part is a brief description of the basic pathophysiology of cerebral ischemia. The third section explores the significance of brain acidosis and what we have termed the acid to base pH "flip-flop." The final section is a glossary of definitions helpful to understanding the material presented in this chapter.

HIGH ENERGY PHOSPHATE AND PHOSPHOLIPID METABOLISM; CEREBRAL BLOOD FLOW AND METABOLISM

High Energy Phosphate and Phospholipid Metabolism

The molecular energy for cellular work in the brain is stored as a high energy phosphate bond of adenosine triphosphate (ATP). ATP is synthesized from glucose by a sequence of biochemical reactions involving glycolysis, Krebs cycle, and oxidative phosphorylation. During glycolysis, a molecule of glucose, two molecules of adenosine diphosphate (ADP), and two molecules of inorganic phosphate (Pi) ultimately yield a net result of two molecules of ATP. When oxygen is absent (anaerobic conditions), the last step of glycolysis produces lactic acid from pyruvic acid. Under aerobic conditions, pyruvic acid is oxidized to form acetyl coenzyme A, which enters the Krebs cycle. The ultimate products of the Krebs cycle are NADH and $FADH_2$, electron-carrying forms of nicotine adenine dinucleotide and flavin adenine dinucleotide. During a pass through the Krebs cycle, six molecules of ATP are produced for each molecule of glucose metabolized during glycolysis. In the mitochondria, NADH and $FADH_2$ transport their electrons, by a chain of respiratory processes, to ADP to form ATP. This process of oxidative phosphorylation consumes oxygen and produces 30 molecules of ATP for every molecule of glucose metabolized at the glycolytic stage. Elevations of ATP cause a reduction in the rate of glycolysis and cause ATP to be stored as phosphocreatine. The rate of phosphocreatine synthesis is partly controlled by the local pH of the tissue. Hexokinase and creatine kinase may function to maintain local levels of ADP by transferring the inorganic phosphate from ATP to creatine or glucose. Lehninger (1975) can be consulted for additional details.

The phospholipids form the main constituents of cell membranes. Two classes of molecules involved in phospholipid metabolism, phosphomonoesters (PMEs) and phosphodiesters (PDEs), can be measured *in vivo* by phosphorus nuclear magnetic resonance (^{31}P NMR) spectroscopy. The PMEs occur primarily in the anabolic phospholipid pathways and are therefore markers of phospholipid synthesis. The PDEs occur primarily in catabolic pathways, reflecting phospholipid breakdown. Major brain phospholipids include diacylglycerophospholipids (phosphatidyl phospholipids) and sphingomyelin. Specific fatty acid moeities of the phospholipids may turn over independently from the whole phospholipid molecule via hydrolytic enzymes within the brain that deacylate phosphatidyl compounds to lysophosphatidyl compounds. For example, phospholipase A deacylates the β position of phosphatidylethamolamine, phosphatidylserine, or lecithin (Suzuki, 1981). Diacylglyceride is used in the anabolic pathways involving both choline and inositol to phospholipids. More information about these pathways can be found in Lehninger (1975).

Cerebral Blood Flow and Metabolism

Under normal physiologic conditions, the rate of blood flow to the brain is determined by the level of neuronal activity (Chien, 1985). The rate of blood flow is therefore coupled to the rate of oxygen and glucose utilization and to changes in pH. As brain perfusion is reduced, total blood volume in a brain region increases as cerebral vessels dilate to maintain the same rate of delivery of glucose and oxygen to a cell. As the limits of this compensation are reached, a further reduction of brain perfusion increases the amount of oxygen extracted from blood (see Chapters 3 and 4). As the upper limits of this oxygen extraction ratio (OER) are exceeded, ATP synthesis must occur under increasingly anaerobic conditions. This mismatch of blood flow and metabolism, a "misery perfusion," has been observed in positron emission tomography (PET) studies of acute stroke patients (Powers and Raichle, 1985). With clinical stroke, the early period of depressed blood flow is generally followed by an increase of flow, producing a state of "luxury perfusion" where the rate of flow exceeds metabolic demand (Chien, 1985; Hakim et al., 1987). The effects of "misery" and "luxury" perfusion on pH remain to be clarified.

BASIC PATHOPHYSIOLOGY OF CEREBRAL ISCHEMIA

About 1 liter of blood—nearly one-fifth of cardiac output—passes through the brain each minute, yielding an overall cerebral blood flow (CBF) of approximately 50 ml/100 g/min. Gray matter CBF (80–100 ml/100 g/min) is approximately three to four times the white matter CBF (20–25 ml/100 g/min). Blood supplies the brain with glucose and oxygen while dispensing the heat and metabolic products of cerebral activity. The brain can tolerate only a brief cessation in delivery of glucose and oxygen, removal of metabolites, or dispersion of heat before neural functioning is disrupted (Chien, 1985). Under normal circumstances, the brain blood flow is autoregulated: There is an intrinsic tendency for cerebral arteriolar dilatation or constriction in response to changes in perfusion pressure to maintain relatively constant CBF (Chien, 1985). Diseases that clog or rupture cerebral vessels, reduce the content of glucose and oxygen in the blood, or affect the autoregulation of blood flow can cause severe neurologic and behavioral deficit.

Metabolic Effects of Complete Cerebral Ischemia

Stroke is the rapid onset of focal neurologic deficit. It is usually caused by cerebrovascular disease, but other diseases (e.g., neoplasm) may present with a stroke-like syndrome. Strokes may be due to cerebral hemorrhage or cerebral ischemia. In the latter, blood flow to neural tissue is insufficient to maintain physiologic function. Cerebral infarction occurs when ischemia is severe enough to produce nerve cell death.

The effects of total cerebral ischemia on cellular metabolism occur rapidly. Within seconds after occlusion of blood flow, glucose metabolism declines until it is 15% of its normal level 30 seconds later (Pulsinelli et al., 1982). Slowing of the electroencephalogram may be observed as soon as 5 seconds after the onset of ischemia, and become isoelectric 20 to 25 seconds later (Gastaut and Meyer, 1961). The alterations in glucose metabolism, as well as the abrupt termination in venous removal of lactic acid and other metabolites, causes acidic pH levels in the brain. This acidosis may alter the excitability of neural tissue. An excess of metabolites may dilate cerebral vessels and lead to a loss of autoregulation (Chien, 1985).

The ability of mitochondria to produce the high energy phosphates necessary to fuel the activities of a nerve cell declines rapidly during the first minute of total ischemia (Welch and Barkley, 1986). Because the distribution of potassium and sodium across the cell membrane depends on active pumps that use high energy phosphates as fuel, these ionic channels collapse and the resting potential dissipates.

Alteration and loss of presynaptic vesicles occur 3 to 4 minutes into the ischemic period. These alterations are accompanied by the release of the neurotransmitters dopamine, serotonin, and norepinephrine into the extracellular space and cerebrospinal fluid (Welch and Barkley, 1986). Disordered cholinergic transmission following acute stroke may add a neurogenic component to metabolic factors causing a disruption of autoregulation (Scremin and Jenden, 1989).

Three zones of differing hemodynamic and metabolic functions in a focus of ischemia have been proposed: (1) a central ischemic zone destined to progress to infarction; (2) a bordering zone in which flow and metabolism fluctuate between conditions adverse or favorable for tissue viability; and (3) a collateral zone in which tissue retains its viability, frequently a site of hyperemia (Welch and Barkley, 1986). The central zone can have zero to minimal flow, usually below 10 ml/100 g brain/min. In this region, there is massive influx of sodium and water into the cell, markedly low to absent oxygen availability, and very low pH due to lactic acid accumulation. The bordering zone, so designated originally by Meyer and colleagues (1962), has been renamed the ischemic penumbra (Astrup et al., 1981). In this zone, flow appears to fluctuate between levels compatible with electrical silence, i.e., below 15 ml/100 g brain/minute, and values regarded as critical for setting up an ischemic infarct, i.e., below 10 ml/100 g brain/min. The residual perfusion in this area supplied sufficient oxygen to maintain near-normal tissue concentrations of ATP, but there is insufficient oxygen to maintain the normally high concentrations of phosphocreatine and low levels of lactate. Some slight elevation in ADP and adenosine monophosphate (AMP) exists so that a degree of energy failure is present in this area. This metabolic and flow state does not always cause tissue infarction but does produce neuronal dysfunction and possibly selective neuronal damage.

An understanding of the critical flow and metabolic alterations that determine cell damage in an ischemic penumbra is important because therapy of patients with acute focal ischemic stroke aims to limit the boundaries of this region. Presumably, the ischemic penumbra and the central zone are first subjected to severe ischemia, but the potential for reperfusion through collateral channels remains. The hemodynamic and metabolic status of the ischemic penumbra is dependent on flow gradients and duration of initial ischemia and their interactions with events that occur during the development of collateral flow or recirculation (Astrup et al., 1981; Welch and Barkley, 1986). Such events include no-reflow and postischemic hypoperfusion due to either hemodynamic factors or limited metabolic demand. Edema is another factor that may limit recovery of function in the ischemic penumbra.

Low ATP and high lactate acid levels in an ischemic focus are markers of potential histopathologic damage, although there is not total agreement on this (Welch and Barkley, 1986). Of the two, lactic acidosis seems to be the most important.

In humans, PET scanning has provided insights into the pathophysiology of cerebral ischemia and infarction in the clinical setting. PET studies have demonstrated that CBF measurements alone are incapable of distinguishing hypoperfusion with and without actual tissue ischemia. Ischemia generally occurs only when the OEF of brain from blood is close to 100% with a subsequent fall in perfusion pressure or increased metabolic demand. The fall in OEF may signal the process of infarction (Powers and Raichle, 1985; Frackowiak, 1986). Within 2 days of clinical onset of stroke, the ischemic cortex is already reperfused in one-third of patients (Hakim et al., 1987). Persistently hypoperfused regions appear acidotic, with alkalosis being associated with reperfusion.

Between the first and fourth hours after complete cerebral ischemia, the blood become stagnant, changes occur in the thin internal lining of the blood vessels, edema develops, and the regional collapse of autoregulation occurs (Kontos, 1986). Blood vessels may undergo structural changes: occlusion by platelet aggregates or by emboli, functional alterations in caliber, and changes in reactivity. Decreased intravascular pressure distal to the occlusion and the reduced CBF may trigger reactive changes in vessel lumen size in occlusive stroke (Kontos, 1986). Ischemic damage to the vascular wall may also occur and can cause breakdown of the blood-brain barrier with consequent loss of fluid into the extravascular compartment. Cerebral edema ensues along with a secondary increase in viscosity and consequent sludging with aggregation of platelets. Vasoactive agents from the ischemic tissue may also be released and act on the vessel wall. All of these secondary vascular factors, which were triggered by the initial ischemia, probably influence the extent of ischemic brain injury and stroke outcome.

Histologic changes continue to develop over the hours and days following ischemia. Late changes include liquefaction and cavitation of the infarcted tissue with a surrounding zone of astrocytic proliferation. The earliest stages of neuronal ischemic pathology include microvasculation, neuronal swelling, and ischemic cell changes. The neurohistopathology of cerebral ischemia is dependent on the severity and size of the initial ischemic episode and on neuronal survival time. Acute macroscopic abnormalities in large infarcts include swollen tissue, hyperemia, and softness of the tissue with diminished structural resolution. Mass effect with shifting of structures may be seen. Gray matter becomes soft and granular within weeks of the infarct. Dead neuronal cytoplasm stains eosinophilic with vacuolation. These early changes—within hours—give way to the more chronic lack of staining and barely detectable cell structure. At 24 hours post-infarct, the edge of the ischemic tissue is infiltrated by polymorphonuclear leukocytes. Nonneuronal components such as microglia, astrocytes, and oligodendroglial begin to swell early in ischemic cell change with subsequent disintegration during the following days. Cystic lesions may appear microscopically in chronic infarctions, and irregular pallor of staining with coagulative necrosis affecting all tissue elements may be seen.

To summarize this section, tissue recovery from ischemia is variable and obviously dependent upon a number of factors, including the completeness of ischemia (paradoxically, incomplete ischemia appears to be more hazardous than complete ischemia), collateral circulation, duration of the ischemic insult, cerebral edema, and other postulated factors such as tissue pH, preischemic glucose content, neurotransmitter dysfunction, generation of free radicals, intracellular calcium, and prostaglandins. Nevertheless, energy failure unquestionably underlies cell damage, even if secondary events take place that are more critical to the irreversibility of cell damage.

ACID-BASE STATUS IN ISCHEMIC STROKE

With cerebral ischemia, a rapid decrease of high energy phosphate intermediates occurs, with a shift toward reduction of mitochondrial respiratory chain metabolites, increased lactic acid, and acidosis in the ischemic focus (Lowry and Passonneau, 1964; Goldberg et al., 1966; Michenfelder and Theye, 1970). Acidosis probably causes or contributes in a major way to cellular damage in ischemic brain (see review by Welch and Barkley, 1986). In clinical studies of acute focal ischemic stroke using the capability of phosphorus nuclear magnetic (^{31}P) spectroscopy to dynamically measure brain pH, we observed a transition from acidosis to alkalosis in ischemic brain as early as 18 hours after onset of stroke (Levine et al., 1987). PET had previously identified alkalosis in clinical studies of subacute and late focal ischemic stroke (Syrota et al., 1985; Hakim et al., 1987). A rapid transition from acidosis to alkalosis had also been observed in experimental stroke models of either focal or global, complete or incomplete ischemia with or without reperfusion (Kogure et al., 1980; Mabe et al., 1983; Paschen et al., 1985; Yoshida et al., 1985).

Brain Acidosis

Disturbances of brain acid-base status are important in the mechanisms of ischemic neuronal damage for the following reasons: (1) pH may control local cerebral blood flow and tissue oxygen delivery (Kuschinsky and Wahl, 1978); (2) there is a pH dependence of membrane transfer mechanisms (Choi and Abramson, 1978; Siesjo, 1978; Lund-Anderson, 1979; Wanke et al., 1979); (3) intracellular hydrogen ion concentration $[H^+]$ controls cytoplasmic enzyme activity, particularly those involved in glycolysis (Siesjo, 1978); and (4) ATP production in mitochondria may be pH-linked (Mitchell, 1961). Regulation of $[H^+]$ is severely stressed by ischemia. The crucial acid-base event in ischemic brain is caused by deterioration of energy status and the ensuing stimulation of anaerobic glycolysis to preserve ATP synthesis at the cost of lactic acid accumulation and CO_2 entrapment, which, together with a relatively minor contribution from ATP hydrolysis, seems primarily responsible for tissue acidosis (Siesjo, 1985a,b). The most important mechanisms whereby H^+ is toxic to neural or glial cells are uncertain and probably diverse. One mechanism is the concurrence of energy failure with brain acidosis and the fact that low pH may prevent recovery of energy phosphates (Welsh et al., 1980; Siesjo, 1981). A second possible toxic mechanism involves the enhancement of membrane breakdown by accelerated free radical reactions at low pH (Siesjo, 1981, 1985b). A third mechanism is loss of cellular volume control perhaps related to glial buffering (Kraig et al., 1985; Siesjo, 1985a).

Brain Alkalosis

The perception that human brain can become alkalotic at certain stages in the evolution of an ischemic insult is relatively recent. It is largely because techniques for measuring brain pH, particularly of the intracellular compartment, have matured only during the immediate past years. Alkalosis was first observed in experimental stroke preparations. After inducing cerebral embolism in the rat, Kogure et al. (1980) observed a permanent decrease of CBF in the ischemic focus, associated initially with acidosis and lactic acid accumulation and later with alkalosis, despite persistence of ischemia and high tissue lactate. ATP was depleted in the same region, but there was hyperoxidation of the mitochondrial electron transport system that suggested to the authors either a flow/metabolism uncoupling or ATP consumption.

After transient middle cerebral artery (MCA) occlusion in the cat, Paschen et al. (1985) found regions of alkalosis associated with complete or partial ATP loss, despite reperfusion. A regional block in the glycolytic pathway was demonstrated in the same regions, postulated by the authors as possibly due to a decrease of NAD^+. Mabe et al. (1983) found transient alkalosis 60 minutes into reperfusion after 15 minutes of transient forebrain ischemia. Reperfusion alkalosis could be seen even after 5 minutes of transient ischemia, and it persisted for as long as 90 minutes after the moment of recirculation at times when lactate levels were still above control. Using a similar model Yoshida et al. (1985) found postischemic alkalosis to be present 4 hours after reperfusion, and to be more pronounced after complete ischemia than after incomplete ischemia. Metabolic recovery was more impaired in regions of greater alkalosis, leading to the authors' speculation that severe tissue alkalosis might be a physicochemical marker of advanced tissue injury.

From these few experimental studies it appears that alkalosis can be found after brief transient ischemia, during which cell damage is not to be expected, or at the other end of the scale when established ischemia progresses to cerebral infarction. Alkalosis may be implicated in recovery mechanisms in the former but may be a marker of cell death in the latter. Thus the mechanisms of alkalosis are probably multifactorial and diverse depending on the conditions of ischemia.

In a small number of patients, PET studies have documented alkalosis in the early period (within 48 hours) (Hakim et al., 1987) and late period (10–14 days) (Syrota et al., 1985) after stroke. Hakim et al. (1987) measured alkaline pH values only in reperfused brain regions. Of interest, these pH shifts correlated with a regional increase in the glucose/oxygen ratio, suggesting ongoing anaerobic glucose metabolism. This finding is somewhat of a paradox, as anaerobic metabolism should generate lactic acid and a lowered tissue pH. Alkalotic pH could therefore be related to intrinsic cellular buffering against lactic acid accumulation, as suggested by the earlier experimental studies conducted by Kogure et al. (1980) and Mabe et al. (1983). In a separate study, alkaline pH values measured 10 to 19 days after acute stroke (Syrota et al., 1985) failed to correlate with CBF, extracellular water, or cerebral oxygen consumption ($CMRO_2$) but did correlate with reduced OER, suggesting a relation to luxury perfusion or tissue metabolic paralysis. Tissue alkalosis therefore seems to be a distinct event in the evolution of clinical stroke. In the dynamic process of deterioration or recovery that takes place over hours or days, there appears to be a dramatic, relatively rapid, switch from the potentially damaging tissue acidosis to an alkaline pH that may persist for days post-stroke.

The mechanisms of ischemic brain alkalosis are currently unknown. The cellular buffering mechanisms of brain can be separated into two processes using time as the basis for separation (Roos and Boron, 1981). The first process occurs within minutes and involves (1) physicochemical buffering, (2) metabolic acid buffering, and (3) sequestration of acid by cellular organelles. The second, slower process is related to active acid efflux from the cell. The precise temporal relations in the mechanisms involved have not been defined. Intracellular alkalosis of the magnitude that has been observed in ischemia occurs in few other conditions (Pelligrino and Siesjo, 1981; McMillan and Siesjo, 1983). The above cellular buffering mechanisms, ATP resynthesis, and temperature effects are causal considerations, the first being probably of most importance and the last unlikely in reperfused brain. Reduced cellular production of acid metabolites and CO_2 due to complete or partially impaired metabolic function in ischemic or infarcted brain in the presence of "luxury" reperfusion may lead to less $[H^+]_i$ accumulation and relative alkalosis. This mechanism was proposed by Syrota et al. (1985) on the basis of PET measurements that showed an indirect correlation between decreased OEF (metabolic impairment) and pH. Reperfusion alkalosis was observed by Hakim et al. (1987) at a time when anaerobic metabolism was stimulated; however, alkalosis is a well established stimulus to glycolysis. Mabe et al. (1983) postulated that with the resumption of tissue circulation and ATP synthesis lactic acidosis can be buffered in part by active energy consuming the efflux of protons from cells. Lactate production is compensated for only in part by its oxidation when other pH buffering mechanisms are active. After ischemia, transient overcompensation and alkalotic pH may result during reperfusion. The greater the lactic acid accumulation or pH fall during ischemia, the more pronounced and protracted this overcompensation is likely to be.

Siesjo (1985a) has argued that the most likely buffering mechanism brought into play under the above circumstances involves an energy-consuming electrosilent Na^+/H^+ antiport system with H^+ extrusion in exchange for Na^+. This process may also be mediated by an agonist–receptor interaction that activates phospholipase C and, in turn, diacylglyceride stimulation of the C-kinase system, which enhances the Na^+/H^+ exchange to increase pH. (Such a process has also been evoked as a stimulus to cell proliferation.) Many cells also contain an electroneutral Cl^-/HCO_3^- antiporter. The linkage of these two antiport systems could result in increased intracellular sodium chloride and alkaline pH. This pH regulation to alkalotic levels occurs at the expense of cell volume control. Alkaline pH shifts in ischemic brain might therefore be a marker of cellular edema.

There is increasing evidence that glia, which occupy one-third of the cellular elements of the neocortex, behave differently than neurons in pH and volume regulation (Kraig et al., 1985; Plum et al., 1985; Siesjo, 1985b; Kempski et al., 1988; Kraig and Petito, 1989). Glial cells also possess antiport systems that can be activated by acidosis with an increase in cell volume and alkalinization. Glia can become alkaline during ischemia, thereby confirming them as a major source of bicarbonate to ischemic brain under normoglycemic conditions (Kraig et al., 1978). Under hyperglycemic conditions, however, glial buffering capacity is more rapidly exhausted and infarction is more pronounced (Kraig and Petito, 1989). Glial acidosis, not alkalosis, was observed at a time of expected glial swelling. Some of the above mechanisms connote ongoing recovery process, from which it may be deduced that the onset of alkalosis may be time-locked with the end of active, acidotic-linked, cell damage or the onset of restorative processes. At least two other scenarios could be heralded by alkalosis, however: (1) irreversible ischemic cell death; and (2) reperfusion injury perhaps leading to cell death. Cell death with membrane breakdown would promote equilibration of the intracellular pH of the brain, which has a higher pH than intracellular fluid. In this instance we would expect to find impaired brain buffering capacity and brain pH that approaches systemic arterial pH. Reperfusion injury, such as may be caused by free radical generation with resultant increase of membrane permeability, may promote passive movement of sodium chloride and HCO_3^- into cells, with resultant cellular edema and alkalosis.

Because of the potential multifactorial causes of ischemic alkalosis it is difficult to derive one mechanism as predominate in any in vivo investigation in patients. Metabolic paralysis, cell death, and intracellular edema with equilibration of intracellular and extracellular HCO_3^- are probably the major biochemical processes in focal ischemic infarction. Independent of mechanism, the acid-to-base shift in ischemic brain appears to be a salutary event that could signify either the beginning of recovery or, more likely, cellular irrecoverability; and as such may be a distinct marker of a particular stage in stroke evolution. Thus it has the potential to indicate a therapeutic window for cell protection as well as serve as a prognostic index.

CLINICAL ^{31}P NUCLEAR MAGNETIC RESONANCE SPECTROSCOPY

In vivo nuclear magnetic resonance (NMR) has afforded the opportunity for noninvasive, dynamic investigation of anatomic, biochemical, and physiologic events in a manner that has not been previously possible. NMR imaging is now a fundamental diagnostic modality in the field of medicine. NMR spectroscopy has provided information about the biochemistry and physiology of numerous pathologic states including cerebrovascular disease. Probably the most significant advantage for in vivo NMR is its noninvasive nature. Thus tissue function (i.e., physiology and biochemistry) can now be assessed on a dynamic biologic time scale without introducing unwanted variables such as traumatic shock or enzymatic decay/catabolism inherent in a secondary or tertiary analysis of the tissue.

In the ensuing paragraphs we describe the use of ^{31}P NMR spectroscopy in stroke patients. The important utility of this technique relative to our thesis is that it provides simultaneous measurement of brain acid-base status with energy and phospholipid metabolism that can be directly correlated with clinical, neurologic, and neuropsychological measures.

The technique we have used to localize the source of the signal for in vivo spectroscopy involves two steps. Traditional magnetic resonance imaging is used to place the brain region of interest into the middle of a sensitive volume. The boundary of this sensitive is sharpened by increasing the homogeneity of the magnetic field within the volume (topical magnetic resonance) for in vivo spectroscopy. A surface coil is used to obtain a good signal-to-noise ratio in the shortest time possible from a reasonably well defined spatial focus. The acquisition time required to obtain ^{31}P spectra with a satisfactory signal-to-noise ratio in brain is approximately 10 to 20 minutes. The total time necessary to perform imaging and spectroscopy currently requires up to 2 hours in the magnet. Figure 2–1 illustrates the use of the technique and explains how pH is calculated.

The ^{31}P NMR technique is currently the only available method for monitoring the adenylate energy status of tissue in vivo. It offers, in addition, an advantage over biochemical techniques that require freeze inactivation of brain, which induces energy breakdown during the process, so that ^{31}P NMR in vivo measurements are probably more physiological. The NMR method is inherently insensitive, however, detecting only millimolar concentrations.

Readily identifiable resonances in the in vivo ^{31}P NMR spectra are commonly labeled: PME, inorganic ortho-phosphate (Pi), PDE, phosphocreatine (PCr), and the γ, α and β phosphate peaks of ATP peaks (Gadian, 1982). The contribution of each of the seven identified peaks of the ^{31}P NMR spectrum to the total phosphorus spectrum is determined by calculating the area under each of the peaks and expressing the result as a percentage (mole percent) of the total phosphorus signal. Bioenergetic ratios can be obtained from spectra that may be useful to characterize the energetic

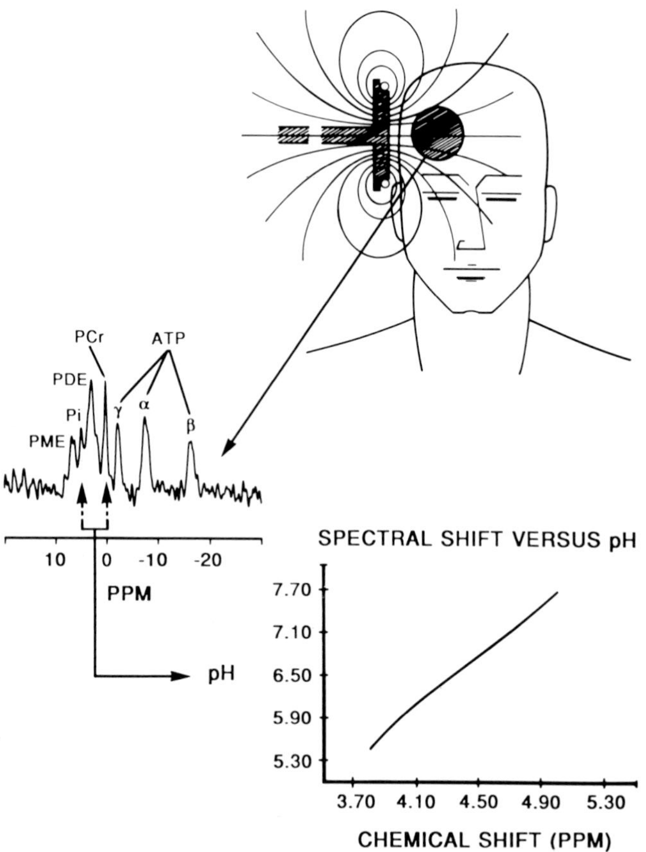

Figure 2–1 Topical magnetic resonance: normal human brain in vivo phosphorus NMR spectra and basis of pH determination calculated from the chemical shift of Pi relative to PCr.

state of the tissue (Gadian, 1982, p. 25). For example, the PCr/Pi ratio is an important index of the phosphorylation potential of the tissue (Atkinson, 1968; Shoubridge et al., 1980; Prichard et al., 1983; Radda, 1986; Mayevsky et al., 1988).

Intracellular pH is calculated from the chemical shift between the PCr and Pi resonances (Petroff et al., 1985) (Figure 1). Because the intracellular compartment of the brain is large relative to the vascular and extracellular fluid compartments, pH estimates within the region of interest principally reflect the intracellular pH (Petroff et al., 1984). The hydrogen ion concentration can be measured to an accuracy of approximately $\pm$ 0.05 pH units (Petroff et al., 1985; Radda, 1986). The PME components are found primarily in phospholipid synthetic pathways (Pettegrew et al., 1985). The PDE components are found only in breakdown pathways. The PME/PDE ratio therefore may be reasonably considered an index of phospholipid turnover reflecting the ratio of synthetic precursors to the breakdown products of phospholipid metabolism. The PMEs are an essential component of neuronal and mitochondrial membranes and are involved in membrane transport processes. Hence this ratio can be viewed as a marker of altered membrane function in ischemic brain.

STROKE STUDIES

We first describe the serial ^{31}P NMR spectroscopy of eight patients: seven with acute focal cortical stroke due to major intracranial artery occlusion and one with transient ischemia. Patients had hemiparesis or hemiplegia and either aphasia (in the case of left hemispheric stroke) or visual spatial disorientation or neglect (in right hemispheric stroke).

Figure 2–2 displays the serial ^{31}P NMR spectra from a patient studied six times within 1 month, the earliest being 18 hours after the ictus (spectra from only four occasions are shown). The PCr/Pi ratio was reduced acutely (within 24 hours) with gradual recovery to normal within 1 month. The pH was acidotic acutely (pH 6.74), shifting to alkalotic values (pH 7.26) subacutely (2–3 days). Intermediate and late pH values continued to show alkalosis (pH 7.20–7.26). There was incomplete recovery of neurologic deficit. Figure 2–3 illustrates a typical series of spectra obtained in a patient studied subacutely and on separate occasions over a 2-month interval. Obliteration of the PCr and ATP peaks with increase of Pi was seen subacutely followed by gradual recovery (somewhat variable and incomplete) toward the normal spectral characteristics of the opposite hemisphere. Alkalotic pH values were obtained at the first time of study. Recovery of neurologic deficit consistently lagged behind the

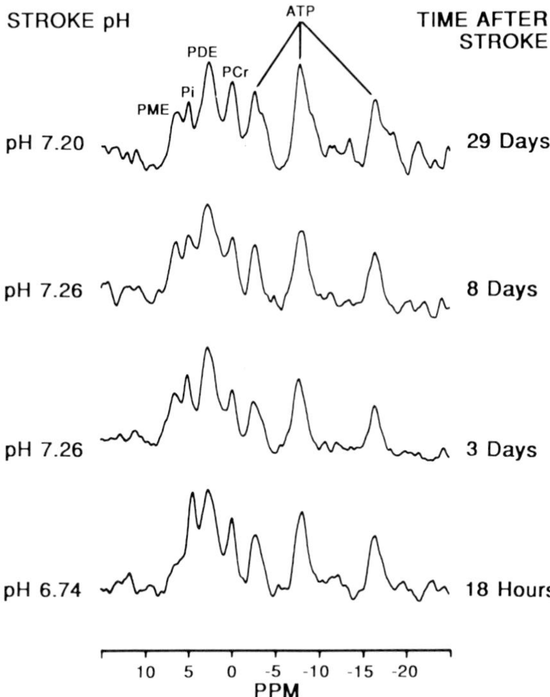

Figure 2–2 Serial in vivo ^{31}phosphorus NMR spectra demonstrating the acidosis to alkalosis pH flip-flop in acute focal human ischemic stroke.

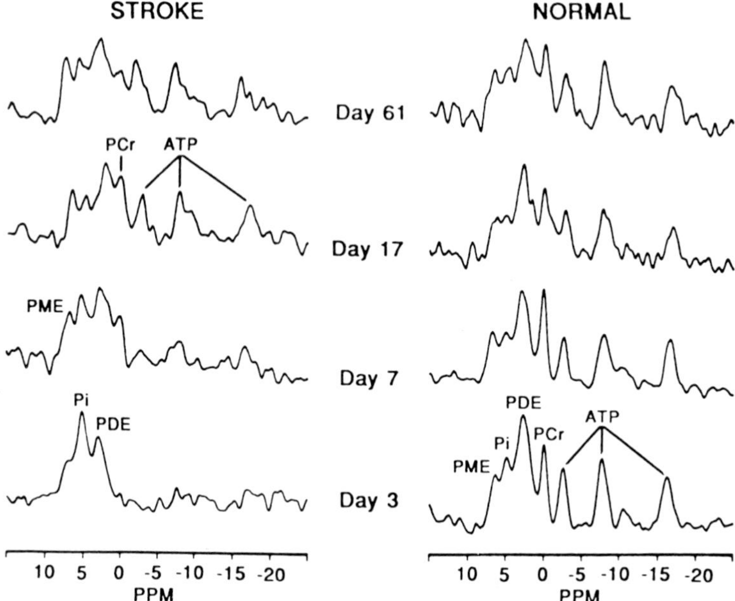

Figure 2–3 Serial in vivo ^{31}phosphorus NMR spectra demonstrating slow recovery of high energy phosphate metabolism over 2 months in a patient with a large MCA territory ischemic infarct.

recovery of cerebral high energy phosphates. The PME value in both cases appeared decreased but recovered with the passage of time.

The mean of the PCr/Pi ratios in six patients studied over time was still significantly reduced, compared with controls, in the ischemic focus 2 to 3 days after onset ($p < 0.02$) (Figure 2–4), but recovered to control values in the ischemic focus 7 to 9 days after onset. The recovery of PCr/Pi occurred despite the persistent neurologic

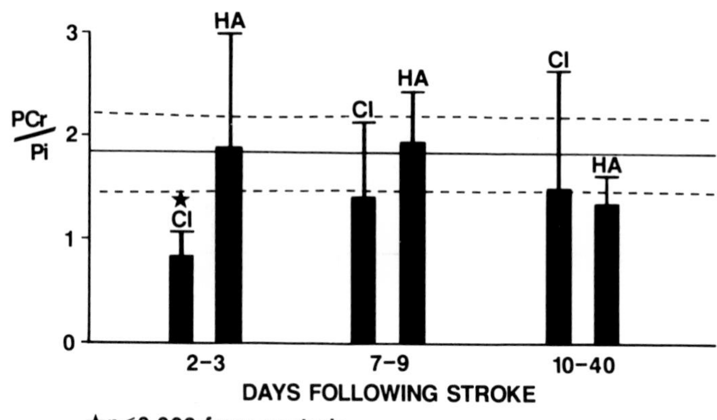

Figure 2–4 Mean brain PCr/Pi data (serial ^{31}P NMR spectroscopy) over time for acute stroke patients (CI = cerebral infarction), the homologous area (HA) of the contralateral hemisphere, and normal controls [solid line ± SD (dotted lines)]. Error bar represents 1 SD. Early reductions in PCr/Pi with recovery to normal levels are demonstrated.

deficit and prominent evidence for infarction on the NMR and computed tomography (CT) scans. This finding is consistent with the concept that, although deterioration of high energy phosphate metabolism is initially responsible for neuronal dysfunction, other factors probably play more important role in causing cell death (Siesjo, 1981). Apart from partial recovery of some neurons, the return of measurable adenine metabolites could also originate from glial cells that are relatively more resistant to ischemia (Kempski et al., 1988) or macrophages that infiltrate the infarct (McCormick and Schochet, 1976). Diaschisis might in part explain a strong trend ($p < 0.06$) toward lower PCr/Pi ratios measured in the contralateral hemisphere 10 days after stroke onset.

Whereas the pH was acidic in the ischemic focus of patients studied acutely, by the time patients were studied during the subacute and intermediate periods (Figure 2–5) the pH was alkalotic compared to the contralateral hemisphere and to normal controls (broken lines, Figure 2–5). Significant alkalotic pH was seen after 24 hours from the onset of the clinical deficit in this group but was present even earlier based on the heterogeneity of infarct pH obtained in one case at 18 hours (Figure 2–2) and in another case of transient ischemia. Spectra in this transient ischemic attack (TIA) patient were obtained from the frontotemporal cortex within 24 hours of the onset of symptoms when the patient was asymptomatic and demonstrated transient, mild alkalosis.

Based on these preliminary data, at some point in the progression of focal ischemia there appears to be a reversal or "flip-flop" in pH from the more immediate acidosis. We consider that this pH flip-flop may define the limit of a therapeutic window.

We have extended our analysis to 44 patients with hemispheric focal ischemia (Table 2–1), and it has substantiated that intracellular pH in ischemic brain progresses through stages of acidosis to alkalosis. Considerable variability in pH and brain energetics exists during the acute (first 24 hours) stages of stroke. When the ischemic brain was acidotic a highly significant elevation of Pi was noted with decrease in ATP but no change in PCr (Table 2–1). The PCr/Pi ratio was reduced as

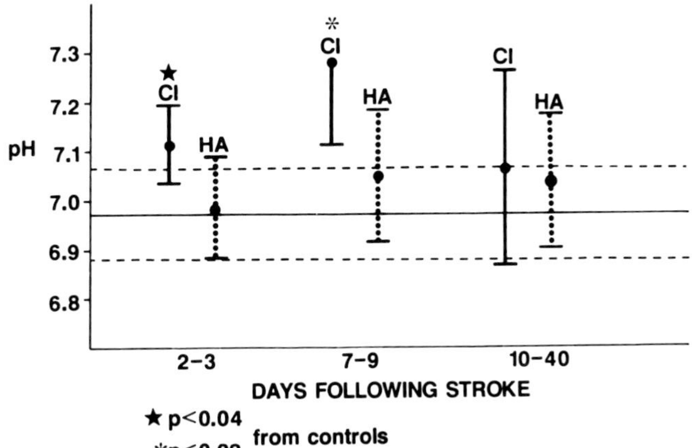

Figure 2–5 Mean brain pH data (serial ^{31}P NMR spectroscopy) over time, demonstrating subacute alkalosis in acute stroke patients' brains. For abbreviations, see Figure 2–4.

Table 2–1 Relations of pH Changes to Energy and Phospholipid Metabolism

Parameter	Control (6.91–7.07)	Acidic (6.91)	Normal (6.91–7.07)	Alkalotic (>7.07)
PCr/Pi	2.2 (0.5)	0.8 (0.9)*	1.7 (0.8)	1.7 (0.9)
PCr/TP	13.1 (2.1)	10.1 (6.5)	14.3 (3.1)	13.7 (3.2)
Pi/TP	6.2 (1.0)	39.5 (38.4)*	9.3 (2.4)*	10.5 (7.4)*
βATP/TP	11.1 (1.5)	7.3 (4.5)*	9.4 (2.2)	10.5 (2.5)
PME/TP	9.1 (1.3)	7.4 (5.2)	11.0 (3.2)	8.9 (2.3)
PDE/TP	29.2 (1.9)	22.4 (13.0)	29.4 (3.1)	27.9 (3.5)
PME/PDE	0.3 (0.1)	0.3 (0.1)	0.4 (0.1)	0.3 (0.1)
	$n = 13$	$n = 9–10$	$n = 11–13$	$n = 19–21$

Different from controls: $^{*}p < 0.05$.

a function of the high Pi. A problem with interpreting these results is that either acid shifts or ischemic metabolism should lead to PCr decrease. Possibly differential recovery rates for the high energy phosphates or the effect of divalent cations such as Mg^{2+} might explain this discrepancy. Alternatively, the inhomogeneity of the ischemic groups in the acute stages of progressing stroke and the wide range of PCr values may make it difficult to achieve a statistically significant decrease in PCr. In fact, a number of patients with acidosis showed obliterated or small PCr spectral peaks (for example see Figure 2–3). When correlation analysis was performed, there were strong correlations with the degree of acidic pH and the reduction of all energy phosphates as well as the Pi increase and PCr/Pi decrease (Table 2–2). Though less marked, changes in the same direction were noted as pH normalized. Pi remained elevated as ischemic brain became alkalotic, but ATP and PCr/Pi recovered. Thus there is ample evidence that acidic pH can account for deterioration or impaired recovery of energy metabolism. The eventual recovery of high energy phosphates as the brain pH normalizes and then becomes alkalotic is a consistent finding and, as discussed above, probably does not reflect neuronal recovery. Neither the mean PME nor the PDE values were altered during acidosis. Nevertheless, in some patients obliteration of peaks was noted, and there were strong correlations between the degree of acidity and the degree of reduction of both PME and PDE (Table 2–2). The PME/PDE ratio was significantly increased as pH normalized owing largely to the increase in the

Table 2–2 Correlations of Acidosis to Energy and Phospholipid Metabolism

Parameter	Correlation Coefficient	N. p value	Two-Tailed
PCr/Pi	0.61	9	>0.08
PCR/TP	0.59	10	>0.07
Pi/TP	−0.70	9	<0.04
β-ATP/TP	0.48	10	>0.15
PME/TP	0.81	9	<0.01
PDE/TP	0.88	9	<0.002
PME/PDE	−0.11	7	>0.81

Note: No significance was found within normal, control, or alkalotic groups.

PME (Table 2–1). These changes subsided during alkalosis. Because PME represents the anabolic phospholipid pathway, elevated levels could reflect a burst of resynthesis of membranes as a reparative measure, particularly because it is time-locked with normalization of pH. Furthermore, the diacylglyceride precursors essential for PME synthesis also stimulate the C-kinase system (Siesjo, 1985a), which in turn activates the cellular Na^+/H^+ antiporter and initiates membrane proliferative processes (Siesjo, 1985b). Thus the observed burst of PME synthesis prior to the development of alkalosis has particular relevance to the hypothesis that alkalosis is due to active cellular buffering mechanisms. Alternatively, PME elevation could be caused by a blockade of enzymic synthesis at a latter step of phospholipid synthesis, perhaps more relevant when alkalosis is due to cellular damage.

Finally, we studied the relation between acid-base status and neurologic outcome. When serial pH measurements were correlated with neurologic deficit (0 = normal, I = mild, II = moderate, III = severe), at the final spectroscopic assessment (7–30 days after onset) there was a slight negative trend for the severity of acidosis versus deficit grade ($n = 28$; $r = 0.204$; $p = 0.29$) but a significant positive correlation with the degree of alkalosis ($n = 28$; $r = 0.383$; $p = 0.044$). These data support the hypothesis that the greater the acidosis, the greater the subsequent alkalosis and the worse the neurological outcome. We can infer from the data that an alkalotic pH, when measured in the ischemic focus of stroke patients, is largely due to metabolic paralysis, cell death, cerebral edema, or all three. The alkalosis associated with active cell buffering is therefore more likely a feature of transient cerebral ischemia (Mabe et al., 1983).

GLUCOSE AND ACID-BASE STATUS

We have proposed that there is a period after stroke when ischemic acidosis causes impaired metabolic function, but with the passage of time a flip-flop to alkalosis occurs. If indeed this flip-flop represents the marker for the closure of a therapeutic window, it should be possible to alter brain function during this time, either favorably or unfavorably by manipulating acidosis. After the establishment of alkalosis, such manipulation should have no effect. We have come some way toward achieving these objectives by examining the influence of systemic glucose levels in ischemic brain metabolism.

It is our theory that the severity of acidosis depends on blood glucose concentration and brain glucose and glycogen stores, which in turn, based on experimental evidence, may dictate neurologic outcome (reviewed in Welch and Barkley, 1986). When glucose delivery to the brain is continued as a result of incomplete ischemia or during reflow, there is apparently further stimulation of glycolytic activity, which provides more metabolic acid at a time when the cell is already stressed to compensate for decreased pH. Myers and Yamaguchi (1976) were able to produce irreversible neurologic deficit in the rhesus monkey when lactate levels exceeded 25 μmol/g. Starvation of the animals increased their resistance to ischemia. As a corollary to these studies, pretreatment of cats with glucose prior to complete ischemia dramatically impaired the restitution of CBF and energy metabolism during the postischemic period, attributed in part to tissue lactic acidosis (Welsh et al., 1980). On the other hand, hypoglycemia markedly attenuates ischemic brain acidosis, reduces infarct size, and decreases ischemic neurologic deficit (Chopp et al., 1988; Nedergaard and Diemer, 1989).

The clinical literature has also suggested that neurologic outcome is worsened by high systemic blood glucose levels at the time of hospital admission for stroke (Melamed, 1976; Asplund et al., 1980; Pulsinelli et al., 1984). It appears to be limited to nonlacunar anterior circulation infarcts (Pulsinelli et al., 1984; Mohr et al., 1985; Berger and Hakim, 1986; Cox and Lorains, 1986; Adams et al., 1988). Furthermore, it appears that it is blood glucose at the time of stroke onset rather than a history of diabetes that is the critical factor (Cox and Lorains, 1986).

From the above clinical data the control of blood glucose levels seems worthwhile in patients with cortical anterior circulation infarcts due to occlusion of major intracranial arteries or large branch occlusion if it can be shown that hyperglycemia does unfavorably affect acidosis, metabolism, and neurologic outcome in these patients (Levine et al., 1988).

Figure 2–6 shows ^{31}P NMR spectroscopy and cerebral pH determination in the ischemic hemisphere and the homologous region of the contralateral hemisphere in one such patient studied first on day 4 and again on days 5 and 6 post-stroke. Throughout the course of the study the serial spectra and pH measurements obtained from the homologous regions of the opposite nonischemic hemisphere were unchanged. In contrast, neither high energy phosphates, PMEs, nor PDEs were

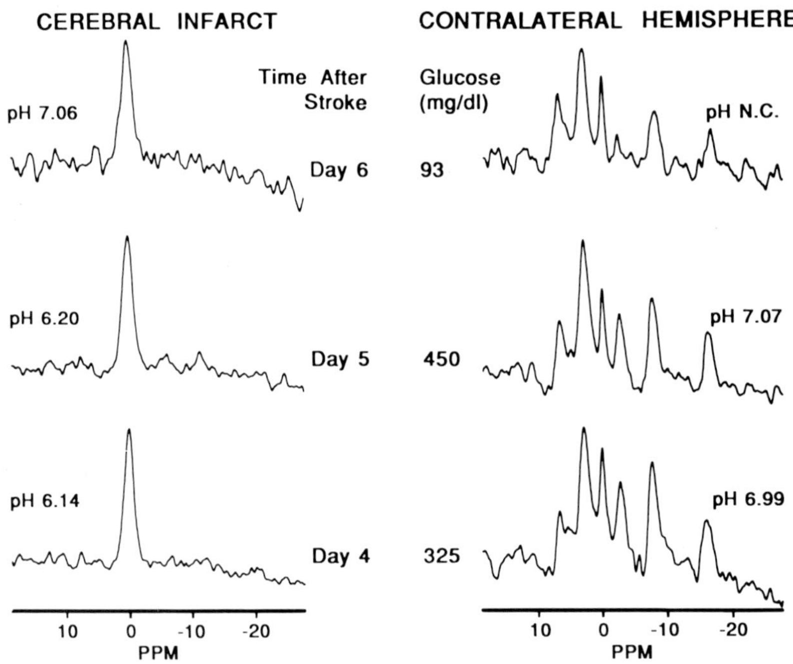

Figure 2–6 Serial in vivo ^{31}phosphorus NMR spectra demonstrating severe depletion of high-energy phosphates and acidosis in a large middle cerebral artery infarction associated with hyperglycemia. Only Pi is apparent. When the severe glucose depletion returned to normal, the acidosis was no longer present.

Table 2–3 Correlation Coefficients of Blood Glucose with Brain pH

Group	No.	Correlation Coefficient	2-Tailed *p* value
Total patients	28	−0.64	<0.001
Acidotic	10	−0.82	<0.004
Normal pH	5	−0.96	<0.001
Alkalotic	13	−0.11	>0.71
Hyperglycemic	10	−0.76	<0.02
Normoglycemic	18	−0.30	<0.22

detected in the serial spectra obtained from the infarct center. The sole spectral peak identified was Pi. Serial examinations failed to show recovery of the high energy phosphates, PME, or PDE components of the spectra. The pH was markedly acidotic (pH 6.14–6.20) so long as the serum glucose levels were high (325–450 mg/dl); but after serum glucose levels were corrected (93 mg/dl) at day 6, the ischemic brain pH did not differ from that of the contralateral hemisphere (pH 7.06). Although this finding could coincide with a shift toward eventual alkalosis, like that observed in stable or recovering patients, this patient died within hours of the last measurement. Furthermore, the total absence of high energy phosphate peaks and severe acidosis persisted well beyond the much earlier return of high-energy phosphate levels and time of alkalotic shifts observed in the normoglycemic stroke patients. As a result of the above case, we proceeded to analyze the relations between pH, energy metabolism and systemic glucose levels obtained upon hospital admission or at a time closest to NMR spectroscopy in patients with focal cortical stroke. There was a significant negative correlation of blood glucose with pH (Table 2–3). Subgroup analysis of the acidotic and normal pH groups or both groups combined revealed additional significant negative correlations (Table 2–4). There was, however, no correlation of blood glucose with pH in the alkalotic group. Furthermore, the hyperglycemic group (glucose $>$ 145 mg/dl) showed a significant negative correlation of systemic glucose with pH, but the normoglycemic group did not. In this group, but not in the normoglycemic group, there were near-significant positive correlations between pH and both the PCr/Pi ratio and β-ATP to support an adverse pH influence on energy

Table 2–4 Relation of pH with Energy and Phospholipid Metabolism in Hyperglycemia and Normoglycemia

	High Glucose (n = 12)		Normal Glucose (n = 22)	
Parameter	*r*	*p*	*r*	*p*
Glucose	−0.76	<0.02	−0.30	>0.22
PCr/Pi	0.62	>0.07	0.33	>0.21
Pi/TP	−0.84	<0.005	−0.62	<0.02
PCR/TP	0.66	<0.04	0.49	<0.05
β-ATP/TP	0.67	<0.04	0.47	<0.05
PME/TP	0.76	<0.02	0.43	>0.08
PDE/TP	0.83	<0.006	0.50	<0.04

metabolism. Thus we now have, hitherto unobtained, metabolic data in patients to support the concept that high systemic glucose levels contribute to brain acidosis and hence potentially poor neurologic outcome (Myers and Yamaguchi, 1976).

CONCLUSION

From our review of the literature and illustrative case series studied by in vivo ^{31}P NMR spectroscopy, we have provided evidence that cerebral ischemia induces intracellular acidosis leading to failure of energy metabolism and damage to the phospholipid components of cell membranes. Acidosis can be made worse by systemic hyperglycemia. At a stage in the progression of the stroke, brain acidosis switches, or flip-flops, to alkalosis, after which time there is little evidence that the tissue pH can be further manipulated. Apparently the worse the ischemic brain acidosis, the worse are the subsequent alkalosis and the neurologic outcome. An alkalotic pH in ischemic infarction probably represents metabolic paralysis, cerebral edema, and death of tissue. The identification of a possible therapeutic window of time, the closure of which may be represented by the pH flip-flop, provides some hope that experimental cerebral protective drugs or other potentially beneficial therapeutic measures may be investigated without the adverse bias of being given when irreversible cellular damage has already been established.

Based on the data just reviewed, it is apparent that in vivo metabolic correlates can be obtained for clinical neurologic phenomena. We can therefore speculate that similar in vivo metabolic correlates (i.e., brain pH and energy metabolism) may be possible for certain neuropsychological and neuropsychometric measures. Based on certain features of presumed transient "uncoupling" of cerebral blood flow and metabolism during specific neurologic/neuropsychological activation procedures (Fox and Raichle, 1986), further studies may allow correlations of brain pH and metabolism with the severity of specific neuropsychological deficits. It may be that brain pH modifies the flow–metabolic coupling and its resulting influence on neuropsychological function.

GLOSSARY

Acidosis: the process of liberating free H^+, reducing pH.

Adenylate energy status:

$$\frac{[\text{ATP}]}{[\text{ADP}][\text{Pi}]} = \frac{[\text{PCr}]K_{eq}[\text{H}^+]}{[\text{Pi}][\text{creatine}]} \text{ (phosphorylation ratio)}$$

equilibrium of high-energy phosphate metabolites as a function of brain pH. ATP = adenosine triphosphate; ADP = adenosine diphosphate; Pi = inorganic orthophosphate; PCr = phosphocreatine; K_{eq} = the equilibrium constant of this chemical reaction.

ATP hydrolysis: the process of converting ATP to ADP or AMP and releasing energy for other chemical reactions.

Bicarbonate (HCO_3^-): a major anionic buffer in the brain.

$$H^+ + HCO_3^- = H_2O + CO_2$$

Therefore the HCO_3^- concentration is dependent on concentration of H^+ and CO_2.

Buffer: the process by which cells and tissues maintain pH and ionic homeostasis.

Carbon dioxide (CO_2): a waste product of cellular metabolism that also regulates many metabolic pathways.

Cl^-/HCO_3^- antiport system: chloride (Cl^-) and bicarbonate (HCO_3^-) are exchanged across membranes to maintain electrostatic charge balance.

Free radicals: metabolic products that are intrinsically unstable in their chemical composition and that may mediate, in part, ischemic cell damage through their adverse effects on mitochondria and membranes.

Na^+/H^+ antiport system: the membrane channel system that allows exchange of sodium ions (Na^+) and protons (H^+) to maintain ionic homeostasis.

pH: − log hydrogen ion (H^+) concentration. Living human brain pH is generally thought to be approximately 6.95 to 7.05. The value is tightly regulated under most, if not all, physiologic, nonpathologic conditions. CO_2 diffuses freely into the brain, whereas H^+ moves across the blood-brain barrier slowly. Consequently, the brain pH reflects blood PCO_2 rather than blood pH.

REFERENCES

Adams, H.P., Olinger, C., Marler, J.R., Biller, J., Brott, T.G., Barsan, W.G., and Banwalt, K. (1988). Comparison of admission serum glucose concentration with neurologic outcome in cerebral infarction. *Stroke,* **19,** 455–458.

Asplund, K., Hagg, E., Helmers, C., Litner, F., Strand, T., and Wester, P-O. (1980). The natural history of stroke in diabetic patients. *Acta Med. Scand.,* **207,** 417–424.

Astrup, J., Siesjo, B.K., and Symon, L. (1981). Thresholds in cerebral ischemia—the ischemic perumbra. *Stroke,* **12,** 723–725.

Atkinson, D.E. (1968). The energy charge of the adenylate pool as a regulatory parameter. *Biochemistry,* **7,** 4030–4034.

Berger, L., and Hakim, A.M. (1986). The association of hyperglycemia with cerebral edema in stroke. *Stroke,* **17,** 865–871.

Chien, S. (1985). Cerebral blood flow and metabolism: appendix IB. In: E.R. Kandel and J.H. Schwartz, (eds.). *Principles of Neural Science,* 2nd ed., pp. 845–852. New York: Elsevier.

Choi, M.U., and Abramson, M.B. (1978). Effects of pH changes and charge characteristics in the uptake of norepinephrine by synaptosomes of rat brain. *Biochim.Biophys. Acta,* **540,** 337–345.

Chopp, M., Welch, K.M.A., Tidwell, C., and Helpern, J.A. (1988). Global cerebral ischemia and intracellular pH during hyperglycemia and hypoglycemia in the cat. *Stroke,* **19,** 1383–1387.

Cox, N.H., and Lorains, J.W. (1986). The prognostic value of blood glucose and glycosylated hemoglobin in patients with stroke. *Postgrad. Med. J.,* **62,** 7–10.

Fox, P.T., and Raichle, M.E. (1986)..Focal physiological uncoupling of cerebral blood flow and oxidative metabolisms during somatosensory stimulation in human subjects. *Proc. Nat. Acad. Sci. USA,* **83,** 1140–1144.

Frackowiak, R.S.J. (1986). PET scanning: can it help resolve management issues in cerebral ischemic disease? *Stroke,* **17,** 803–807.

Gadian, D.G. (1982). *Nuclear Magnetic Resonance and Its Applications to Living Systems.* New York: Oxford University Press.

Gastaut, H., and Meyer, J.S., eds. (1961). *Cerebral Anoxia and the Electroencephalogram.* Springfield: Charles C Thomas.

Goldberg, N.D., Passonneau, J.V., and Lowry, O.H. (1966). Effects of changes in brain metabolism on the levels of citric acid cycle intermediates. *J. Biol. Chem.,* **241,** 3997–4003.

Hakim, A.M., Pokrupa, R.P., Villanueva, J., Diksic, M., Evans, A.C., Thompson, C.J., Meyer, E., Yamamoto, Y.L., and Feindel, W.H. (1987). The effect of spontaneous reperfusion on metabolic function in early human cerebral infarcts. *Ann. Neurol.*, **21**, 279–289.

Kempski, O., Staub, F., Jansen, M., Schodel, F., and Baethmann, A. (1988). Glial swelling during extracellular acidosis in vitro. *Stroke*, **19**, 386–392.

Kogure, K., Busto, R., Schwartzman, R.J., and Scheinberg, P. (1980). The dissociation of cerebral blood flow, metabolism, and function in the early stages of developing cerebral infarction. *Ann. Neurol.*, **8**, 278–290.

Kontos, H.A. (1986). Cerebral microcirculation in stroke. In: H.J.M. Barnett, B.M. Stein, J.P. Mohr, and F.M. Yatsu, eds., *Stroke: Pathophysiology, Diagnosis, and Management*, Vol. 1, pp. 91–95. New York: Churchill Livingstone.

Kraig, R.P. and Petito, C.K. (1989). Interrelation of proton and volume regulation in astrocytes. Ginsberg, M.D., and Dietrich, W.D., eds. In: *Cerebrovascular Disease: Sixteenth Research (Princeton) Conference*, pp. 239–246. New York: Raven Press.

Kraig, R.P., Pulsinelli, W.A., and Plum, F. (1985). Heterogeneous distribution of hydrogen and bicarbonate ions during complete brain ischemia. *Prog. Brain Res.*, **63**, 155–166.

Kraig, R.P., Pulsinelli, W.A., and Plum, F. (1985). Behavior of brain bicarbonate ions during complete ischemia. *J. Cereb. Blood Flow Metab.*, **5**(suppl. 1), S227–S228.

Kuschinsky, W., and Wahl, M. (1978). Local chemical and neurogenic regulation of cerebral vascular resistance. *Physiol. Rev.*, **58**, 656–689.

Lehninger, A.L. (1975). *Biochemistry*, 2nd ed. New York: Worth Publishers.

Levine, S.R., Welch, K.M.A., Bruce, R., and Smith, M.B. (1987). Brain intracellular pH "flip-flop" in human ischemic stroke identified by ^{31}P NMR. *Ann. Neurol.*, **22**, 137.

Levine, S.R., Welch, K.M.A., Helpern, J.A., Chopp, M., Bruce, R., Selwa, J., and Smith, M.B. (1988). Prolonged deterioration of ischemic brain energy metabolism and acidosis associated with hyperglycemia: human cerebral infarction studied by serial ^{31}P NMR spectroscopy. *Ann. Neurol.*, **23**, 416–418.

Lowry, O.H., and Passonneau, J.V. (1964). The relationship between substrates and enzymes of glycolysis in brain. *J. Biol. Chem.*, **239**, 31–42.

Lund-Anderson, H. (1979). Transport of glucose from blood to brain. *Physiol. Rev.*, **59**, 305–352.

Mabe, H., Blomqvist, P., and Siesjo, B.K. (1983). Intracellular pH in the brain following transient ischemia. *J. Cereb. Blood Flow Metab.*, **3**, 109–114.

Mayevsky, A., Nioka, S., Subrammanian, V.H., and Chance, B. (1988). Brain oxidative metabolism of the newborn dog: correlation between ^{31}P NMR spectroscopy and pyridine nucleotide redox state. *J. Cereb. Blood Flow Metab.*, **8**, 201–207.

McCormick, W.F., and Schochet, S.S., Jr. (1976). *Atlas of Cerebrovascular Disease*. Philadelphia: Saunders.

McMillan, V., and Siesjo, B.K. (1983). The effect of phenobarbitone anesthesia upon some organic phosphates, glycolytic metabolites and citric acid cycle-associated intermediates of the rat brain. *J. Neurochem.*, **20**, 1669–1681.

Melamed, E. (1976). Reactive hyperglycemia in patients with acute stroke. *J. Neurol. Sci.*, **29**, 267–275.

Meyer, J.S., Gotoh, F., and Tazaki, Y. (1962). Metabolism following experimental cerebral embolism. *J. Neuropathol. Exp. Neurol.*, **21**, 4–24.

Michenfelder, J.D., and Theye, R.A. (1970). The effects of anesthesia and hypothermia on canine cerebral ATP and lactate during anoxia produced by decapitation. *Anesthesiology*, **33**, 430–439.

Mitchell, P. (1961). Coupling of phosphorylation to electron and hydrogen transfer by a chemiosmotic type of mechanism. *Nature*, **191**, 144–148.

Mohr, J.P., Rubenstein, L.V., Tatemichi, T.K., Nichols, F.T., Caplan, L.R., Hier, D.B., Kase,

C.S., Price, T.R., and Wolf, P.A. (1985). Blood sugar and acute stroke: the NINCDS pilot stroke data bank. *Stroke,* **16,** 143.

Myers, R.E., and Yamaguchi, M. (1976). Tissue lactate accumulation as cause of cerebral edema. *Neurosci. Abstr.,* **2,** 1042.

Nedergaard, M., and Diemer, N.H. (1989). Hypoglycemia reduces infarct size in experimental focal cerebral ischemia. In: M.D. Ginsberg and W.D. Dietrich, eds., *Cerebrovascular Disease: Sixteenth Research (Princeton) Conference,* pp. 259–264. New York: Raven Press.

Paschen, W., Sato, W., Pawlik, G., Umbach, C., and Heiss, W.D. (1985). Neurologic deficit, blood flow and biochemical sequelae of reversible focal cerebral ischemia in cats. *J. Neurol. Sci.,* **68,** 119–134.

Pelligrino, D., and Siesjo, B.K. (1981). Regulation of extra- and intracellular pH in the brain in severe hypoglycemia. *J. Cereb. Blood Flow Metab.,* **1,** 85–96.

Petroff, O.A.C., Prichard, J.W., Behar, K.L., Alger, J.R., and Shulman, R.G. (1984). In vivo phosphorus nuclear magnetic resonance spectroscopy in status epilepticus. *Ann. Neurol.,* **16,** 169–177.

Petroff, O.A.C., Prichard, J.W., Behar, K.L., Alger, J.R., den Hollander, J.A., and Shulman, R.G. (1985). Cerebral intracellular pH by ^{31}P nuclear magnetic resonance spectroscopy. *Neurology,* **35,** 781–788.

Pettegrew, J.W., Kopp, S.J., Minshew, N.J., et al. (1985). ^{31}P nuclear magnetic resonance studies of phosphoglyceride metabolism in developing and degenerating brain: preliminary observations. *J. Neuropathol. Exp. Neurol.,* **46,** 419–430.

Plum, F., Cooper, A.J.L., Kraig, R.P., Petito, C.K., and Pulsinelli, W.A. (1985). Glial cells: the silent partners of the working brain. *J. Cereb. Blood Flow Metab.,* **5,** S1–S4.

Power, W.J., and Raichle, M.E. (1985). Positron emission tomography and its application to the study of cerebrovascular disease in man. *Stroke,* **16,** 361–376.

Prichard, J.W., Alger, J.R., Behar, K.L., Petroff, O.A.C., and Shulman, R.G. (1983). Cerebral metabolic studies in vivo by ^{31}P NMR. *Proc. Nat. Acad. Sci. USA.* **80,** 2748–2751.

Pulsinelli, W.A., Levy, D.A., and Duffy, T.E. (1982). Regional cerebral blood flow and glucose metabolism following transient forebrain ischemia. *Ann. Neurol.,* **11,** 499–509.

Pulsinelli, W., Sigsbee, B., Rawlinson, D., et al. (1984). Experimental hyperglycemia and diabetes mellitus worsen stroke outcome. *Ann. Neurol.,* **8,** 91.

Radda, G.K. (1986). The use of NMR spectroscopy for the understanding of disease. *Science,* **223,** 640–645.

Roos, A., and Boron, W.F. (1981). Intracellular pH. *Physiol. Rev.,* **61,** 296–434.

Scremin, O.U., and Jenden, D.J. (1989). Focal ischemia enhances choline output and decreases acetylcholine output from rat cerebral cortex. *Stroke,* **20,** 92–95.

Shoubridge, E.A., Briggs, R.W., and Radda, G.W. (1980). ^{31}P NMR saturation transfer measurements of the steady state rates of creatine kinase and ATP synthetase in the rat brain. *FEBS Lett.,* **140,** 288–292.

Siesjo, B.K. (1978). *Brain Energy Metabolism.* New York: Wiley.

Siesjo, B.K. (1981). Cell damage in the brain: a speculative synthesis. *J. Cereb. Blood Flow Metab.,* **1,** 155–185.

Siesjo, B.K. (1985a). Acid-base homeostasis in the brain: physiology, chemistry, and neurochemical pathology. *Prog. Brain Res.,* **63,**121–154.

Siesjo, B.K. (1985b). Acidosis and brain damage: possible molecular mechanisms. *J. Cereb. Blood Flow Metab.,* **5,** S225–S226.

Suzuki, K. (1981). Chemistry and metabolism of brain lipids. In: G.J. Siegel, R.W. Albers, B.W. Agranof, and R. Katzman, eds., *Basic Neurochemistry,* 3rd ed., pp. 355–370. Boston: Little, Brown.

Syrota, A., Samson, Y., Boullais, C., Wajnberg, P., Loc'h, C., Crouzel, C., Maziere, B., Soussaline, F., and Baron, J.C. (1985). Tomographic mapping of brain intracellular pH and extracellular water space in stroke patients. *J. Cereb. Blood Flow Metab.,* **5,** 358–368.

Wanke, E., Carbone, E., and Testa, P.L. (1979). K^+ conductance modified by a titratable group accessible to protons from the intracellular side of the squid axon membrane. *Biophys. J.,* **26,** 319–324.

Welch, K.M.A., and Barkley, G.L. (1986). Biochemistry and pharmacology of cerebral ischemia. In: H.J.M. Barnett, J.P. Mohr, B.M. Stein, and F.M. Yatsu, eds., *Stroke: Pathophysiology, Diagnosis, and Management,* Vol. 1, pp. 75–90. New York: Churchill-Livingstone.

Welsh, F.A., Ginsberg, M.D., Rieder, W., et al. (1980). Deleterious effect of glucose pretreatment on recovery from diffuse cerebral ischemia in the cat. *Stroke,* **11,** 355–363.

Yoshida, S., Busto, R., Martinez, E., and Ginsberg, M.D. (1985). Regional energy metabolism after complete versus incomplete cerebral ischemia in the absence of severe lactic acidosis. *J. Cereb. Blood Flow Metab.,* **5,** S233–S234.

3

Xenon 133 Cerebral Blood Flow: Review of Methods and Utility in Cerebrovascular Disease

BRETT E. SKOLNICK

The measurement of regional cerebral blood flow (rCBF) with noninvasive xenon 133 methods has permitted the direct study of the brain's response to neurologic insult (stroke or hemorrhage). Also, rCBF methods have been used to determine the effects of various challenges to the central nervous system (hyperventilation, vasodilatory agents, cognitive tasks). These various approaches have enhanced our understanding of brain physiology and have made possible comprehensive investigations of brain-behavior relations. As such, rCBF measurements and their extension to three-dimensional imaging techniques offers a unique view of the dynamic brain.

WHY STUDY CBF MEASURED BY XENON 133?

The Xenon 133 (^{133}Xe) methods provide a number of advantages compared to other methods of measuring cerebral blood flow, e.g. positron emission tomography (PET), single photon emission computed tomography (SPECT), and stable xenon computed tomography. The ^{133}Xe method is a noninvasive procedure that requires no arterial sampling. The radiation exposure for the ^{133}Xe studies is considered negligible, in contrast with PET and SPECT studies. The ^{133}Xe methods typically expose the lung to less than 200 millirad per study. The ^{133}Xe method is well documented with established quantification procedures; and although there are a number of methods for analysis of the clearance curve, there is good correspondence between methods (Risberg et al., 1975; Obrist and Wilkinson, 1980; Ryding, 1989). The Xenon 133 method also provides excellent reproducibility within a session as well as over time (Warach et al., 1988). These features distinguish the ^{133}Xe method from other methods of determining regional cerebral blood flow. In addition, the ^{133}Xe method provides demonstrated sensitivity to regional neuronal activation obtained by either simple sensory stimulation or cognitive tasks (Risberg and Ingvar, 1973; Gur and Reivich, 1980; Gur et al., 1982b).

The method, however, is not without some disadvantages. It provides only two-dimensional data and is limited principally to measurement of the outer cortical mantle. The ^{133}Xe method provides a measure only of cerebral blood flow; it does not measure oxygen metabolism unless concurrent measurements are made of oxygen from arterial and venous supplies of the brain. The method also depends on the validity of the assumed partition coefficients for uptake of ^{133}Xe by the gray and white matter of the brain (see the ^{133}Xe CBF method section below for a discussion of partition coefficients). Although these coefficients are stable in normal brain, they may be less stable in pathologic brain. Finally, the problem of "look-through" has the potential to limit the stability of the measurement, especially in ischemia. This phenomenon occurs in low flow conditions when the scintillation detectors tend to "look through" the pathologic tissue to the normal tissue in the homotopic region of the opposite hemisphere. Each of these factors must be acknowledged and carefully attended to in order to provide a meaningful interpretation of the resulting measurements. These issues are described more completely in the ^{133}Xe CBF method section of this chapter.

Alternative methods are available for measuring rCBF, including PET (Reivich, 1985), SPECT (Bonte et al., 1988), and stable xenon computed tomography (CT) (Gur et al., 1982b). A complete discussion of these methods and a critical review of their respective advantages and disadvantages is beyond the scope of this chapter. However, a brief review of each method and a number of points of comparison to the ^{133}Xe method are outlined below.

Single Photon Emission Computed Tomography

Computed tomography of isotope distribution is based on principles pioneered by Kuhl and colleagues (1976) and is conducted using SPECT. This method provides the capability of three-dimensional detection of ^{133}Xe uptake and washout, thereby providing determination of cerebral blood flow (Stokely et al., 1980).

SPECT is based on the use of a high sensitivity fast rotating gamma ray detection system developed specifically to allow dynamic studies. The high sensitivity is achieved by a large crystal area consisting of 64 separate crystals typically arranged in four banks of 16. The fast rotation of the detector arrangement at a continuous speed allows sampling of a complete set of projections. Because of the counting requirements, several sets of projections must be recorded. At present, the measurements are principally limited to qualitative assessment. A variety of other isotopes can be used for imaging, including ^{99}technetium, ^{123}iodine, and ^{123}I-isopropyliodo-amphetamine (IMPN). Additional information can be obtained on SPECT methods by referring to Vorstrup and colleagues (1986).

Positron Emission Tomography

Positron (dual-photon) emission computed tomography provides another method for determining cerebral blood flow and enables measurement of cerebral blood volume and glucose and oxygen utilization. PET uses short-lived isotopes, typically requiring preparation in a cyclotron. It makes possible the quantitative measurement of local tissue concentrations of injected or inhaled biologically compatible radioactive tracers. The technique is based on the simultaneous detection of two paired photons traveling in opposite directions and provides uniform resolution and high accuracy (see Chapter 4). The absorbed radiation dose in the patient/volunteer is high, however, and thus imposes strict limitations on the frequency of studies undertaken in the same individual. Also, the high cost of technology, isotope production, and associated short half-lives of the isotopes restricts the use of PET to a select group of large medical centers. For a comprehensive review see Phelps and associates (1982). A more specific review of PET as it relates to aphasia is provided in Chapter 4 of this book.

Stable Xenon Computed Tomography

The stable xenon CT method (Gur et al., 1982b) represents another technique for measuring CBF in man. It has had only limited acceptance, the principal reason being that the concentration of stable xenon (Xe_s) administered during the typical study is 30 to 40%. This level of Xe_s has been demonstrated to alter CO_2 reactivity and the electroencephalographic (EEG) spectrum as well as CBF levels in both baboon (Hartmann et al., 1987) and man (Obrist et al., 1985). In addition, concerns have been raised regarding volume averaging and low signal-to-noise ratios and apparent violation of the indicator dilution principles.

Each of these three-dimensional techniques provides enhanced brain representation when compared to ^{133}Xe techniques, but each also requires greater radiation exposure and better patient cooperation during the setup and measurement phases. Quantification has been a subject of much concern; studies (Bartlett et al., 1988) using PET, however, have demonstrated high test-retest reliability (within 24 hours) for global (changes less than 7%) and regional changes (less than 1%) using scaled data based on the first session values, although larger variability has been found with 2-week intervals (Duara et al., 1987). Quantification is a special problem for the SPECT method, although one study suggested that reliable quantification using IMP-SPECT is possible (Podreka et al., 1989). Variations between laboratories have remained a problem.

The influence of subject/patient anxiety on the measurement of CBF is an additional problem, common to all CBF techniques, including the ^{133}Xe method. Variations in anxiety provide a possible source for some of the between-subject and between-session variability. Gur and colleagues (1987a) reported a significant negative correlation between self-report measures of anxiety (Spielberger's State-Trait Anxiety Inventory) and cortical metabolism. Also, Bartlett and colleagues (1988) reported that relatively higher anxiety, reflected as higher pulse rates, was associated with relatively lower metabolism. Other studies (Mountz et al., 1989; Reiman et al., 1989; Rodrigues et al., 1989; Zohar et al., 1989) have examined aspects of anxiety in both patient and normal populations using blood flow measures obtained by either PET or ^{133}Xe techniques. The results are suggestive of lateralized and localized abnormalities being detected (with the exception of the Mountz et al. study). These isolated studies have only explored, in a limited manner, the contribution of patient state on the dependent variable(s) of interest. Further exploration of the interrelation between autonomic measures and regional brain metabolism may aid in accounting for some of the variability of the measures of cerebral blood flow and metabolism.

HISTORICAL PERSPECTIVE ON CBF METHODOLOGY

The CBF methods, using a diffusible tracer, are based on the Fick principle, which is a restatement of the law of conservation of matter. The Fick principle states that the quantity of a metabolically inert substance taken up by tissue in a unit time is equal to the quantity brought to the tissue by the arterial blood minus the quantity carried away by the venous blood. The assumptions are that the tracer is metabolically inert and diffuses rapidly between blood and tissue, that arterial flow is equal to venous flow, and that the blood and tissue form only a small percentage of the total tissue volume. The Fick equation is as follows:

$$\frac{dQ_t}{d_t} = F \times (C_a - C_v)$$

where dQ_t represents the quantity of tracer in tissue at time t, dQ_t/d_t is the change in tracer quantity with time, F is blood flow (measured as ml/100 g/min), and C_a and C_v are the tracer concentrations in arterial and venous blood, respectively.

A variety of techniques over the past four decades have extended this general method for measuring cerebral blood flow. The first of these methods measured oxygen uptake in the brain (Lennox and Gibbs, 1932) and provided an initial view of the working brain. The inert gas method of Kety and Schmidt (1945) using nitrous oxide provided a major advance in methodology. The method was considered invasive, required arterial and jugular punctures, and depended on the administration of low concentrations of nitrous oxide by inhalation for a 10-minute equilibrium period. At the termination of nitrous oxide delivery, the concentrations of nitrous oxide in arterial blood, tissue, and venous blood were approximately equal. Following nitrous administration, a series of blood samples were taken from the jugular vein and the carotid artery. These blood samples were analyzed, and nitrous oxide content was determined. Global cerebral blood flow could then be calculated using an integrated form of the Fick equation.

$$C_i(T) = \frac{F_i}{W_i} \int_0^t (C_a - C_v)\, d_t$$

The method provided the foundation for extension of these general principles to the measurement of CBF using radioactive gases, with calculations being made during the desaturation phase. The specifics of this alternative method are discussed below.

Intraarterial Injection of Inert Gas

The principles for measuring CBF by intraarterial injection of an inert gas were proposed by Lassen and Ingvar (1961). Krypton (^{85}Kr) was injected as a bolus into the internal carotid artery, and the beta radiation from the exposed cortex of experimental animals was measured. Desaturation of the tracer in tissue over time (tracer washout) provided the physiologic model for determining rCBF. A variety of indices were derived, including F_1, a measure of fast-clearing tissue compartment, presumably representing gray matter tissue clearance; F_2, a measure of slow-clearing tissue compartment, presumably representing white matter and extracerebral tissue clearance; CBF_{15}, a measure of the height-over-area of the clearance curve, representing an average gray and white matter flow independent of partition coefficients; and W_1, a percent measure of relevant size of the fast-clearing compartment. The intracarotid injection method was extended by Mallet and Veall (1963; Veall and Mallett, 1966). Their contribution was to extend the intracarotid injection principles to the less invasive intravenous injection of the isotope, which also enabled bihemispheric measurements. This initial work was further extended and refined by Obrist and coworkers, as described below.

XENON 133 CBF METHOD

The noninvasive ^{133}Xe (inhalation and intravenous) methods are an extension of the intraarterial injection methods. The ^{133}Xe method, like most tracer kinetic methods, is based on the theoretical and empirical work conducted by Kety and Schmidt (1945). The tracer, in this case an inert gamma-emitting gas, is introduced into the systemic circulation by inhalation or intravenous injection. It reaches the brain in the arterial blood and diffuses into the parenchyma from the capillaries in accordance with its concentration gradient and partition coefficient. The partition coefficient is a ratio of the solubilities of the tracer in the blood and the tissue, with a theoretically ideal tracer having a partition coefficient of 1. Clearance of the tracer is monitored for 10 to 15 minutes, and the results are calculated through fitting a theoretical biexponential function by the least-squares method (Obrist et al., 1975).

Adequate compartmentalization requires that distinct blood flow components be resolved using biexponential analyses. This situation has been demonstrated to be accurate in healthy subjects, where gray and white matter have two distinctly different distributions of flow (Reivich et al., 1969). Repeated measurements with a high degree of reliability and reproducibility (Obrist and Wilkinson, 1980) can be made with this method.

The intracarotid injection method was compared with the inhalation ^{133}Xe method by Reivich and colleagues (1975). Eleven patients with cerebrovascular disease undergoing cerebral angiography were studied using the intracarotid technique and the inhalation method. On the basis of this study, it was concluded that the ^{133}Xe inhalation technique compared favorably with the ^{133}Xe intracarotid injection method. This conclusion was demonstrated to be valid even in the low flow situation (not less than 33 ml/100 g/min).

The model used for the calculation of cerebral blood flow in the inhalation studies employs a convolution integral, where an input (arterial or end-tidal ^{133}Xe concentration) is convoluted with an exponential function to yield the tissue concentration.

$$C(t) = \sum_{i=1}^{2} P_i \int_0^t Ca(u)e^{-Ki(t-u)}\,du$$

The process of convolution is represented by the sum of the products of the arterial concentration with the exponential for each time interval. Given an observed tissue concentration [C(t)] obtained from extracranial monitoring and the ^{133}Xe input function [C_a (t)] obtained from the end-tidal curve, the above equation yields a solution for four unknowns: P1 and P2 (weight coefficients) and K1 and K2 (clearance rates). Two compartments are assumed: a fast-clearing (principally gray matter) component and a slow-clearing (principally white matter) component, which because of extracerebral contamination also includes a component of scalp flow. The computed parameters are generally determined by a least-squares curve fitting procedure, although maximum likelihood methods are also available (Ewing et al., 1977). Two types of indices are typically calculated: separate estimates for each of the two compartments and estimates of the mean CBF for the combined compartments. Compartmental indices include F_1, which has been widely used and is applicable for description of normal gray matter CBF, where the assumption of separate gray and white matter compartments is reasonable; and F_2, a measure of principally white matter flow, which contains a small unknown amount of scalp flow, thereby limiting its interpretability. Both F_1 and F_2 are subject to instability in grossly pathologic tissue, where compartment separation is no longer in accordance with anatomic designations or where low signal-to-noise ratios, represented as low count rates, are obtained.

Noncompartmental indices provide estimates of mean CBF for combined fast- and slow-clearing compartments, assuming a mean partition coefficient. Two principal indices have been used: height-over-area to infinity (CBF_∞) and a height-over-area to 15 minutes (CBF_{15}). In addition, two other noncompartmental indices have been developed: the initial slope index (ISI) of Risberg (Risberg et al., 1975) and the initial slope (IS) of Obrist (Obrist and Wilkinson, 1980). Neither of these measures requires an assumption of the partition coefficients, but they are nevertheless derived from the four parameters computed by the biexponential analysis. The ISI index can be defined as the slope between minutes 2 and 3 of the recirculation-corrected curve. This index has been found to be exceptionally stable in pathologic conditions (Risberg et al., 1975), a characteristic that has resulted in its widespread use. The index, however, is not particularly sensitive to high flow rates and depends on the shape and duration of the input function (Obrist et al., 1987). Reformulations of the ISI measure have been described that attempt to correct these problems (Prohovnik et al., 1985). In contrast, the IS measure is sensitive to high flow owing to its being heavily weighted by the fast tissue compartment. The measure is the initial slope at time zero of the equivalent unit-impulse curve. It is comparable to F_1 but has the advantage that it is highly stable and has been found to be particularly useful in the study of psychological activation (Gur et al., 1982b).

A critical component of the rCBF analysis is the determination of the recirculation of isotope. The concentration of ^{133}Xe in arterial blood entering the brain (arterial input function) is estimated by measuring the ^{133}Xe concentration in the mouth at the end of each nominal exhalation. This method provides an end-tidal estimate for the ^{133}Xe gas concentration curve that is believed to be a reliable estimate of the arterial ^{133}Xe concentration because in most cases it is representative of the arterial blood leaving the lungs, which are in a diffusion equilibrium with ^{133}Xe in the alveoli of the lungs. In patients with pulmonary disease these estimates are inaccurate. Methods for more reliably estimating this arterial input function have been suggested (Jaggi and Obrist, 1981; Hazelrig et al., 1985; Allison et al., 1988). The method suggested by Allison and colleagues (1988) makes use of the concentration of CO_2 in the respiratory gases sampled at the mouth to provide greater certainty in the estimates of the arterial input function. This method provides an automated means of determining optimal exhalations and inhalations and does not depend on the discretion of the technician. Figure 3–1 provides a representation of the ^{133}Xe system.

A number of other potential limitations exist with the noninvasive ^{133}Xe methods, including issues of "look-through," which limits the sensitivity of the method to detect ischemia. Previous work (Wyper and Booke, 1977) demonstrated that approximately 30% of the recorded counts originate in the contralateral hemisphere. This phenomenon, called cross-talk, provides a source of potential artifact, but is of little significance in normal brain, where blood flow distributions are fairly homogeneous. For cases in which focal asymmetry exists (e.g., stroke) cross-talk potentially could obscure the results. Jaggi and Obrist (1987) empirically determined the degree of functional cross-talk, defined as the ratio of contralateral/ipsilateral detector sensitivity for a given lesion of various sizes and depths using a computer-simulated model (Jaggi, 1985). The model simulated normal and abnormal ^{133}Xe distribution in brain and demonstrated that functional cross-talk is dependent on lesion depth. Superficial lesions demonstrate minimal cross-talk (less than 10%) whereas deep lesions demonstrate greater cross-talk (15–30%). The degree of cross-talk was relatively independent of lesion size.

The same computer model has been used to evaluate the sensitivity of the various rCBF parameters to detect focal lesions. Lesions of different sizes were modeled with flow levels for gray and white tissue compartments. Simulated head curves were developed with varying flow levels for the two compartments. CBF changes obtained from the standard biexponential analysis remained proportional to modeled flows in the lesion. In extreme flow reductions of more than 45%, fast clearance measures (F_1 and IS) were no longer proportional.

REGULATION OF CBF

Regulation of CBF in normal brain is determined by a variety of intrinsic control mechanisms. Despite wide variations in blood flow throughout the body, the brain

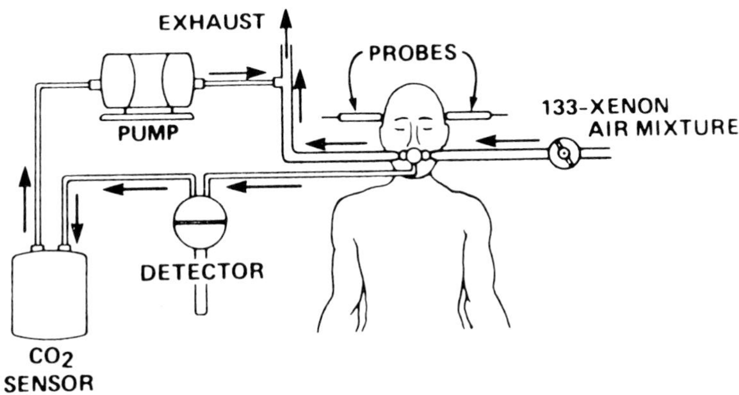

Figure 3–1 Cerebral blood flow system that enables inhalation studies to be performed.

extracts the amount of blood required for its tissue nutrition and for ensuring homeostasis. There are four basic intrinsic control mechanisms of cerebral blood flow.

Autoregulation

The concept of autoregulation implies that CBF remains relatively constant even when changes in cerebral perfusion pressure (CPP), within certain limits, have occurred (Harper, 1966; Fitch et al., 1975). It is a result of the active countermeasures of vasoconstriction and vasodilation initiated by the precapillary resistance vessels, which alter cerebrovascular resistance (CVR). Autoregulation ensures that a supply of oxygen, glucose, and other essential nutrients are maintained, and that capillary pressure is kept within normal limits. Control of the cerebrovascular resistance is maintained by the sympathetic nervous system and provides a means for the vasculature to tolerate increases in blood pressure without arterial overstretching, blood-brain barrier leakage, and edema formation (Strandgaard et al., 1975; Berne et al., 1981). When increasing blood pressure exceeds the compensatory vasodilation capacity, autoregulation fails and CBF is no longer independent of cerebral perfusion pressure. The relation of CBF to blood pressure beyond the limit of autoregulation is complex and heterogeneous (Burke et al., 1987). At this point the brain is capable of increasing its oxygen extraction when the oxygen supply is diminished in regions of decreased CBF (Schmidt et al., 1945; Raichle et al., 1976a,b). One mechanism for this change in oxygen extraction fraction is the change in oxygen-hemoglobin affinity in the setting of high concentrations of CO_2. One study (Aaslid et al., 1989) using a novel set of procedures demonstrated the dynamic nature of autoregulation. The rapid autoregulatory response was argued to be mediated by metabolic mechanisms, partially supported by the fact that cerebral autoregulatory action is much faster than the baroreceptor reflex, which regulates arterial blood pressure.

Chemical Control

Variations in arterial pCO_2 exert a profound influence on CBF. Hypercapnia causes cerebrovasodilation, whereas hypocapnia produces marked intracerebral vasoconstriction. At normal pCO_2 levels CBF changes by approximately 3.0 to 4.0% for every 1% change in pCO_2 (Obrist et al., 1975; Davis et al., 1983) although other proportional changes have been reported (Maximilian et al., 1980). Accurate measurements of pCO_2 are consequently important for proper evaluation of CBF levels. The arteriolar response that follows changes in pCO_2 is believed to be mediated by pH variations in the extracellular fluid surrounding resistance vessels in the brain (Skinhoj and Paulson, 1969; Pannier et al., 1972).

Carbon dioxide response has also been explored as a method for assessing cerebrovascular functional reserve in patients with cerebrovascular disease (Norrving et al., 1982; Bullock et al., 1985; Brown et al., 1986) and has been shown to be altered by the normal aging process (Yamaguchi et al., 1979; Yamamoto et al., 1980). This type of challenge has been demonstrated to be of significant value in the assessment of cerebrovascular reserve in patients with carotid artery disease (reviewed below).

Metabolic Control

Early methods for measuring CBF in man evaluated large tissue masses for fairly long intervals of time. These analyses suggested that CBF was reasonably constant during variations of neuronal activity. As methods for determining CBF have improved, more dynamic conditions have been revealed that demonstrate that enhanced neuronal function is associated with increased metabolic activity and cerebral blood flow (Raichle et al., 1976a,b).

Cerebral metabolism is a critical factor in the control of CBF. The brain is considered to be an "obligatory aerobe" in that it derives all of its energy from the metabolism of oxygen and glucose. The brain uses 25% of the total body oxygen consumption per minute and 10% of the glucose (Siesjo, 1978), which translates to 45 to 55 ml of oxygen and 60 to 80 mg of glucose per minute. By means of glycolysis via the Embden-Meyerhof pathway and the Krebs cycle, as well as by means of oxidative phosphorylation, high energy phosphate bonds are produced in the form of ATP. The chemical pathway for glucose and oxygen metabolism to produce water, CO_2, and energy is as follows:

$$6O_2 + C_6H_{12}O_6 \rightarrow 6H_2O + 6CO_2 + \text{energy}$$

Because the amount of water is roughly equal to the CO_2 produced, the respiratory quotient (O_2/CO_2) is near 1.0. In summary, the cerebral blood flow in normal brain is regulated by metabolic demands of the brain tissue as it adjusts to the functional needs of the brain. Evidence (Fox and Raichle, 1986), however, has provided a demonstration in which the normal coupling between flow and metabolism may be lost under certain physiologic conditions in which local neuronal activity is increased.

Neurogenic Control

Neurogenic mechanisms probably play a small role in controlling cerebral circulation. Although the specific mechanism(s) still remains somewhat of an enigma, anatomic studies have demonstrated the existence of an extensive nerve supply to the extracranial and intracranial cerebral vessels. Sympathetic postganglionic fibers arise from the superior cervical and sympathetic ganglia and form a sympathetic plexus on the internal carotid and vertebral arteries. Nerve branches continue within the vasculature covering the surface of the brain, as well as penetrating deep within the brain. Intracerebral arterioles as small as 25 μm have extensive perivascular nerve supplies. Blockade of the stellate sympathetic ganglia bilaterally using procaine in either normotensive or hypertensive patients with cerebrovascular disease failed to influence blood flow measured by nitrous oxide methods. Parasympathetic stimulation, however, produced a 16% ipsilateral cerebral vasodilation of the pial arteries. Sokoloff and Kety (1960) concluded that there was no evidence, to date, of a resting neurogenic vasoconstrictor or vasodilatory state mediated through their respective autonomic pathways. There is experimental support (Heistad, 1980) that sympathetic innervation plays a modulating role during acute hypertensive episodes resulting in vasoconstriction of the cerebral vasculature. This observation supports the possibility that a neurogenic mechanism has some role in adjusting total or regional CBF and vasomotor tone. This role appears to be more pronounced in hypertensive states than in hypotensive states or normotensive states.

Summary

Two of the four intrinsic control mechanisms thus play an important but limited role in normal brain function (autoregulation, neurogenic). Chemical factors, in particular CO_2 levels, play a regulatory role on CBF and necessitate that continuous and accurate measurements of CO_2 be obtained during the assessment of CBF. In addition, cortical metabolism has a direct influence on CBF, and activation paradigms that provide selective cortical involvement have been shown to result in localized CBF alterations. The use of multiple detectors, to be described below, enable the measurement of discrete alterations in CBF that provide the ability to determine the relative metabolic demands for the underlying tissue by measurement of CBF.

PATHOPHYSIOLOGY OF ISCHEMIA

Adequate CBF or tissue perfusion is necessary for efficient energy metabolism and maintenance of brain pH and metabolic homeostasis. CBF supplies the energy substrates to the brain and removes the metabolic end-products. The interdependence between CBF and energy production is complex and dynamic in cerebral ischemia (Frackowiak, 1985). Cerebral ischemia and the risk for subsequent infarction is a complicated process that results from alterations in local cerebral hemodynamics as well as disturbances in local cellular biochemistry (Siesjo, 1981). The available evidence suggests that the process of ischemia that leads to tissue infarction occurs within hours to 1 to 2 days (Wise et al., 1983; Hakim et al., 1987) and that disruption of the normal coupling between CBF and metabolism occurs within areas of cerebral infarction (Wise et al., 1983). The development of infarction in man is preceded by a fall in CBF compensated by an increased in blood volume. Consequently, cerebral metabolism is preserved. A fall in CBF below the level compensated by increased blood volume is associated with an increased rate of extraction of oxygen by the blood. The ischemic process has been characterized by an initial phase of maximally raised oxygen extraction sufficient to maintain normal levels of metabolism. This phase is followed by a fall in oxygen extraction, which occurs with the onset of cell death and is dependent on the duration and severity of the ischemia (Wise et al., 1983). Disruption of the plasma membrane and internal cytoarchitecture can lead to complex alterations in cellular biochemistry, including ionic shifts, prostaglandin activation, disturbed calcium homeostasis, and other potentially disruptive events (Siesjo, 1981; Plum, 1983; Raichle, 1983). These cellular processes are not yet detectable by current in vivo cerebral imaging techniques. However, CBF, oxygen and glucose consumption, and cerebral blood volume can be measured by PET techniques, which provide a sensitive tool for enhancing our understanding of the underlying pathophysiologic processes.

Oxidative phosphorylation is the process that provides most of the energy demand required for brain function (Raichle, 1983). Early studies with the Kety-Schmidt method demonstrated that the rate of necessary substrate delivery exceeded normal cerebral metabolic demand (Kety and Schmidt, 1945). In normal brain, homeostatic mechanisms maintain CBF levels at a relatively constant level over a wide range of cerebral perfusion pressures (Harper and Glass, 1965). This process, described above and called autoregulation is a function of the interaction of perfusion pressure, cerebrovascular resistance, and CBF. For constant levels of CBF to be maintained when perfusion pressure is reduced, a compensatory vasodilatory response in the cerebrovascular bed is needed. At the point of maximal vasodilation, CBF declines as a linear function of perfusion pressure. Beyond the range of autoregulation, other compensatory mechanisms are available to attempt to maintain cerebral metabolism despite reductions in CBF (Gibbs et al., 1984). This state of preserved metabolism during declining levels of cerebral perfusion has been described as "critical perfusion" (Frackowiak and Wise, 1983) or "misery-perfusion" (Baron et al., 1981). Normal levels of oxidative metabolism are maintained by an increase in oxygen extraction efficiency from the residual CBF. At maximal oxygen extraction rates, oxygen delivery to the tissue cannot be further increased and oxidative metabolism is placed at risk. It is at this point, where CBF and the cerebral metabolic rate for oxygen vary directly, that true ischemia is defined. Ischemia can thus be defined as the point where no further compensatory mechanisms can counteract the further decreases in CBF (Jones et al., 1981). When ischemia is prolonged and energy production is disrupted, the brain tissue is at risk for membrane ion-pump failure and resulting cytotoxic damage or infarction. At this stage the residual metabolism is no longer a function of CBF level and "luxury perfusion" is possible (Lassen, 1966). Figure 3–2 provides a representation of this continuum.

The usefulness of CBF measurements lies in the assessment of these changes in global and regional perfusion during the various phases of ischemia and the potential for possible therapeutic interventions. The remainder of this chapter is directed toward describing the ^{133}Xe literature as applied to the evaluation of cerebral ischemia and concludes with an example of the possible utility of serial rCBF measures for monitoring the efficacy of a therapeutic intervention (e.g., a calcium channel antagonist).

A comprehensive review of the use of noninvasive rCBF methods in cerebrovascular disease is a difficult task owing to the various methods applied (intracarotid, intravenous, or inhalation), use of different indices (F_1, ISI, CBF_{15}), differences in time delay between symptom onset and the rCBF study, and the possibility of various pathophysiologic processes leading to similar clinical symptoms. An attempt is made here to review the experience with principally noninvasive rCBF studies dealing with transient ischemic attacks (TIAs), followed by a review of studies conducted during the acute phase of a stroke and in patients during the chronic phase of stroke. For contrast, patients with carotid artery occlusion are discussed. The aim of this section is to demonstrate the potential utility of noninvasive rCBF methods, within the previous described constraints, to provide useful information in stroke management.

TRANSIENT ISCHEMIC ATTACKS

The early and repeated study of patients with TIAs is limited, to my knowledge, to two known reports: ^{133}Xe SPECT study by Vorstrup and colleagues (1983) and a

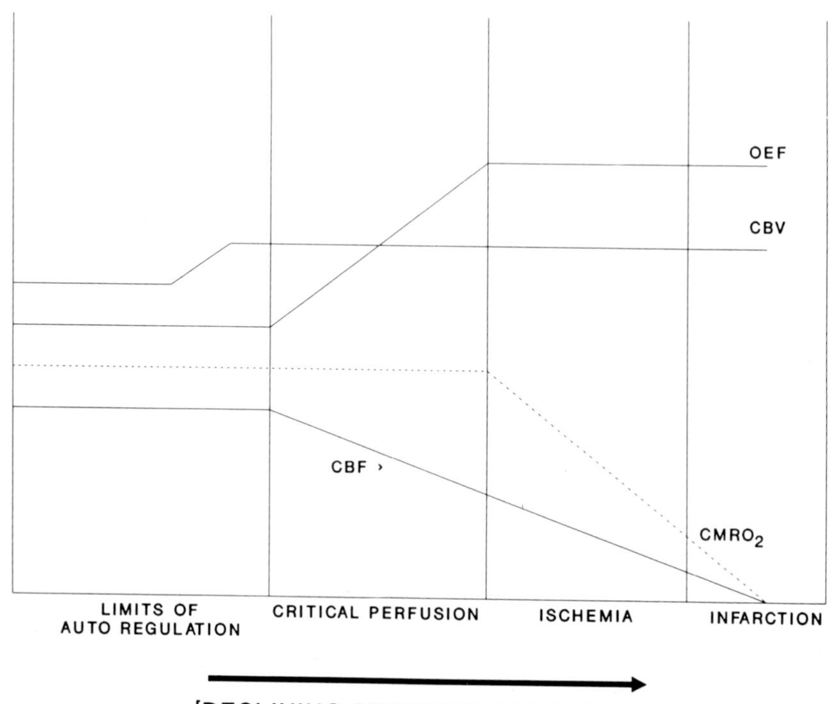

Figure 3–2 Relation between a number of physiologic parameters, including cerebral blood flow (CBF), cerebral blood volume (CBV), oxygen extraction fraction (OEF), and cerebral metabolic rate ($CMRO_2$) during changes in perfusion pressure. At the limits of autoregulation, CBF remains stable as a result of compensatory vasodilation with concomitant decreases in cerebral vascular resistance and an increase in CBV. At maximal vasodilation further decreases in perfusion pressure are accompanied by decreased CBF; $CMRO_2$ may remain stable owing to increased oxygen extraction. Further decreases in CBF result in increases in OEF until the ischemic threshold is reached, at which point $CMRO_2$ falls as a function of decreased CBF with no further increases in OEF being possible. An extension in the duration of the ischemia or the level of perfusion pressure results in an infarct.

noninvasive rCBF study by Hartmann (1985). The SPECT study evaluated rCBF in 14 patients with TIAs and demonstrable arteriosclerotic disease of the carotid or vertebral arteries. Studies were conducted from day 2 through day 90 after the most recent event. Patients with normal CT scans presented with normal CBF tomography, whereas three patients without CT evidence of infarction demonstrated abnormal CBF. These patients had either significant stenosis or occlusion of the internal carotid artery and demonstrated focal reductions in rCBF. This focal reduction of rCBF did not change following technically successful reconstructive vascular surgery, suggesting the presence of a cerebral infarct with transient signs.

Hartmann extended these observations using the noninvasive ^{133}Xe method and performed follow-up studies in patients with TIAs either during or immediately after ictus. Nineteen patients with unilateral TIAs in the carotid territory, 13 of whom were studied during the event, were evaluated. The involved hemisphere demonstrated reduced global CBF compared to the uninvolved hemisphere or when compared to an appropriate control group. No changes in CBF measures were noted in the uninvolved hemisphere with studies conducted at days 2 and 7, whereas the involved hemisphere demonstrated an increase in CBF from day 1 to 2. A more detailed analysis of regional CBF patterns demonstrated a more complex picture of significant deviation from the global CBF (either ischemic or hyperemic). The relative ischemia or hyperemia normalized over the 7 days, suggesting that, although overall CBF is within normal limits, regional patterns of ischemia and hyperemia are present that tend to recover to normal levels.

STROKE

The first noninvasive ^{133}Xe study in stroke was conducted by Rao and colleagues (1974). The principal finding was that regional abnormalities were detectable and could be followed serially in the acute setting. Slater and coworkers (1977) extended these observations using ^{133}Xe inhalation methods to assess alterations in the uninvolved hemisphere. Measurements were conducted on 15 patients, with most of the patients being studied within 72 hours; measurement was limited to a maximum of eight probes, and the ISI index was used. They demonstrated a bilateral progressive decline in rCBF during the first week after ictus and argued that the decline could be partially explained by loss of autoregulation but appeared unrelated to level of consciousness, clinical status, or CO_2 level.

Yamamoto and colleagues (1980) described levels of rCBF in patients with varying risk factors and determined their vasodilatory response to hypercarbia. Ten subjects with risk factors, 20 with vertebrobasilar insufficiency, and 11 with cerebrovascular disease were evaluated. Cerebrovascular reactivity was mildly impaired with normal aging, moderately impaired in subjects with stroke risk factors, and most impaired in patients with a history of cerebrovascular disease. Studies during the acute phase have been conducted by Meyer and coworkers (1978), who reported on the effect of diaschisis and "steal" in 32 patients with unilateral infarction and 19 patients with TIAs. At 3 weeks after ictus, all patients demonstrated reduced CBF in both the involved and the uninvolved hemispheres. In chronic patients (studied after 4 weeks), only the involved hemisphere had reduced CBF. It was noted that, in the regional analysis, areas contralateral to the involved areas had depressed flow levels similar to their values at 3 weeks, providing support for diaschisis.

Attempting to extend these early observations, Halsey and coworkers (1981) evaluated the sensitivity of the most commonly used indices. Maximum sensitivity was found to be obtained with ISI when combined with the infrequently used fractional flow index. The F_1 and W_1 measures in isolation were limited in their sensitivity to correctly lateralize the lesion. Ewing and colleagues (1981) studies 40 acute patients (average time 3.3 days) as well as eight TIA patients using only the ISI index. Both patient groups presented with lower flows than age-matched controls. Hemispheric blood flow asymmetries were consistent with the lateralized clinical signs. This effect was demonstrated in 79% of the stroke sample and 88% of the TIA sample. The rCBF technique was demonstrated to be sensitive to the ischemic infarct.

Demeurisse and coworkers (1983) studied 30 stroke patients at days 15, 30, 60, and 90 post-ictus using the ISI index. Clinical improvement was not accompanied by improvement in CBF during resting conditions. These investigators concluded that CBF at rest has no predictive value in regard to clinical evolution. There are a number of possible explanations for this result. One is the use of the ISI index, a measure that has been found to be stable, although not particularly sensitive, to gray matter flow. A study by Gur and colleagues (1987b) evaluated rCBF in 15 patients with unilateral infarction (eight left-sided and seven right-sided) and 12 matched controls. Measurements were made while at rest, while performing a right hemisphere activation task (spatial line orientation), and while performing a left hemisphere activation task (verbal analogies). rCBF was lower in the patient groups, and regional activation patterns were different from controls. Left hemisphere infarct patients failed to activate to the verbal task and had only slight increases in the right hemisphere for the spatial task, whereas right hemisphere infarct patients demonstrated rCBF relative increases in the left hemisphere to the verbal and spatial tasks. This finding suggests that a more systematic regional analysis conducted on a larger sample would provide a clearer picture of areas of impairment.

In all of the studies reviewed above, it should be noted that the CBF study was confounded by a number of factors: issues of spatial resolution, which is restricted by the number of probes available; patient selection criteria; elapsed time after ictus, and the specific rCBF index used for analysis. The uniform agreement in the results of the rCBF methods in the stroke patient population provides support for the sensitivity of the noninvasive method to brain ischemia and infarction.

A study by Hojer-Pedersen and Petersen (1989) demonstrated the sensitivity of the rCBF technique in both cortical and subcortical infarctions. These investigators studies 26 patients with symptoms of unilateral disease in the MCA distribution in which CT confirmed the presence of a nonhemorrhagic infarct. Sixteen patients had deep cerebral infarcts without cortical involvement, and 10 patients had cortex affected. Of the 16 patients with subcortical infarcts, 14 demonstrated focal areas of decreased rCBF in the symptomatic hemisphere. A similar effect was found for the ten patients with cortical infarcts, with slightly more pronounced hemispheric asymmetry when compared to subcortical patients. These results demonstrate that the rCBF technique is sensitive to infarcts in both superficial cortex and deep structures. In addition, reductions in rCBF of cortical tissue as a result of subcortical infarcts appear to provide some explanation for the clinical effects found with subcortical infarction (Metter et al., 1981; Damasio et al., 1982).

CAROTID ARTERY DISEASE

In patients with carotid artery disease, rCBF studies provide a slightly more consistent picture. Bullock and coworkers (1985) evaluated 74 patients with varying cerebrovascular symptoms (e.g., TIAs, reversible ischemic neurologic deficits, minor strokes) who underwent carotid angiography, rCBF studies at rest and with hypercapnia, CT and serial neurologic examinations. The rCBF measurements at rest and during hypercapnia were correlated with angiographic findings. Patients with carotid artery stenosis (60% or greater) had normal resting flows but reduced responsiveness to a CO_2 challenge (7% PCO_2 added to room air). Patients with an occluded vessel had reduced resting flows and reduced CO_2 responsiveness. It was concluded that the normal effect of CO_2 was reduced as a function of increased severity of carotid artery disease. These results suggest the possibility of using noninvasive rCBF methods to determine if patients have hemodynamically significant carotid artery disease. These results have been confirmed and extended by others (Norrving et al., 1982; Brown et al., 1986).

In general, it can be seen that the rCBF methods have utility for assessing alterations in brain perfusion in cerebrovascular disease. It is of greater importance, however, to evaluate the utility of these measures for assessing the effectiveness of clinical therapies aimed at improving outcome from stroke. A brief review of one such area demonstrates the potential contribution of noninvasive rCBF methods in this setting. In this context a calcium channel blocker now under investigation for its utility in reducing stroke morbidity and mortality is briefly reviewed.

TREATMENT OF ACUTE STROKE

Therapies under current investigation for their potential role in modifying the clinical deficits following stroke include the calcium channel blockers, which are proposed on the basis at least partially of their vasodilatory effect. Their administration may lead to reperfusion of ischemic areas. CBF techniques are therefore important in that pretreatment measurements may provide a measure of the initial level of perfusion and allow determination of the percent change in CBF as a function of therapy.

There is a recognized need for an effective treatment that minimizes tissue destruction in acute ischemic brain infarction. Nimodipine, a calcium channel blocker with a predilection for cerebral circulation, has been demonstrated to have beneficial effects in animal models of severe cerebral ischemia. Cerebral ischemia is thought to induce a cascade of pathophysiologic reactions, including a massive influx of calcium into the neuron that results in catabolism and cell necrosis due to calcium overload. Calcium antagonists can act to block this reuptake of calcium as well as have the effect of increasing CBF. Nimodipine has been shown to be of particular effectiveness in ameliorating the delayed postischemic hypoperfusion of the brain with the prevention of neurologic deficits and death (Hoffmeister et al., 1979; Kazda and Towart, 1982). An early study (Gelmers, 1982), using the intracarotid ^{133}Xe injection procedure, demonstrated a dose-related increase in CBF with Nimodipine. A second study using noninvasive ^{133}Xe methods (Gaab et al., 1985) demonstrated similar increases in CBF after either oral or intravenous doses of Nimodipine.

European trials (Gelmers, 1984; Gelmers et al., 1988) have demonstrated significant neurologic improvement following ischemic strokes in patients treated with nimodipine. This prospective double-blind, placebo-controlled trial measured morbidity and mortality and demonstrated fewer deaths for the Nimodipine treated group, as well as significantly greater improvement in scales used to measure neurologic deficit. A large multicenter double-blind placebo-controlled trial is currently being conducted in the United States in an attempt to substantiate these early results.

SUMMARY

The isolated rCBF measurement of global flow provides only limited information about the state of the cerebral circulation in any given state of health or disease. It is critical to evaluate regional levels of CBF and to provide appropriate stress on the system in order to measure the system's ability to respond to changing physiologic conditions. The responsiveness of the cerebrovasculature can be assessed in response to a number of stressors, including hypercapnia, cognitive stimulation, and pharmacologic challenges. The practical problems encountered with individual patient cooperation are recognized, and effort is needed to select appropriate challenges to the nervous system that ensure substantial alterations in CBF without unnecessary risk to the patient. These strategies are of particular importance as innovative therapies are developed for the treatment of cerebrovascular disease. As new therapies are developed it is of increased importance to be able to quantify both global and regional CBF so as to provide reliable indications of the effects of the specific therapy in the acute care setting. In addition, the assessment of vascular reserve may also prove useful for tailoring these new therapies. It is possible that patients with globally low flows with an intact capability to respond to alterations in metabolic demands are not good candidates for certain therapeutic interventions, whereas patients without an intact perfusion reserve may benefit.

REFERENCES

Aaslid, R., Lindegaard, K., Sorteberg, W., and Nornes, H. (1989). Cerebral autoregulation dynamics in humans. *Stroke,* **20,** 45–52.

Allison, J.D., Kingsbury, T.B. IV, and Goode, J.J. (1988). Inhalation regional cerebral blood flow: the use of tidal CO_2 data to find radionuclide activity associated with exhaled alveolar gas. *Med. Phys.,* **15,** 874–878.

Baron, J.C., Bousser, M.G., Guillard, A., Comar, D., and Castaigne, R. (1981). Reversal of focal "misery-perfusion syndrome" by extra-intracranial arterial bypass in hemodynamic cerebral ischemia. *Stroke,* **12,** 454–459.

Bartlett, E.J., Brodie, J.D., Wolf, A.P., Christman, D.R., Laska, E., and Meissner, M. (1988). Reproducibility of cerebral glucose metabolic measurements in resting human subjects. *J. Cereb. Blood Flow Metab.,* **8,** 502–512.

Berne, R.M., Winn, H.R., and Rubio, R. (1981). The local regulation of cerebral blood flow. *Prog. Cardiovasc. Dis.,* **24,** 243–260.

Bonte, F.J., Devous, M.D., and Stokely, E.M. (1988). Tomographic imaging of regional cerebral blood flow with diffusible tracers. In A. Gottschalk, P.B. Hoffer, and E.J. Potchen, eds., *Diagnostic Nuclear Medicine,* pp. 914–926. Baltimore: Williams & Wilkins.

Brown, M.M., Wade, J.P.H., Bishop, C.C.R., and Russell, R.W. (1986). Reactivity of the cerebral circulation in patients with carotid occlusion. *J. Neurol. Neurosurg. Psychiatry,* **49,** 899–904.

Bullock, R., Mendelow, A.D., Bone, I., Patterson, J., Macleod, W.N., and Allardice, G. (1985). Cerebral blood flow and CO_2 responsiveness as an indicator of collateral reserve capacity in patients with carotid arterial disease. *Br. J. Surg.,* **72,** 348–351.

Burke, A.M., Greenberg, J.H., Sladky, J., and Reivich, M. (1987). Regional variation in cerebral perfusion during acute hypertension. *Neurology,* **37,** 94–99.

Damasio, A.R., Damasio, H., Rizzo, M., Varney, N., and Gersh, F. (1982). Aphasia with non-hemorrhagic lesions in the basal ganglia and internal capsule. *Arch. Neurol.,* **39,** 15–20.

Davis, S.M., Ackerman, R.H., Correia, J.A., Alpert, N.M., Chang, J., Buonanno, F., Kelley, R.E., Rosner, B., and Taveras, J.M. (1983). Cerebral blood flow and cerebrovascular CO_2 reactivity in stroke-age normal controls. *Neurology,* **33,** 391–399.

Demeurisse, G., Verhas, M., Capon, A., and Paternot, J. (1983). Lack of evolution of the cerebral blood flow during clinical recovery of a stroke. *Stroke,* **14,** 77–81.

Duara, R., Gross-Glenn, K., Barker, W.W., Chang, J.Y., Apicella, A., Lowenstein, D., and Boothe, T. (1987). Behavioral activation and the variability of cerebral glucose metabolic measurements. *J. Cereb. Blood Flow Metab.,* **7,** 266–271.

Ewing, J.R., Sheehe, P., and Chipman, P. (1977). The precision of flow estimates in a clinical study of stroke patients. *Acta Neurol. Scand.* [Suppl. 64], **56,** 466–467.

Ewing, J.R., Keating, E.G., Sheehe, P.R., Hodge, C.J., Chipman, M., and Brooks, C.T. (1981). Concordance of inhalation rCBFs with clinical evidence of cerebral ischemia. *Stroke,* **12,** 188–195.

Fitch, W., MacKenzie, E.T., and Harper, A.M. (1975). Effects of decreasing arterial blood pressure on cerebral blood flow in the baboon. *Circ. Res.,* **37,** 550–557.

Fox, P.T., and Raichle, M.E. (1986). Focal physiological uncoupling of cerebral blood flow and oxidative metabolism during somatosensory stimulation in human subjects. *Proc. Nat. Acad. Sci. USA,* **83,** 1140–1144.

Frackowiak, R.S.J. (1985). Pathophysiology of human cerebral ischemia: studies with positron tomography and oxygen-15. *Res. Publ. Assoc. Res. Nerv. Ment. Dis.,* **63,** 139–162.

Frackowiak, R.S.J., and Wise, R.J.S. (1983). Positron tomography in ischemic cerebrovascular disease. *Neurol. Clin.,* **1**:183–200.

Gaab, M.R., Haubitz, I., Brawanski, A., Korn, A., and Czech, T. (1985). Acute effects of nimodipine on the cerebral blood flow and intracranial pressure. *Neurochirurgia (Stuttg.),* **28,** 93–99.

Gelmers, H.J. (1982). Effect of Nimodipine (Bay e 9736) on postischaemic cerebrovascular reactivity, as revealed by measuring regional cerebral blood flow (rCBF). *Acta Neurochir. (Wien),* **63,** 283–290.

Gelmers, H.J. (1984). The effect of nimodipine on the clinical course of patients with acute ischemic stroke. *Acta Neurol. Scand.,* **69,** 232–239.

Gelmers, H.J., Gorter, K., De Weerdt, C.J., and Wiezer, H.J.A. (1988). A controlled trial of nimodipine in acute ischemic stroke. *N. Engl. J. Med.,* **318,** 203–207.

Gibbs, J.M., Wise, R.J.S., Leenders, K.L., and Jones, T. (1984). Evaluation of cerebral perfusion reserve in patients with carotid-artery occlusion. *Lancet,* **1,** 310–314.

Gur, D., Wolfson, S.K., Yonas, H., Good, W.F., Shabason, L., Latchaw, R.E., Miller, D.M., and Cook, E.E. (1982a). Progress in cerebrovascular disease: local cerebral blood flow by xenon enhanced CT. *Stroke,* **13,** *750–757.*

Gur, R.C., Gur, R.E., Obrist, W.D., Hungerbuhler, J.P., Younkin, D., Rosen, A., Skolnick, B.E., and Reivich, M. (1982). Sex and handedness differences in cerebral blood flow during rest and cognitive activity. *Science,* **217,** 659–661.

Gur, R.C., Gur, R.E., Resnick, Ṡ.M., Skolnick, B.E., Alavi, A., and Reivich, M. (1987a). The effect of anxiety on cortical cerebral blood flow and metabolism. *J. Cereb. Blood Flow Metab.,* **7,** 173–177.

Gur, R.C., Gur, R.E., Silver, F.L., Obrist, W.D., Skolnick, B.E., Kushner, M., Hurtig, H.I., and Reivich, M. (1987b). Regional cerebral blood flow in stroke: hemispheric effects of cognitive activity. *Stroke,* **18,** 776–780.

Gur, R.C., and Reivich, M. (1980). Cognitive task effects on hemispheric blood flow in humans: evidence for individual differences in hemispheric activation. *Brain Lang.,* **9,** 78–92.

Hakim, A.M., Pokrupa, R.P., Villanueva, J., Diksic, M., Evans, A.C.,Thompson, C.J., Meyer, E., Yamamoto, Y.L., and Feindel, W.H. (1987). The effect of spontaneous reperfusion on metabolic function in early human cerebral infarcts. *Ann. Neurol.,* **21,** 279–289.

Halsey, J.H., Jr., Nakai, K., and Wariyar, B. (1981). Sensitivity of rCBF to focal lesions. *Stroke,* **12,** 631–635.

Harper, A.M. (1966). Autoregulation of cerebral blood flow: influence of the arterial blood pressure on the blood flow through the cerebral cortex. *J. Neurol. Neurosurg. Psychiatry,* **29,** 398–403.

Harper, A.M., and Glass, H.I. (1965). The effect of alterations in the arterial carbon dioxide tension on the blood flow through the cerebral cortex at normal and low arterial blood pressures. *J. Neurol. Neurosurg. Psychiatry,* **28,** 449–452.

Hartmann, A. (1985). Is it possible to measure regional cerebral blood flow in patients with acute cerebral ischemia. In: A. Hartmann and S. Hoyer, eds., *Cerebral Blood Flow and Metabolism Measurement,* pp. 98–108. Berlin: Springer-Verlag.

Hartmann, A., Wassman, H., Czernicki, Z., Dettmers, C., Schumacher, H.W., and Tsuda, Y. (1987). Effect of stable xenon in room air on regional cerebral blood flow and electroencephalogram in normal baboons. *Stroke,* **18,** 643–648.

Hazelrig, J.B., Halsey, J.H., Jr., Wilson, E.M., and Wills, E.L. (1985). Comparison of external lung monitoring with end-tidal air detection using the 133-xenon inhalation method. *Stroke,* **16,** 964–968.

Heistad, D.D. (1980). Protection of cerebral vessels by sympathetic nerves. *Physiologist,* **23**(5), 44–49.

Hoffmeister, F., Kazda, S., and Krause, H.P. (1979). Influence of nimodipine (Bay e 9736) on the post-ischemic changes of brain function. *Acta Neurol. Scand.,* **72,** 358–359.

Hojer-Pedersen, E., and Petersen, O.F. (1989). Changes of blood flow in the cerebral cortex after subcortical ischemic infarction. *Stroke,* **20,** 211–216.

Jaggi, J.L. (1985). Analysis of the spatial resolution of noninvasive xenon-133 cerebral blood flow measurements (doctoral dissertation, University of Pennsylvania, 1985). *Dissertations Abstracts International,* (abstract).

Jaggi, J.L., and Obrist, W.D. (1981). External monitoring of the lung as a substitute for end-tidal 133-Xe sampling in non-invasive CBF studies: preliminary findings. *rCBF Bull.,* **2,** 25–27.

Jaggi, J.L., and Obrist, W.D. (1987). Regional cerebral blood flow determined by ^{133}xenon clearance. In: J.H. Wood, ed., *Cerebral Blood Flow: Physiologic and Clinical Aspects,* pp. 189–201. New York: McGraw-Hill.

Jones, T.H., Morawetz, R.B., Crowell, R.M., Marcoux, F.W., Fitzgibbon, S.J., DeGirolami, U., and Ojemann, R.G. (1981). Thresholds of focal cerebral ischemia in awake monkeys. *J. Neurosurg.,* **54,** 773–782.

Kazda, S., and Towart, R. (1982). Nimodipine, a new calcium antagonistic drug with a preferential cerebrovascular action. *Acta Neurochir. (Wien),* **63,** 259–265.

Kety, S.S., and Schmidt, C.F. (1945). The determination of cerebral blood flow in man by use of nitrous oxide in low concentrations. *Am. J. Appl. Physiol.,* **143,** 53–66.

Kuhl, D.E., Edwards, R.Q., and Ricci, A.R. (1976). The Mark IV system for radionuclide computed tomography of the brain. *Radiology,* **121,** 405–413.

Lassen, N.A. (1966). The luxury-perfusion syndrome and its possible relation to acute metabolic acidosis localised within the brain. *Lancet,* **2,** 1113–1115.

Lassen, N.A., and Ingvar, D.H. (1961). The blood flow on the cerebral cortex determined by radioactive krypton-85. *Experientia,* **17,** 42–45.

Lennox, W.G., and Gibbs, E.L. (1932). The blood flow in the brain and the leg of man, and the changes induced by alterations of blood gases. *J. Clin. Invest.,* **11,** 1155–1177.

Mallett, B.L., and Veall, N. (1963). Investigation of cerebral blood flow in hypertension, using radioactive-xenon inhalation and extracranial recording. *Lancet,* **1,** 1081–1082.

Maximilian, V.A., Prohovnik, I., and Risberg, J. (1980). Cerebral hemodynamic response to mental activation in normo and hypercapnia. *Stroke,* **11,** 342–347.

Metter, E.J., Wasterlein, C.G., Kuhl, D.E., Hansson, W.R., and Phelps, M.E. (1981). ^{18}FDG positron emission computed tomography in a study of aphasia. *Ann. Neurol.,* **10,** 173–183.

Meyer, J.S., Naritomi, H., Saskai, F., Ishihara, N., and Grant, P. (1978). Regional cerebral blood flow, diaschisis, and steal after stroke. *Neurol. Res.,* **1,** 101–119.

Mountz, J.M., Modell, J.G., Wilson, M.W., Curtis, G.C., Lee, M.A., Schmaltz, S., and Kuhl, D.E. (1989). Positron emission tomographic evaluation of cerebral blood flow during state anxiety in simple phobia. *Arch. Gen. Psychiatry,* **46,** 501–504.

Norrving, B., Nilsson, B., and Risberg, J. (1982). rCBF in patients with carotid occlusion: resting and hypercapnic flow related to collateral pattern. *Stroke,* **13,** 155–162.

Obrist, W.D., and Wilkinson, W.E. (1980). The non-invasive Xe-133 method: evaluation of CBF indices. In: G. Geraud and A. Bes, eds., *Cerebral Circulation,* pp. 119–124. Amsterdam: Excerpta Medica.

Obrist, W.D., Thompson, H.K., Jr., Wang, H.S., and Wilkinson, W.E. (1975). Regional cerebral blood flow estimated by 133-xenon inhalation. *Stroke,* **6,** 245–256.

Obrist, W.D., Jaggi, J.L., Harel, D., and Smith, D.S. (1985). Effect of stable xenon inhalation on human CBF. *J. Cereb. Blood Flow Metab.,* **5,** S557–S558.

Obrist, W.D., Wilkinson, W.E., Wang, H.S., and Harel, D. (1987). The noninvasive 133-Xe method: influence of the input function on computed rCBF values. In: S. Knezevic, V.A. Maximilian, Z. Mubrin, Z. Prohovnik, and J. Wade, eds., *Handbook of rCBF.* Hillsdale, NJ: Lawrence Erlbaum.

Pannier, J.L., Weyne, J., and Leusen, I. (1972). Effects of changes in acid-base composition in the cerebral ventricles on local and general cerebral blood flow. *Eur. Neurol.,* **6,** 123–126.

Phelps, M.E., Mazziotta, J.C., and Huang, C. (1982). Study of cerebral function with positron computed tomography. *J. Cereb. Blood Flow Metab.,* **2,** 113–162.

Plum, F. (1983). What causes infarction in ischemic brain? The Robert Wartenberg lecture. *Neurology,* **33,** 222–233.

Podreka, I., Baumgartner, C., Suess, E., Muller, C., Brucke, T., Lang, W., Holzner, F., Steiner, M., and Deecke, L. (1989). Quantification of regional cerebral blood flow with IMP-SPECT. *Stroke,* **20,** 183–191.

Prohovnik, I., Knudsen, E., and Risberg, J. (1985). Theoretical evaluation and simulation test of the initial slope index for noninvasive rCBF. In: A. Hartmann and S. Hoyer, eds., *Cerebral Blood Flow and Metabolism Measurement,* pp. 56–60. Berlin: Springer-Verlag.

Raichle, M.E. (1983). The pathophysiology of brain ischemia. *Ann. Neurol.* **13,** 2–10.

Raichle, M.E., Grubb, R.L., Jr., Eichling, J.O., and Ter-Pogossian, M.M. (1976a). Measurement of brain oxygen utilization with radioactive oxygen-15: experimental verification. *J. Appl. Physiol.,* **40,** 638–640.

Raichle, M.E., Grubb, R.L., Mokhtar, H.G., Eichling, J.O., and Ter-Pogossian, M.M. (1976b). Correlation between regional cerebral blood flow and oxidative metabolism. *Arch. Neurol.,* **33,** 523–526.

Rao, N., Ali, Z., Omar, H., and Halsey, J.H. (1974). Regional cerebral blood flow in acute stroke: preliminary experience with xenon inhalation method. *Stroke,* **5,** 8–12.

Reiman, E.M., Fusselman, M.J., Fox, P.T., and Raichle, M.E. (1989). Neuroanatomical correlates of anticipatory anxiety. *Science,* **243,** 1071–1074.

Reivich, M. (1985). Cerebral glucose consumption: methodology and validation. In: M. Reivich and A. Alavi, eds., *Positron Emission Tomography,* pp. 131–151. New York: Alan R. Liss.

Reivich, M., Slater, R., and Sano, N. (1969). Further studies on exponential models of cerebral clearance curves. In: M. Brock, C. Fieschi, D.H. Ingvar, N.A. Lassen, and K. Schurmann, eds., *Cerebral Blood Flow: Clinical and Experimental Results,* pp. 8–10. New York: Springer-Verlag.

Reivich, M., Obrist, W.D., Slater, R., Greenberg, J., and Goldberg, H.I. (1975). A comparison of the Xe 133 intracarotid injection and inhalation techniques for measuring regional cerebral blood flow. In: E.M. Harper, W.B. Jennett, J.D. Miller, and J.O. Rowan, eds., *Blood Flow and Metabolism in the Brain. Proceedings of the Seventh International Symposium on Cerebral Blood Flow and Metabolism,* pp. 8.3–8.11. Edinburgh: Churchill Livingstone.

Risberg, J., and Ingvar, D.M. (1973). Patterns of activation in the gray matter of the dominant hemisphere during memorization and reasoning. *Brain,* **96,** 737–756.

Risberg, J., Ali, Z., Wilson, E.M., Wills, E.L., and Halsey, J.H. (1975). Regional cerebral blood flow by 133-xenon inhalation: preliminary evaluation of an initial slope index in patients with unstable flow compartments. *Stroke,* **6,** 142–148.

Rodrigues, G., Cogorno, P., Gris, A., Marenco, S., Mesiti, C., Nobili, E., and Rosadini, G. (1989). Regional cerebral blood flow and anxiety: a correlation study in neurologically normal patients. *J. Cereb. Blood Flow Metab.,* **9,** 410–416.

Ryding, E. (1989). Estimation of error limits for cerebral blood flow values obtained from xenon-133 clearance curves. *Stroke,* **20,** 205–210.

Schmidt, C.F., Kety, S.S., and Pennes, H.H. (1945). The gaseous metabolism of the brain of the monkey. *Am. J. Physiol.,* **143,** 33–52.

Siesjo, B.K. (1978). *Brain Energy Metabolism.* New York: Wiley.

Siesjo, B.K. (1981). Cell damage in the brain: a speculative synthesis. *J. Cereb. Blood Flow Metab.,* **1,** 155–185.

Skinhoj, E., and Paulson, O.B. (1969). Carbon dioxide and cerebral circulatory control. *Arch. Neurol.,* **20,** 249–252.

Slater, R., Reivich, M., Goldberg, H., Banka, R., and Greenberg, J. (1977). Diaschisis with cerebral infarction. *Stroke,* **8,** 684–690.

Sokoloff, L., and Kety, S.S. (1960). Regulation of cerebral circulation. *Physiol. Rev.,* **40,** 38–44.

Stokely, E.M., Sveinsdottir, E., Lassen, N.A., and Rommer, P. (1980). A single photon dynamic computer-assisted tomography (DCAT) for imaging brain function in multiple cross-sections. *J. Comput. Assist. Tomogr.,* **4,** 230–240.

Strandgaard, S., Sengupta, D., MacKenzie, E.T., Rowan, J.O., Olesen, J., Skinhoj, E., and Lassen, N.A. (1975). The lower and upper limits of autoregulation of cerebral blood flow. In: T.W. Langfitt, L.C. McHenry, Jr., M. Reivich, and J. Wollman, eds., *Cerebral Circulation and Metabolism.* New York: Springer Verlag.

Veall, N., and Mallet, B.L. (1966). Regional cerebral blood flow determination by 133-Xe inhalation and external recording: the effect of arterial recirculation. *Clin. Sci.,* **30,** 353–369.

Vorstrup, S., Hemmingsen, R., Henriksen, L., Lindewald, H., Engell, H.C., and Lassen, N.A. (1983). Regional cerebral blood flow in patients with transient ischemic attacks studied by xenon-133 inhalation and emission tomography. *Stroke,* **14,** 903–910.

Vorstrup, S., Paulson, O.B., and Lassen, N.A. (1986). Cerebral blood flow in acute and chronic ischemic stroke using xenon-133 inhalation tomography. *Acta Neurol. Scand.,* **74,** 439–451.

Warach, S., Gur, R.C., Gur, R.E., Skolnick, B.E., Obrist, W.D., and Reivich, M. (1988). The reproducibility of the 133-xenon effects in healthy young adults. *J. Cereb. Blood Flow Metab.,* **7,** 702–708.

Wise, R.J., Bernardi, S., Frackowiak, R.S., Legg, N.J., and Jones, T. (1983). Serial observations on the pathophysiology of acute stroke: the transition from ischaemia to infarction as reflected in regional oxygen extraction. *Brain,* **106,** 197–222.

Wyper, D.J., and Booke, M.B.D. (1977). Compensating for hemisphere cross-talk when measuring CBF. *Acta Neurol. Scand.,* **56,** 470–471.

Yamaguchi, F., Meyer, J.S., Sakai, F., and Yamamoto, M. (1979). Normal human aging and cerebral vasoconstrictive responses to hypocapnia. *J. Neurol. Sci.,* **44,** 87–94.

Yamamoto, M., Meyer, J.S., Sakai, F., and Yamaguchi, F. (1980). Aging and cerebral vasodilator responses to hypercarbia: responses in normal aging in persons with risk factors for stroke. *Arch. Neurol.,* **37,** 489–496.

Zohar, J., Insel, T.R., Berman, K.F., Foa, E.B., Hill, J.L., and Weinberger, D.R. (1989). Anxiety and cerebral blood flow during behavioral challenge. *Arch. Gen. Psychiatry,* **46,** 505–510.

4

Behavioral Correlates of Abnormalities of Metabolism in Stroke Patients

E. JEFFREY METTER

Cerebral infarctions and hemorrhages are frequently associated with behavioral changes. Studies correlating these behavioral changes with pathologic anatomy have contributed to our general understanding of brain-behavior relations in humans. One example is the anatomically based model for classifying aphasia (Benson, 1979; Benson and Geschwind, 1985). This model emphasizes the importance of specific cortical regions and cortical-cortical connections. With the advent of computed tomography, the model has been expanded to encompass subcortical structures such as the thalamus (Brown, 1975; Mohr et al., 1975; Van Buren, 1975; Crosson, 1984) and basal ganglia (Benson, 1979; Damasio et al., 1982; Darley, 1982; Naeser et al., 1982) as relevant for language processes. This model has several shortcomings, including the fact that it fails to classify many aphasic patients. Moreover, although specific aphasic syndromes suggest a lesion site with better-than-chance accuracy, a specific structural lesion does not predict the nature of the aphasia with such accuracy (Benson, 1979; Basso et al., 1985). This lack suggests that the traditional anatomic approach is limited for explaining the neuropathology of language. The imperfections of such constrained anatomic models is understandable in view of our current recognition that brain lesions have dynamic effects and may influence the function of anatomically intact but remote brain regions. Such lesions might cause diffuse physiologic or biochemical changes in the brain with widespread alterations of behavioral function, or they could produce focal physiologic changes in specific distant regions (Metter et al., 1985a). Varying combinations of diffuse and distant focal effects are also possible. Understanding these patterns of physiologic and biochemical changes remote from a focal lesion might provide new insights about brain function and behavior.

This chapter discusses the application of positron emission tomography (PET) in studying correlations between behavior and physiologic or biochemical changes in cerebral infarction. Although some basic metabolic and blood flow characteristics of acute infarction are reviewed, the primary focus is on the effects of chronic infarction on language. PET methodology can be used to study cerebral blood flow (CBF), glucose and oxygen metabolism, and receptor distribution. It is argued here that the combination of information available from PET allows the incorporation of physiologic and biochemical parameters into a broad understanding of the consequences of focal structural brain damage.

POSITRON EMISSION TOMOGRAPHY

Imaging techniques are distinguished by the location of the energy source in relation to the object to be imaged. The energy can arise from either internal (emission) or external (transmission) sources. Transmission techniques include the x-ray methods of standard radiography and computed tomography (CT) (see Chapter 5). Emission sources involve radionuclides injected intravenously or intraarterially, or taken by inhalation. A second internal energy source is the radiofrequency (rf) signals that resonate from tissue activated in a high magnetic field by an external rf source (Gadian, 1982). Emission techniques include PET, single photon emission computed tomography (SPECT), xenon rCBF using multiple detectors, and nuclear magnetic resonance (NMR or MRI). The meaning and distribution of the signal from radionuclides within the body are based on the physiologic and biochemical properties of the radioactive tracer. The meaning and distribution of rf signal from magnetic resonance studies depend on the frequency of the external rf signal and its site of application.

PET uses radioisotopes that emit positrons, positively charged particles with the mass of an electron. When emitted, positrons combine with negatively charged electrons, and both are annihilated. This process creates two high-energy photons or gamma rays, which travel in directions nearly 180 degrees apart. A pair of detectors, which send a signal when photons are detected coincidentally, can identify the line of transit of the pair of particles. Using a circular array of pairs of detectors, an image can be constructed similar to that of CT. The limiting factor for resolution becomes the size of the detectors and how closely they can be packed. The ability to image a structure depends on the size, shape, and influence of neighboring regions, as well as the resolution (Mazziotta et al., 1981b).

A number of positron-emitting isotopes are available, including ^{15}Oxygen, ^{13}Nitrogen, ^{11}Carbon, ^{77}Krypton, and ^{18}Fluorine, which have half-lives of 2 minutes to 110 minutes. A variety of physiologic and biochemical processes can be studied depending on the molecule carrying the isotope. The ability to study several physiologic and biochemical processes has made PET an attractive investigative tool. The primary limitation for its widespread use is the short half-life of the radionuclides, which require a readily available cyclotron for isotope production.

Models

Interpretation of positron images requires knowledge of the meaning of the distribution of the isotope under study. Currently, the most frequently studied processes are cerebral blood flow (CBF) and oxygen and glucose metabolism. Several models exist for the measurement of regional cerebral blood flow (rCBF) by either inhalation or intravenous injection of (^{15}O)-water or (^{15}O)-CO_2 (Jones et al., 1976; Alpert et al., 1977; Baron et al., 1979; Frackowiak et al., 1980; Lammertsma et al., 1981; Huang et al., 1982). When the oxygen extraction ratio (OER), the amount of oxygen taken up by the brain, is also measured using ^{15}O, oxygen metabolism can then be calculated. The advantages of blood flow and oxygen metabolism studies include simplicity and a short scanning time. The latter makes CBF measures ideal for activation studies. The major disadvantage is poor resolution, which limits detail in the images.

Another biochemical function frequently measured is glucose metabolism. Models are based on the deoxyglucose (DG) method (Sokoloff et al., 1977) that was extended to use in man with ^{18}F-fluorodeoxyglucose (FDG) (Phelps et al., 1979; Reivich et al., 1979). 2-Deoxyglucose is a competitive substrate for glucose; i.e., it is transported and metabolized as though it were glucose. Once transported into a cell, DG is phosphorylated but cannot be metabolized further, essentially being trapped within the cell. The amount of DG accumulated is proportional to the amount of glucose utilized by the cell. FDG behaves similarly to DG and has been modeled using a three-compartment system (Phelps et al., 1979; Huang et al., 1980).

Based on the model, regional glucose utilization can be calculated in two ways. Repeated scans can be made over time after injection to calculate a metabolic rate. This approach is accurate but labor-intensive and limited in the number of tomographic planes that can be studied. In the standard method, FDG is injected intravenously, and arterialized venous blood samples are obtained to create a blood curve needed for the calculation. Scanning is started after 40 minutes when FDG has reached a steady state in the brain. Local cerebral metabolic rates of glucose (LCMRGlc) are then calculated using standardized constants. This method is relatively simple and is the most commonly used. The accuracy of the second approach depends on the stability of the kinetic constants and the lump constant, which examines the differences between glucose and FDG in terms of transportation and phosphorylation. The kinetic constants and the lump constant are assumed to be normal and were originally derived from young control subjects. The other constants in the model were likewise derived from previous studies in humans or animals.

Several features of the DG model are controversial. The first issue has been the assumption that phosphorylated DG remains unaltered (Partridge, 1983; Sacks et al., 1983). The model developed by Phelps and Huang for use in man accounts for this possibility. The second issue is the stability of the equation constants in damaged brain. Relative stability of the constants have been shown in man (Reivich et al., 1985), during aging (Hawkins et al., 1983), in ischemic regions after stroke (Hawkins et al., 1981), and in dementia (Friedland et al., 1983). With severe ischemia the standard method can underestimate the actual metabolic values for a region by as much as 50%. This error, though, represents only a 10 to 20% difference when comparing abnormally low metabolic rates in pathologic states with normal values, as the actual and the standard calculations for LCMRGlc are frequently less than 14 to 30% of normal for the severely ischemic region. The major advantage of the FDG method is that multiple high resolution images can be obtained after a single injection.

Behavioral States

Glucose and oxygen are natural energy sources used by the brain and are utilized as the brain works. It has been shown that neurons increase their utilization of glucose in direct proportion to their activity (Freygang and Sokoloff, 1958; Salford et al., 1973; DesRosiers et al., 1974; Yarowsky et al., 1983). We can assume, therefore, that changes in glucose utilization reflect changes in tissue functional activity. In normal brain the rate of oxygen and glucose utilization is coupled to the CBF, so that changes in neuronal activity influence the rate of CBF.

Resting Studies

A number of strategies can be used for applying PET to the study of brain-behavior relations. Selection of a strategy depends on the specific questions under study, the availability of appropriate radionuclides, and the appropriate testing paradigms. The simplest application is to study patients with a specific pathology in the resting (uncontrolled) state, either at one time or at repeated intervals. Normal LCMRGlc values for various brain regions during rest in man have been determined (Reivich et al., 1979; Kuhl et al., 1980; Mazziotta et al., 1981a) and can be compared to pathological states. Similar normative data have been presented for rCBF and oxygen metabolism (Frackowiak et al., 1980). As a general rule, regional variability between studies in a single individual and with repeated measures of the same region in a single study is approximately 10%. A small decline in global and cortical glucose metabolism with increasing age has been demonstrated in subjects with a normal health history (Kuhl et al., 1982). However, other investigators have not found this decline (Duara et al., 1984). The blood flow rates agree closely with measurements made with xenon and multiple surface detectors.

Mazziotta and coworkers (1982a) examined differences in glucose metabolic patterns in several resting states by systematically plugging the ears, covering the eyes, or both. Under resting conditions with eyes and ears open, cerebral glucose metabolism was symmetric in the left and right hemispheres. Changing the resting state by plugging both ears and covering the eyes resulted in significant right $<$ left hemisphere asymmetry that was not apparent when only eyes or ears were occluded. In addition, there was a significant progressive decline in global glucose metabolism comparing eyes and ears unoccluded, eyes closed, ears closed, and both eyes and ears closed. This study demonstrated that all resting states are not equivalent and that general cerebral activation is state-dependent. PET studies of stroke patients in resting states are discussed later in this chapter.

Activation Studies

An alternative strategy is to study patients during the performance of specific tasks. The advantage of this approach is that there can be some control over ongoing behavior during the study, which makes intersubject comparisons easier. Nevertheless, activation strategies are not without their limitations. In a sense, all PET studies are activation studies, as the brain remains active whether the subject is resting or engaged in a task. To understand the patterns of cerebral activity associated with a specific task, it is necessary to perform both resting and activation studies. In such studies, we assume that all individuals use similar cognitive processes during the task, an assumption which may not hold true (Mazziotta et al., 1982b). Likewise, when using activation tasks in pathologic states, such as in stroke patients, interpretation may be difficult. For example, a pattern of activation in a stroke patient that differs from normal may imply transfer of the specific function under study (e.g., auditory processing) to another region or involvement of other cognitive processes not generally involved with normal processing. Task difficulty and complexity may affect regions differentially. As an example, consider a regional metabolic response to a task that has three levels of difficulty and assume the following for normal subjects: For the simplest task, there is a 20% increase in regional glucose metabolism (GMRGlc), for the moderate task a 40% increase, and for the most difficult task a 60% increase. In the stroke patient, assume that we observe for the simplest task a 40% increase in regional GMRGlc. Based on such an observation, we could conclude that the region compensates for structural damage and has increased its activity in a functional way to do the simple task. Alternatively, we could argue that the difficulty of doing the simple task by the stroke patient was equivalent to the moderate task for the normal subject, so the regional change was a "normal" response based on difficulty. Finally, we could argue that the simple task was a very difficult task for the aphasic subject and that the 40% increase was less than the 60% increase that occurred for the most difficult level in normal subjects. As can be seen, all three interpretations are plausible, making a final judgment difficult. Despite such limitations, activation studies may prove useful for understanding brain-behavior relations in brain-damaged individuals.

Activation studies in normal subjects are being pursued. Auditory tasks have been shown to cause different metabolic patterns depending on the nature of the stimulus and the perceptual or cognitive strategy employed when doing the task (Mazziotta et al., 1982b). Verbal stimuli produced diffuse left hemisphere plus focal bilateral superior and posterior temporal increases in glucose metabolism. Nonverbal stimuli (chords) produced diffuse right temporal and bilateral inferior parietal activation. Tone sequences produced variable responses, depending on the subject's probable strategy for analyzing the data. Subjects using highly analytic strategies had greater left posterior temporal activations, whereas those using nonanalytic strategies had greater right-sided activation. These studies demonstrated that FDG can be used to identify differential patterns of metabolism that reflect both task and strategy.

Bartlett and colleagues (1987) examined the performance of normal subjects on a phoneme discrimination task. No specific changes in regional glucose metabolism were found between subjects doing the task and other subjects who acted as controls in a resting state. However, an increase in the number of strong interregional correlations in the left hemisphere, particularly with Broca's area, when doing the task was reported. That is, although measurable regional activity did not change, regions in the left hemisphere tended to co-vary in subjects performing the task.

Other studies (Peterson et al., 1988; Posner et al., 1988) have advocated the use of subtraction techniques to compare the baseline and activation states. In these studies statistically significant point by point differences between the activation and baseline states are imaged. The concept is to select an activation state that adds one psychological component to the state studied at the baseline. The assumption is that the difference in the activation versus the baseline represents brain regions that are critical for the added psychological function. This approach has been used to study single-word processing when presented auditorially and visually (Peterson et al., 1988). The observations supported a concept of parallel routes for processing auditory and visually presented material. The most striking finding was the absence of task-specific activation of inferior parietal regions (including supramarginal and angular gyrus) during single-word processing. This observation appears to be inconsistent with lesion data that suggest an important role for the parietal cortex in word processing.

The subtraction technique proposed by these investigators is totally dependent on the validity of the assumption of additivity of response. For some brain regions and tasks, this assumption is probably reasonable. For other regions and tasks, additivity may not exist. It is conceivable that a brain region is equally activated by a baseline and an activated state and yet be critical for the added feature. In the latter situation, no change would be noted using the subtraction technique. This type of study is laying the groundwork for a major expansion and application of such procedures (Posner et al., 1988).

Studies of the visual system have also been completed. Phelps and colleagues (1981) have shown that with increasing complexity of visual stimuli greater increases in occipital glucose metabolism occur with a broadening of the area of activation. Fox and associates (1986) have shown, using more focal activation in the visual field measuring CBF and analyzing images by subtraction techniques, that small localized cortical occipital areas can be identified that are specific for where the visual field is stimulated.

Roland (1984) has shown that specific hand movements differentially activate precentral, premotor, and supplementary motor areas depending on the complexity of the task. Similarly, Ginsberg and co-investigators (1987) have shown that somatosensory tasks requiring active perceptual participation caused contralateral somatosensory activation. Similar activation was achieved by vigorous sensory stimulation but not by passive stimulation. Few activation studies have been done in stroke patients. One such study is discussed below, in the section on recovery and prognosis.

METABOLIC CHANGES AND BEHAVIORAL STUDIES IN STROKE

Metabolic Changes: Acute Stroke

With acute stroke it has been observed that blood flow and metabolic changes occur in regions with and without structural damage. In addition, in acute stages following a cerebral infarction, blood flow and glucose/oxygen metabolism may not correspond. These discrepancies may reflect different potentials for recovery of ischemic tissue and may represent the physiologic demonstration of the penumbra (i.e., ischemia surrounding infarction).

Studies in patients during the first few days after acute ischemic events have focused on understanding the pathophysiology of the process. Most studies have compared various parameters with major emphasis on relations between blood flow, oxygen metabolism, and oxygen extraction (Ackerman et al., 1981), and others have also examined glucose metabolism (Kuhl et al., 1980; Baron et al., 1982; Wise et al.,

1983a,b), and pH (Syrota et al., 1983). In ischemic or hypoxic tissue, there are different patterns of changes in CBF, OER, and oxygen metabolism, which have different implications for the degree and extent of brain damage. Frackowiak (1985) has summarized a number of these relations and argued for a descriptive nomenclature (Table 4–1). Immediately after an infarction, oxygen extraction increases in the infarcted region and then declines over the following week. This decline is associated with a marked reduction of oxygen metabolism. Blood flow over time either remains low or returns toward normal. The apparent pathophysiology involves the progression of ischemia to infarction (Wise et al., 1983a,b). Ackerman and co-investigators (1981) noted that oxygen metabolism correlated better with tissue survival than did blood flow, and that PET changes were observable prior to changes on CT.

These data suggest a spectrum of pathophysiologic consequences of cerebral infarction that may have differential effects on the nature or extent of behavior deficit, rate or extent of recovery, and prognosis. They also may indicate treatment strategies and be predictive of surgical outcome (Powers et al., 1984; Hakim et al., 1987).

Behavioral Studies: Aphasia

The emphasis in this discussion is on studies of aphasic patients. Resting FDG PET studies with eyes open and ears unoccluded have demonstrated that cerebral metabolic abnormalities extend beyond the zone of infarction determined by CT (Kuhl et al., 1980; Metter, 1981). In our experience with 60 to 70 aphasic patients, metabolic abnormalities in the affected hemisphere always exceeded the limits of symptomatic structural lesions. These metabolic changes persist following a stroke (up to 15 years in some patients we have studied) (Metter et al., 1981), though an evolution in the metabolic pattern occurs. We believe that persistent metabolic alterations accompanies structural lesions and causes clinical symptoms. In fact, we have found that regional glucose metabolism had more consistent correlations to behavioral measures than did structural damage (Metter et al., 1984a). Also, we have identified six apparently clinically silent lesions, none of which demonstrated measurable glucose metabolic abnormalities beyond the structural lesion. One subject (Figure 4–1) was a normal volunteer who was found incidentally to have a small structural lesion on CT. Extensive evaluation included normal neurologic, memory, linguistic, and neuropsychological evaluations. The pattern suggests that for a structural lesion to be associated with a persistent clinical deficit it must affect other brain regions. Lesions with little influence in other regions are asymptomatic.

Explanations for why regions without structural damage are metabolically reduced were examined in a case report (Metter et al., 1985b). A 69-year-old man was studied with PET 1 month after a stroke with a left hemiparesis; he died 10 days later from a gastrointestinal hemorrhage. Figure 4–2 shows corresponding brain and FDG scan sections. The patient had lacunes in the basal ganglia region of both hemispheres. On the left, where a lacune destroyed the anterior limb of the internal capsule, the subcortical lesion was associated with decreased glucose metabolism in the overlying frontal cortex. The anterior limb of the internal capsule contained fibers that represented afferent and efferent tracts to the metabolically depressed frontal cortex. Destruction of the tract disconnected the cortex with many of its connections. Histologic evaluation of the metabolically involved frontal cortex showed no statis-

Table 4–1 Stages of Progression from Ischemia to Infarction Demonstrated by PET

Stage	Pathophysiology	Blood Flow	Blood Volume	Oxygen Extraction	Oxygen Metabolism	Symptomatology	Tissue Recovery
Decreased perfusion rate	Vasodilatation	Normal	Increased	Normal	Normal	Subtle, cognitive, memory	Good
Mild ischemia	Desaturation	Decreased	Increased	Increased	Normal	Subtle	Good
Moderate ischemia	Ischemia	Decreased further	Increased	Decreased	Decreased	Symptomatic	Variable
Severe ischemia	Infarction	Decreased to absent	—	Decreased	Decreased	Persistent	Poor

Source: Modified from Frackowiak and Wise (1983).

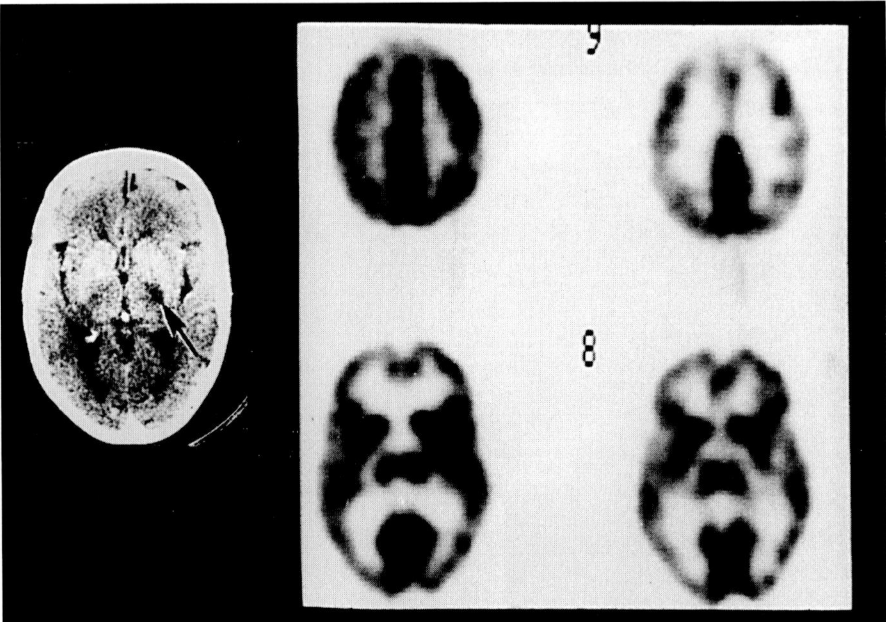

Figure 4–1 Normal volunteer with a structural lesion and a normal fluorodeoxyglucose (FDG) PET scan. The arrow points to a small lesion in the posterior limb of the right internal capsule on x-ray CT. Other than the site of infarction, the FDG PET study was normal, with symmetric FDG uptake between homologous structures in the left and right hemispheres. The blacker a region, the greater is the uptake of FDG. (Reproduced with permission from Metter, 1987.)

tically significant loss of neuronal elements, compared to the right frontal region, to account for the metabolic decline. Rather, this patient demonstrated a functionally significant lacunar infarct that disconnected the left frontal region from deep structures by destroying principal fiber tracts. The resulting metabolic effect was a reduction of glucose utilization in the frontal region. This finding extends the disconnection concept discussed by Geschwind (1965) to the level of metabolism. Lacunes in the right basal ganglia spared the internal capsule and seemingly preserved frontal metabolic function. The slight difference in location of the left and right lesions resulted in a distinctly different frontal metabolic effect.

Pappata and colleagues (1987) compared MRI and PET of either oxygen consumption or glucose utilization in patients with chronic infarctions. In all patients, remote effects (hypometabolism in apparently nondamaged brain) were found on PET that were not observed with MRI. These observations further support the hypothesis that remote metabolic effects reflect functional changes occurring in undamaged brain tissue.

Traditional Aphasic Syndromes

We have identified four patterns of metabolic abnormalities associated with structural lesions in our aphasic patients (Metter et al., 1985a, 1986a,b). Kushner and coinvestigators (1987) have found similar distributional changes in a more general study of stroke patients.

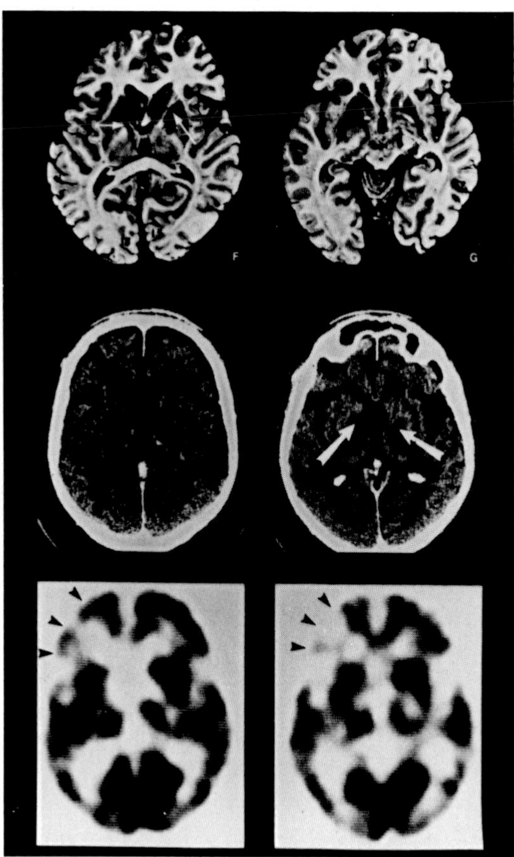

Figure 4–2 Patient with multiple brain infarctions and a lesion consistent with a disconnection syndrome. (A) Brain section from postmortem examination demonstrated multiple infarcts (arrows). An infarct in the genu of the left internal capsule was associated with degeneration of the anterior limb of the internal capsule. The infarcts in the right hemisphere were in the lenticular nuclei and spared the internal capsule. (B) CT scans demonstrating the same sections. Arrows point to the subcortical infarcts bilaterally. (C) FDG scan corresponding to the postmortem sections in (A). Note the marked metabolic asymmetry in the left inferior frontal region compared to the same region on the right (arrowheads). This patient demonstrated a functionally significant lacunar infarct that disconnected the left frontal region from deep structures by destroying the principal fiber tracts. The resulting metabolic effect was a reduction of glucose utilization in the frontal region. (Reproduced with permission from Metter et al., 1985b.)

To examine the behavioral consequences of metabolic and structural dysfunction after strokes, we investigated three traditional anatomically related aphasic syndromes: Wernicke's, Broca's, and conduction aphasias. Typical examples of CT and PET studies of each syndrome are shown in Figures 4–4 to 4–6. Quantitative observations on these patients have been published elsewhere (Metter et al., 1986c, 1989). We studied 11 Broca's, 10 conduction, and 7 Wernicke's aphasic patients with PET and CT. The structural lesions tend to differ in the depth of the lesions for the three syndromes. Patients with Broca's aphasia showed slightly more anterior lesions but, more importantly, had deeper extension into the lenticular nuclei and internal capsules than those with Wernicke's or conduction aphasia. Comparing Broca's aphasic patients to other aphasic patients with similar lesions but other types of aphasia, the critical structural difference appeared to be in the extent of damage to the posterior internal capsule (Metter et al., 1987a). Conduction aphasia patients showed no structual involvement of the lenticular nuclei and basal ganglia, but lesions often involved the insula. Patients with Wernicke's aphasia occupied a middle ground in terms of the extent of lesion depth. Wernicke's and conduction aphasic patients tended to have lesions that extended farther posteriorly into posterior temporal and lateral occipital lobes than did those with Broca's aphasia.

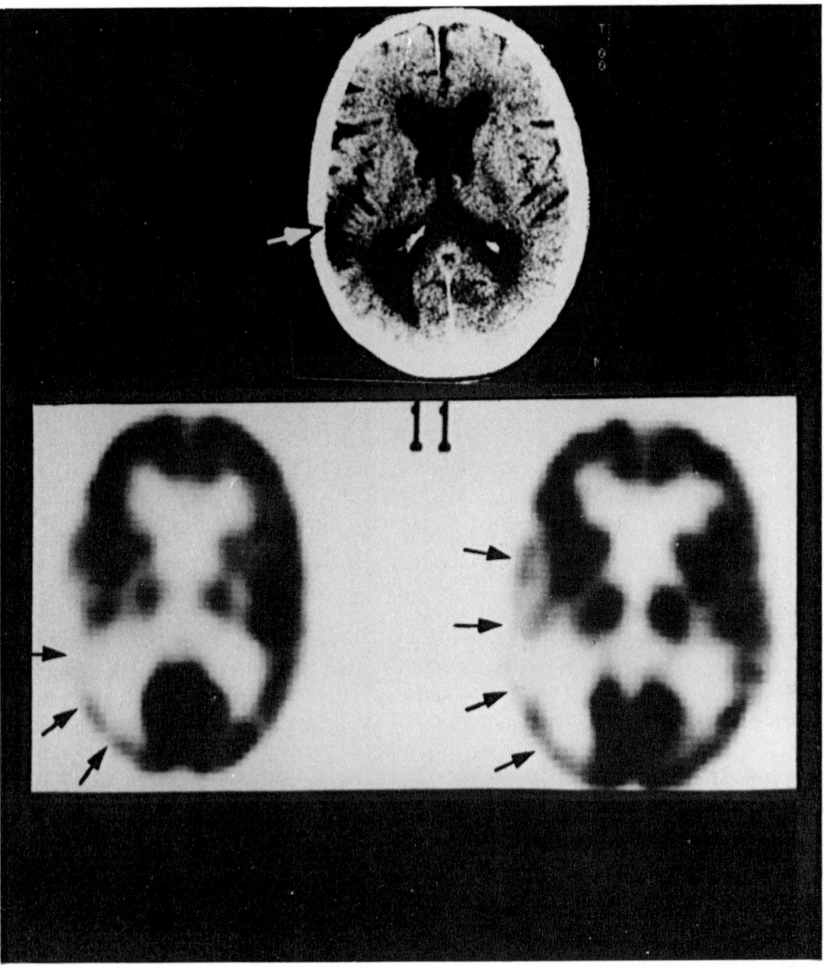

Figure 4–3 Patient with a conduction aphasia. This 55-year-old man was studied 6 months after his stroke, when he had mild conduction aphasia based on the Western Aphasia Battery. His x-ray CT scan showed a left superior temporal gyrus infarct (white arrow) and generalized atrophy, and the PET demonstrated hypometabolism in the lesion and adjacent temporoparietal regions, including more posteroinferior temporal and inferoparietal areas (black arrows). No metabolic changes were found frontally. (Reproduced with permission from Metter, 1987.)

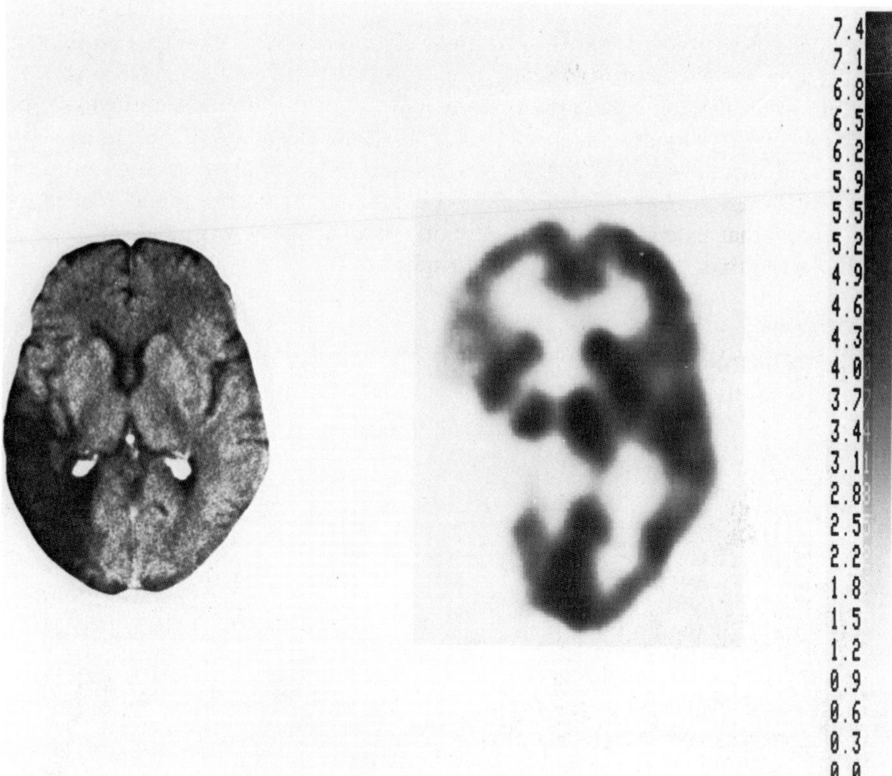

Figure 4–4 Patient with Wernicke's aphasia. CT (left) demonstrates a left temporal and parietal lesion with extensive damage to Wernicke's area. FDG PET (right) demonstrates reduced glucose metabolism throughout the left temporal lobe and frontal lobe. The gray scale on the right gives glucose metabolism in grams per 100 grams of tissue per minute.

The left hemisphere glucose metabolic patterns were different among the three aphasic syndromes. They demonstrated similar metabolic asymmetry in the temporoparietal regions but differed in the extent of asymmetry in some frontal regions (i.e., Broca's region and prefrontal cortex). The prefrontal abnormalities were independent of structural damage to these regions. Conduction aphasia (Figure 4–3) showed mild Broca's region metabolic asymmetry and none in prefrontal regions. Wernicke's aphasia (Figure 4–4) showed mild to moderate glucose metabolic asymmetry in both Broca's and prefrontal regions. Broca's aphasia (Figure 4–5) had severe glucose metabolic asymmetry in both areas.

Anatomy of Metabolic Effects in Aphasia

Prefrontal Regions. The prefrontal metabolic changes were interesting because they distinguished the three syndromes, showed no consistent structural damage, and have not in the past been recognized as contributing to discrimination of these three syndromes. In Broca's aphasia, frontal hypometabolism was frequently as severe as is observed in moderate to severe structural damage, suggesting that normal frontal function may have been disrupted. It may explain some aspects of the patients'

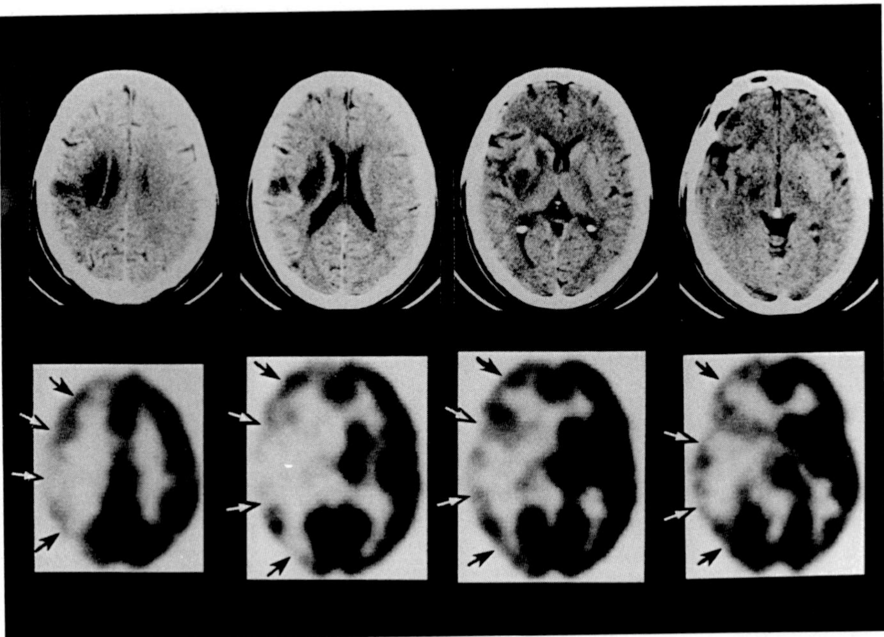

Figure 4–5 Patient with Broca's aphasia. This 43-year-old man had a stroke with Broca's aphasia, as diagnosed by the Western Aphasia Battery. He was studied 2 months after onset. A repeat study 6 months later was similar. CT showed a lesion in the basal ganglia that extended into the cortex. The PET study showed extensive metabolic changes (arrows) throughout much of the left hemisphere compared to the right hemisphere. (Reproduced with permission from Metter, 1987.)

behavior, including slow, difficult motoric features and some of the difficulties they had sequencing materials, as seen in transcortical motor aphasias (Luria and Hutton, 1977; Friedman et al., 1984) and with frontal lobe lesions (Stuss and Benson, 1984). In Wernicke's and conduction aphasia, prefrontal hypometabolism was less apparent and suggested less modification (or loss) of normal frontal function than is seen with Broca's aphasia. Because prefrontal changes in Wernicke's aphasia are not prominent, frontal cortical function may in general be preserved. What may be lost is information normally received from the temporal region and the loss of the ability to send specific integrated information to other brain regions. Thus prefrontal cortex may have lost at least part of its influence on cerebral function. In Wernicke's aphasia, it may be part of the reason for jargon speech. In these individuals the frontal lobes may function with little assistance from the left temporoparietal language regions, so that when speech is required the frontal lobe talks but without normal control and feedback supplied by the temporal lobe.

Comparing all the aphasic patients we studied, measurable metabolic abnormalities were restricted to the temporoparietal regions in about 45%. Structural lesions that caused this pattern tended to spare the lenticular nuclei and internal capsule. Measurable metabolic abnormalities in both left temporoparietal and prefrontal regions were found in the remaining 55% of aphasic patients. The structural lesions tended to be larger and to extend deeper into the lenticular and internal capsule.

In a study examining cerebellar asymmetry, we found data that directly relates to the functional significance of prefrontal asymmetry in aphasia (Metter et al., 1987b). In a principal components analysis, the first component (consisting of all frontal measures, caudate, thalamus, and contralateral cerebellum) accounted for 62% of the metabolic variance. The second component was made up of the temporal regions. Parietal cortex loaded on both components. The observations suggested the presence of two overlapping systems: a frontoparietal system and a temporoparietal system. These anatomic systems agree with classic behavioral dichotomies in aphasia (e.g., fluent/nonfluent, motor/nonmotor, frontal/posterior) and with previous observations we have made in normal subjects (Metter et al., 1984c). Comparison of aphasic patients with and without frontal asymmetry (Metter et al., 1987a) revealed that the asymmetric frontal group had greater hemiparesis as well as poorer fluency and writing. These findings are consistent with a motoric role for the frontal lobe. Other studies have suggested a variety of roles for frontal regions involving motor control, including initiation and maintenance of movements, temporal planning and sequencing, and executive planning, i.e., decisions as to importance, goals, and so on (see Fuster, 1989, and Stuss and Benson, 1984, for reviews). Relative impairment of such "executive" functions could account for some of the behavioral differences.

Caudate and thalamus. Another observation of interest is the strong association of metabolic asymmetry of the head of the caudate and thalamus to the frontal and parietal regions. Pathoanatomic studies have demonstrated the presence of aphasic syndromes with subcortical lesions, particularly in the region of lenticular nuclei and the thalamus (Damasio et al., 1982; Naeser et al., 1982). Previous studies using FDG PET have shown that such lesions can be associated with temporoparietal hypometabolism (Metter et al., 1981, 1983), particularly with posterior internal capsule and posterior lenticular nuclei lesions. On close scrutiny, the left thalamic hypometabolism seemed more involved with memory tasks involving language, whereas the head of the caudate was more closely associated with frontal metabolism and more basic functions underlying but probably not specific to language.

In some patients, small thalamic lesions produced mild metabolic changes throughout the ipsilateral hemisphere. This pattern has been seen in several patients, including patient N.A. (Metter et al., 1983). Baron and associates (1986) have studied patients with similar lesions and found similar general cortical metabolic changes. We believe that such cortical changes are independent of specific behavior. Rather, these changes reflect a general thalamic influence on ipsilateral cortex, which causes a relatively uniform degree of metabolic asymmetry throughout much of the hemisphere. These mild generalized changes appear to have functional consequences different from the focal temporoparietal hypometabolism found in other thalamic lesions. The differences presumably have to do with the thalamic nuclei that were damaged. Damage to the dorsomedial nucleus (as in N.A.) resulted in the generalized pattern.

To better understand the role of subcortical structural damage in producing language abnormalities, we have used pathway analysis to build a model from observations of glucose metabolism in aphasia (Figure 4–6) (Metter et al., 1988). The model was intended to answer the question of whether subcortical structural damage had an effect on behavior that could be separated from effects on cortex. The data clearly showed both a direct and an indirect effect of subcortical damage on word

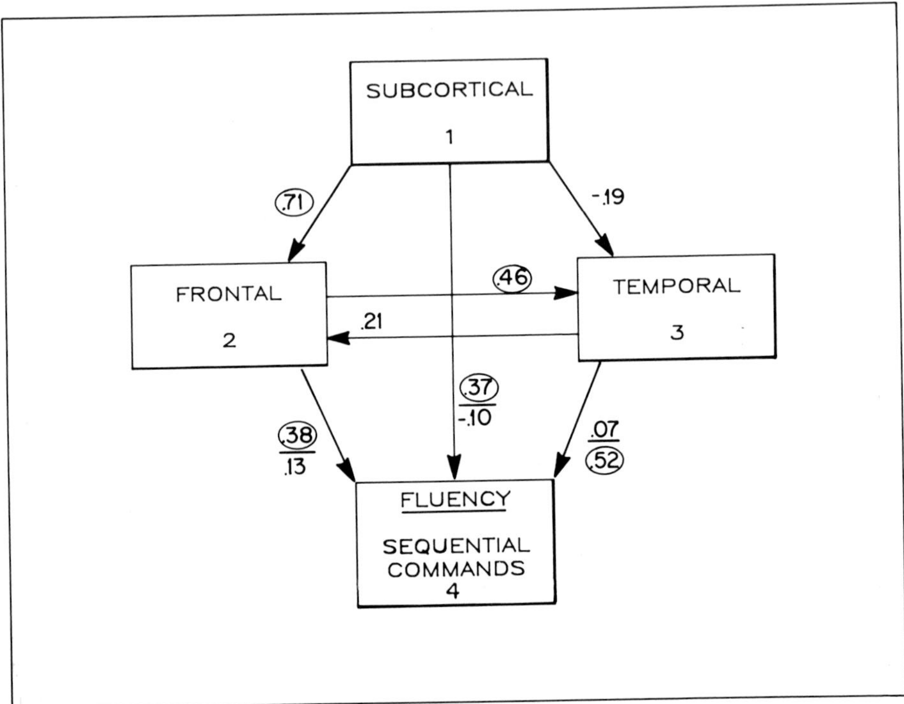

Figure 4–6 Path analysis model of the effect of subcortical structural damage on fluency and sequential command scores from the Western Aphasia Battery. Arrows represent relations between boxes, with direction implying the causal relation. The number next to each arrow is an estimate of the association between the two boxes. Numbers that are circled are considered to represent important connections. The analysis showed that subcortical structural damage has a direct effect on fluency but not sequential commands. In addition, it has an indirect affect on fluency through its action on the frontal lobe. (Reproduced with permission from Metter et al., 1988.)

fluency. The results indicated that a primary effect of subcortical damage on some aspects of linguistic behavior can be separated from secondary effects associated with a depression of cortical metabolism.

Studies of diseases that primarily damage subcortical structures, e.g., Huntington's (HD) and Parkinson's diseases, have implications for understanding cortical-subcortical relations. The two diseases were found to show fewer cortical-cortical regional metabolic intercorrelations than in normal subjects, suggesting a role for the basal ganglia in directing cortical to cortical communication (Metter et al., 1984b). Mazziotta et al. (1985) had normal volunteers repeatedly write their name or do a novel finger sequence task after the injection of FDG. With writing, prominent increases were found in striatal metabolism as well as contralateral sensorimotor cortex, whereas with the novel task only cortical activation occurred. HD subjects showed no striatal activation similar to controls during the novel sequence task. The authors argued that loss of striatal function caused HD patients to lose the semiautomated processes controlled by the basal ganglia requiring the use of motor system functions usually reserved for novel acts. Likewise, in progressive supranuclear palsy, a disease with basal ganglia pathology, FDG PET studies have shown prominent metabolic reduction in the frontal lobes, indicating important relations between these structures (D'Antona et al., 1985). Patients with progressive supranuclear palsy show a "subcortical dementia" characterized by slowness of thought and response, with delayed recall, apathy, but no aphasia or apraxia (Albert et al., 1974). These observations and the strong correlation between caudate nucleus and frontal metabolism suggest a strong cortical-subcortical interrelation in the executions of specific behaviors.

Temporal lobe. So far, the focus has been on the frontal and subcortical regions that were found to differ between some aphasic syndromes. Another observation concerns changes occurring in temporoparietal metabolism. In Wernicke's, Broca's, and conduction aphasia, a similar degree of left temporoparietal hypometabolism was found in all three syndromes. In fact, in all aphasic patients we have studied (approximately 65 subjects, all right-handed with left hemisphere lesions), the common finding was the constant presence of left temporoparietal hypometabolism. At present, we have not found any aphasic patient who did not have metabolic changes in the left temporoparietal region. The presence of similar metabolic dysfunction in all aphasic patients argues for some commonality of features in all these individuals (Metter et al., in press).

A major debate, dating from at least Dejerine and Marie, has been whether aphasia is a unitary phenomena or multiple types of aphasia exist. Differences in the two views depend on whether you focus on features that appear to be similar in all aphasic patients (regardless of severity) or on features that are somewhat different. The PET observations support both viewpoints. Common changes in temporoparietal glucose metabolic asymmetry are consistent with aphasia as a unitary abnormality, whereas differences in prefrontal regions were associated with different aphasic syndromes. Thus both sides of the traditional debate can be supported, and the advantages of each might profitably be integrated to create a more realistic model of brain-behavior relations.

Another theory suggests that conduction aphasia results from damage to the arcuate fasciculus with disconnection of intact Wernicke's and Broca's regions. Conceptually, with a disconnection, metabolic asymmetry would be expected in both Broca's and Wernicke's regions. Of ten conduction aphasic patients, six were found to have a mild degree of metabolic asymmetry in Broca's area (Kempler et al., 1986). Both Wernicke's and Broca's aphasias appear to disrupt frontal-posterior communications to a much greater extent than does conduction aphasia. These data suggest that perhaps two mechanisms produce the syndrome, one of which involves disconnections.

An alternate model (Levine and Calvanio, 1982) argues that language function is mediated by tightly integrated auditory and sensorimotor centers that functionally partially overlap primarily in the parietal area. Damage to overlapping regions with preservation of most of each center causes the conduction aphasia. This model does not rely on disconnection. The absence of prominent Broca's metabolic asymmetry in conduction aphasia argues that, if a disconnection is responsible, the critical pathway (arcuate fasciculus) appears to be minor in terms of distant effects on Broca's region, rather than the major one argued by traditional theorists.

Recovery and Prognosis

PET should also prove useful for investigations of the process of recovery. Brain function during recovery has been measured by blood flow and metabolism changes, but there have been few PET studies to date. Bosley et al. (1987) studied the recovery of homonymous hemianopsia after cerebral infarction and showed that improvement of the visual field is accompanied by normalization of occipital brain metabolism. Stroke recovery has been studied using xenon to measure regional CBF with multiple external detectors (see Metter and Hanson, 1985, for review). In one study (Yamaguchi et al., 1980), patients with "good prognosis for recovery" had increased regional blood flow in the "area homologous to Broca's area in the nondominant hemisphere." In another study (Knopman et al., 1984), aphasic patients were tested with a stimulation paradigm ("purposeful listening") during early and late stages of recovery from word comprehension deficits. The patients with better recovery overall showed diffuse right hemisphere activation at the early session (within the first 100 days of the stroke). However, these patients showed a greater increase in posterior left activation at the later session (approximately 100 days later), suggesting "restitution of left posterior temporal-inferior parietal function following early impairment," and that right hemisphere compensation may be important for recovery.

In our studies, global glucose metabolic rates were found to change by 20 to 40% from the first to the seventh month post-stroke. This change involved all brain regions, representing a generalized response to stroke that does not appear to be directly related to behavior but, rather, to physiologic phenomena or to factors within the FDG model. In addition, relative regional changes can occur that are correlated to improvement or decline in aspects of performance (Jackson et al., 1987).

Consequences of Remote Effects

Alterations in regional metabolism in nondamaged brain regions clearly occur, but such effects can be associated with a number of biochemical, cellular, and regional changes that could affect behavior differently. Contributions to regional metabolism include the metabolic activity of neurons, glia, and dendritic innervation. The innervation of dendrites derives from cell–cell interactions within a region, short-distance connections from adjacent brain regions, and long fibers arising from more distant regions. Measured metabolism depends on the summation of these individual contributions. Regional hypometabolism can result from damage to one or more of these components. Alternatively, changes in the neuronal firing patterns within the region can occur that would result from increases or decreases in either excitatory or inhibitory inputs to the region. Structural damage in one region can result in metabolic changes in a distant region based on damage to the message sent from the first to the second region.

Such region-to-region information transfer is not uniform. It is clear that hemisphere lesions are associated with contralateral cerebellar hypometabolism, which is a transsynaptic process. On the other hand, transcallosal fibers are not associated with significant persistent changes in the contralateral hemisphere despite the enormous number of fibers crossing the corpus callosum. The most prominent remote effects appear to be intrahemispheric. Although distant effects can be indirect (decreased dendritic activity), it is possible that some are direct due to loss of neuronal firing secondary to unsuspected injury or even transsynaptic neuronal loss. The contribution from each of these factors is difficult or impossible to determine.

The influence of remote metabolic changes on behavior may be distinctly different from that of direct structural damage. Structural lesions have a probability of causing specific behavioral changes based on the degree of disruption of the structural integrity and connections within the region. When damage is severe, regional function is lost. Remote metabolic changes caused by a lesion may cause functional loss similar to what would be observed in the case of direct damage. Conversely, the functional integrity of the remote region may not be lost but, rather, only modified in its ability to carry out its goals. That is, the distant region may operate in a normal way but without information normally received from the structurally damaged area. Thus a 50% loss of metabolic activity at a structural lesion site may manifest differently behaviorally from a 50% metabolic reduction at a remote site with no structural damage. New concepts are needed to understand how remote metabolic effects are similar to and different from direct local effects of structural damage.

CONCLUSION

The PET studies reviewed above demonstrate that current anatomic-behavioral models need to be expanded. Structural damage to the language system, for example, affects other functional brain systems, including a "prefrontal system." Furthermore, temporoparietal metabolic changes were found in all aphasic patients. We have hypothesized that the common language abnormalities in aphasia are associated with the temporoparietal changes. In contrast, the distinguishing features among syndromes are associated with the extent and nature of changes occurring in other brain regions, including subcortical structures and prefrontal regions.

Clearly, other physiologic systems exist that interact with language functions. They can be considered physiologically and behaviorally. Not all physiologic systems manifest behaviorally. PET reveals a complex interplay within the damaged brain. Both resting studies and activation studies will help to unravel the complex interactions between brain regions; for example, our data suggest that undamaged but modified frontal systems require extensive investigation. The challenge is to expand existing models to account for the multiple interactions that are needed for even simple tasks. In this way PET will improve our understanding of brain-behavior relations in language and other behavior.

REFERENCES

Ackerman, R.H., Correia, J.A., Alpert, H.M., Baron, J.C., Gouliamos, A., Grotta, J.C., Brownell, G.L., and Taveras, J.M. (1981). Positron imaging in ischemic stroke disease using compounds labelled with oxygen-15. *Arch. Neurol.*, **38,** 537–543.

Albert, M.L., Feldman, R.G., and Willis, A.L. (1974). The "subcortical dementia" of progressive supranuclear palsy. *J. Neurol. Neurosurg. Psychiatry,* **37,** 121–130.

Alpert, M.M., Ackerman, R.H., Correia, J.A., Baron, J.C., Brownell, G.L., and Taveras, J.M. (1977). Measurement of rCBF and $rCMRO_2$ by continuous inhalation of ^{15}O-labelled CO_2 and O_2. *Acta Neurol. Scand.*, [*Suppl 72*], **56,** 186–187.

Baron, J.C., Comar, D., Soussaline, F., Todd-Pokropek, A., Bousser, M.G., Castaigne, P., and Kellershohn, C. (1979). Continuous ^{15}O inhalation technique: an attempt to quantify CBF, EO_2 and $CMRO_2$. *Acta Neurol. Scand.* [*Suppl 72*], **60,** 194–195.

Baron, J.C., Lebrun-Grandie, P., Collard, P., Crouzel, C., Mestelan, G., and Bousser, M.G. (1982). Noninvasive measurement of blood flow, oxygen consumption and glucose utilization in the same brain regions in man by positron emission tomography: concise communication. *J. Nucl. Med.,* **23,** 391–399.

Baron, J.C., D'Antona, R., Pantano, P., Serdaru, M., Samson, Y., and Bousser, M.G. (1986). Effects of thalamic stroke on energy metabolism of the cerebral cortex. *Brain,* **109,** 1243–1259.

Bartlett, E.J., Brown, J.W., Wolf, A.P., and Brodie, J. (1987). Correlations between glucose metabolic rates in brain regions in healthy male adults at rest and during language stimulation. *Brain Lang.,* **32,** 1–18.

Basso, A., Lecours, A.R., Moraschini, S., and Vanier, M. (1985). Anatomoclinical correlations of the aphasias as determined through computerized tomography: exceptions. *Brain Lang.,* **26,** 201–229.

Benson, D.F. (1979). *Aphasia, Alexia, Agraphia.* New York: Churchill Livingstone.

Benson, D.F., and Geschwind, N. (1985). The aphasias and related disturbances. In: A.B. Baker and R.J. Joynt, eds., *Clinical Neurology,* pp. 1–34. Philadelphia: Harper & Row.

Bosley, T.M., Dann, R., Silver, F.L., Alavi, A., Kushner, M., Chawluk, J.B., Savino, P.J., Sergott, R.C., Schatz, N.J., and Reivich, M. (1987). Recovery of vision after ischemic lesions: positron emission tomography. *Ann. Neurol.,* **21,** 444–450.

Brown, J.W. (1975). On the neural organization of language: thalamic and cortical relationships. *Brain Lang.,* **2,** 18–30.

Crosson, B. (1984). Role of the dominant thalamus in language: a review. *Psychol. Bull.,* **9,** 491–517.

Damasio, A.R., Damasio, H., Rizzo, M., Varney, N., and Gersch, F. (1982). Aphasia with nonhemorrhagic lesions in the basal ganglia and internal capsule. *Arch. Neurol.,* **39,** 15–20.

D'Antona, R., Baron, J.C., Samson, Y., Serdaru, M., Viader, F., Agid, Y., and Cambier, J. (1985). Subcortical dementia: frontal cortex hypometabolism detected by positron tomography in patients with progressive supranuclear palsy. *Brain,* **108,** 785–799.

Darley, F.L. (1982). *Aphasia.* Philadelphia: Saunders.

DesRosiers, M.H., Kennedy, C., Patlak, C.S., Pettigrew, K.D., Sokoloff, L., and Reivich, M. (1974). Relationship between local cerebral blood flow and glucose utilization in the rat. *Neurology,* **24,** 389.

Duara, R., Grady, C., Haxby, J., Ingvar, D., Sokoloff, L., Margolin, R.A., Manning, R.G., Cutler, N., and Rapoport, S. (1984). Human brain glucose utilization and cognitive function in relation to age. *Ann. Neurol.,* **16,** 702–713.

Fox, P.T., Mintun, M.A., Raichle, M.E., Miezin, F.M., Allman, J.M., and Van Essen, D.C. (1986). Mapping human visual cortex with positron emission tomography. *Nature,* **323,** 806–809.

Frackowiak, R.S.J. (1985). A new perspective obtained with positron tomography. *Q. J. Med.,* **57,** 713–727.

Frackowiak, R.S.J., and Wise, R.J.S. (1983). Positron tomography in ischemic cerebrovascular disease. *Neurol. Clin.,* **1,** 183–201.

Frackowiak, R.S.J., Lenzi, G.L., Jones, T., and Heather, J.D. (1980). Quantitative measurement of regional cerebral blood flow and oxygen metabolism in man using ^{15}O and positron emission tomography: theory, procedure and normal values. *J. Comput. Assist. Tomogr.,* **4,** 727–736.

Freygang, W.H., and Sokoloff, L. (1958). Quantitative measurement of regional circulation in the central nervous system by use of radioactive inert gas. *Adv. Biol. Med. Physiol.*, **6**, 263–279.

Friedland, R.P., Budinger, T.F., Yano, Y., Huesman, R.H., Knittel, B., Derenzo, S.E., Koss, B., and Ober, B.A. (1983). Regional cerebral metabolic alterations in Alzheimer-type dementia: kinetic studies with 18-fluorodeoxyglucose. *J. Cereb. Blood Flow Metab.*, **3**(suppl 1), S510–S511.

Friedman, M., Alexander, M.P., and Naeser, M.A. (1984). Anatomic basis of transcortical motor aphasia. *Neurology*, **34**, 409–417.

Fuster, J. (1989). *The Prefrontal Cortex: Anatomy, Physiology, and Neuropsychology of the Frontal Lobe.* Second edition. New York: Raven Press.

Gadian, D.G. (1982). *Nuclear Magnetic Resonance and Its Applications to Living Systems.* New York: Oxford University Press.

Geschwind, N. (1965). Disconnection syndromes in animals and man. I and II. *Brain*, **88**, 237–294, 585–644.

Ginsberg, M.D., Yoshi, F., Vibulsresth, S., Chang, J.Y., Duara, R., Barker, W.W., and Boothe, T.E. (1987). Human task-specific somatosensory activation. *Neurology*, **37**, 1301–1308.

Hakim, A.M., Pokrupa, R.P., Villaneuva, J., Diksic, M., Evans, A.C., Thompson, C.J., Meyer, E., Yamamoto, Y.L., and Feindel, W.H. (1987). The effects of spontaneous reperfusion on metabolic functions in early human cerebral infarcts. *Ann. Neurol.*, **21**, 279–289.

Hawkins, R.A., Phelps, M.E., Huang, S.C., and Kuhl, D.E. (1981). Effect of ischemia on quantification of local cerebral glucose metabolic rate in man. *J. Cereb. Blood Flow Metab.*, **1**, 37–51.

Hawkins, R.A., Mazziotta, J.C., Phelps, M.E., Huang, S.C., Kuhl, D.E., Carson, R.E., Metter, E.J., and Riege, W.H. (1983). Cerebral glucose metabolism as a function of age in man: influence of the rate constants in the fluorodeoxyglucose method. *J. Cereb. Blood Flow Metab.*, **3**, 250–253.

Huang, S.C., Phelps, M.E, Hoffman, E.J., Sideris, K., Selin, C.J., and Kuhl, D.E. (1980). Noninvasive determination of local cerebral metabolic rate of glucose in man. *Am. J. Physiol.*, **238**, E69–E82.

Huang, S.C., Carson, R.E., and Phelps, M.E. (1982). Measurement of local blood flow and distribution volume with short-lived isotopes: a general input technique. *J. Cereb. Blood Flow Metab.*, **2**, 99–108.

Jackson, C.A., Kempler, D., Metter, E.J., Hanson, W.R., Mazziotta, J., and Phelps, M.E. (1987). Recovery of language comprehension in aphasia. Presented at the Annual Meeting of American Speech & Hearing Association.

Jones, T., Chesler, D.A., and Ter-Pogossian, M.M. (1976). The continuous inhalation of oxygen-15 for assessing regional oxygen extraction in the brain of man. *Br. J. Radiol.*, **49**, 339–343.

Kempler, D., Metter, E.J., Jackson, C.A., Hanson, W.E., Phelps, M.E., and Mazziotta, J. (1986). Conduction aphasia: sub-groups based on behavior, anatomy and physiology. In: R.H. Brookshire, ed., *Clinical Aphasiology*, Vol. 16, pp. 105–115. Minneapolis: BRK Publishers.

Knopman, D., Rubens, A., Selnes, O., Klassen, A.C., and Meyer, M.W. (1984). Mechanisms of recovery from aphasia: evidence from serial xenon 133 cerebral blood flow studies. *Ann. Neurol.*, **15**, 530–535.

Kuhl, D.E., Phelps, M.E., Kowell, A.P., Metter, E.J., Selin, C., and Winter, J. (1980). Effect of stroke on local cerebral metabolism and perfusion: mapping by emission computed tomography of ^{18}FDG and $^{13}NH_3$. *Ann. Neurol.*, **8**, 47–60.

Kuhl, D.E., Metter, E.J., Riege, W.H., and Phelps, M.E. (1982). Effects of human aging on patterns of local cerebral glucose utilization determined by the (^{18}F) fluorodeoxyglucose method. *J. Cereb. Blood Flow Metab.,* **2,** 163–171.

Kushner, M., Reivich, M., Fieschi, C., Silver, F., Chawluk, J., Rosen, M., Greenberg, J., Burke, A., and Alavi, A. (1987). Metabolic and clinical correlates of acute ischemic infarction. *Neurology,* **37,** 1103–1110.

Lammertsma, A.A., Jones, T., Frackowiak, R.S.J., and Lenzi, G.L. (1981). A theoretical study of the steady-state model for measuring regional cerebral blood flow and oxygen utilization using oxygen-15. *J. Comput. Assist. Tomogr.,* **5,** 544–550.

Levine, D.N., and Calvanio, R. (1982). Conduction aphasia. In: H.S. Kirshner, and F.R. Freeman, eds., *The Neurology of Aphasia,* pp. 79–111, Lisse: Swets & Zeitlinger.

Luria, A.R., and Hutton, J.T. (1977). A modern assessment of the brain forms of aphasia. *Brain Lang.,* **4,** 129–151.

Mazziotta, J.C., Phelps, M.E., Miller, J., and Kuhl, D.E. (1981a). Tomographic mapping of human cerebral metabolism: normal unstimulated state. *Neurology,* **31,** 503–516.

Mazziotta, J.C., Phelps, M.E., Plummer, D., and Kuhl, D.E. (1981b). Quantitation in positron emission computed tomography. 5. Physical-anatomical effects. *J. Comput. Assist. Tomogr.,* **5,** 734–743.

Mazziotta, J.C., Phelps, M.E., Carson, R.E., and Kuhl, D.E. (1982a). Tomographic mapping of human cerebral metabolism: sensory deprivation. *Ann. Neurol.,* **12,** 435–444.

Mazziotta, J.C., Phelps, M.E., Carson, R.E., and Kuhl, D.E. (1982b). Tomographic mapping of human cerebral metabolism: auditory stimulation. *Neurology,* **32,** 921–937.

Mazziotta, J.C., Phelps, M.E., and Wapenski, J. (1985). Metabolic differences of motor system responses found between normal subjects and patients with basal ganglia disease. *Neurology,* **32***(Suppl. 1), 110.*

Metter, E.J. (1987). Neuroanatomy and physiology of aphasia: evidence from positron emission tomography. *Aphasiology,* **1,** 3–33.

Metter, E.J., and Hanson, W.R. (1985). Brain imaging as related to speech and language. In: J. Darby, ed., *Speech Evaluation in Neurology,* pp. 123–160. Orlando: Grune & Stratton.

Metter, E.J., Wasterlain, C.G., Kuhl, D.E., Hanson, W.R., and Phelps, M.E. (1981). ^{18}FDG positron emission computed tomography in a study of aphasia. *Ann. Neurol.,* **10,** 173–183.

Metter, E.J., Riege, W.H., Hanson, W.R., Kuhl, D.E., Phelps, M.E., Squire, L.R., Wasterlain, C.G., and Benson, D.F. (1983). Comparisons of metabolic rates, language and memory in sub-cortical aphasias. *Brain Lang.,* **19,** 33–47.

Metter, E.J., Riege, W.R., Hanson, W., Camras, L., Kuhl, D.E., and Phelps, M.E. (1984a). Correlations of cerebral glucose metabolism and structural damage to language function in aphasia. *Brain Lang.,* **21,** 187–207.

Metter, E.J., Riege, W.H., Kameyama, M., Kuhl, D.E., and Phelps, M.E. (1984b). Cerebral metabolic relationships for selected brain regions in Alzheimer's, Huntington's and Parkinson's disease. *J. Cereb. Blood Flow Metab.,* **4,** 500–506.

Metter, E.J., Riege, W.H., Kuhl, D.E., and Phelps, M.E. (1984c). Cerebral metabolic relationships for selected brain regions in healthy adults. *J. Cereb. Blood Flow Metab.,* **4,** 1–7.

Metter, E.J., Hanson, W.R., Riege, W.H., Jackson, C., Mazziotta, J., Phelps, M.E., and Kuhl, D.E. (1985a). Remote metabolic effects in aphasia stroke patients. In: R.H. Brookshire, ed., *Clinical Aphasiology,* Vol. 15, pp. 126–135. Minneapolis: BRK Press.

Metter, E.J., Mazziotta, J.C., Itabashi, H.H., Mankovich, N.J., Phelps, M.E., and Kuhl, D.E. (1985b). Comparison of x-ray CT, glucose metabolism and post-mortem data in a patient with multiple infarctions. *Neurology,* **35,** 1695–1701.

Metter, E.J., Jackson, C.A., Kempler, D., Hanson, W.R., Mazziotta, J.C., and Phelps, M.E.

(1986a). Remote glucose metabolic patterns in chronic stroke lesions. *Neurology,* **36**(suppl 1), 349.

Metter, E.J., Jackson, C., Kempler, D., Riege, W.H., Hanson, W.R., Mazziotta, J.C., and Phelps, M.E. (1986b). Left hemisphere intracerebral hemorrhages studied by (F-18)-fluorodeoxyglucose positron emission tomography. *Neurology,* **36,** 1155–1162.

Metter, E.J., Kempler, D., Jackson, C., Hanson, W.R., Mazziotta, J.C., and Phelps, M.E. (1986c). Cerebral glucose metabolism: differences in Wernicke's, Broca's and conduction aphasias. In: R.H. Brookshire, ed., *Clinical Aphasiology,* Vol. 16, pp. 97–104. Minneapolis: BRK Publishers.

Metter, E.J., Kempler, D., Jackson, C.A., Hanson, W.R., Mazziotta, J.C., and Phelps, M.E. (1987a). A study of Broca's aphasia by ^{18}F-fluorodeoxyglucose positron emission tomography. *Ann. Neurol.,* **22,** 134.

Metter, E.J., Kempler, D., Jackson, C.A., Hanson, W.R., Riege, W.H., Camras, L., Mazziotta, J.C., and Phelps, M.E. (1987b). Cerebellar glucose metabolism in chronic aphasia. *Neurology,* **37,** 1599–1606.

Metter, E.J., Riege, W.H., Hanson, W.R., Jackson, C.A., Kempler, D., and Van Lancrera, D. (1988). Subcortical structures in aphasia: an analysis based on (F-18)-fluorodeoxy: positron emission tomography, and computed tomography. *Arch. Neurol.,* **45,** 1229–1234.

Metter, E.J., Kempler, D., Jackson, C., Hanson, W.R., Mazziotta, J.C., and Phelps, M.E. (1989). Cerebral glucose metabolism in Wiernicke's, Broca's and conduction aphasia. *Arch. Neurol.,* **46,** 27–34.

Metter, E.J., Hanson, W.R., Jackson, C.A., Kempler, D., and Van Lancker, D. (in press). Temporoparietal cortex: the common substrate for aphasia. In: T. Prescott, ed., *Clinical Aphasiology,* Vol. 19. San Diego: College-Hill.

Mohr, J.P., Watters, W.C., and Duncan, G.W. (1975). Thalamic hemorrhage and aphasia. *Brain Lang.,* **2,** 3–17.

Naeser, M.A., Alexander, M.P., Helm-Estabrooks, N., Levine, H.L., Laughlin, S.A., and Geschwind, N. (1982). Aphasia with pre-dominantly subcortical lesion sites. *Arch. Neurol.,* **39,** 2–14.

Pappata, S., Tran Dinh, S., Baron, J.C., Cambon, H., and Syrota, A. (1987). Remote metabolic effects of cerebrovascular lesions: magnetic resonance and positron tomography imaging. *Neuroradiology,* **29,** 1–6.

Partridge, W. (1983). Brain metabolism: a perspective from the blood-brain barrier. *Physiol. Rev.,* **63,** 1481–1535.

Peterson, S.E., Fox, P.T., Posner, M.I., Mintum, M., and Raichle, M.E. (1988). Positron emission tomographic studies of the cortical anatomy of single-word processing. *Nature,* **331,** 585–589.

Phelps, M.E., Huang, S.C., Hoffman, E.J., Selin, C.S., Sokoloff, L., and Kuhl, D.E. (1979). Tomographic measurement of local cerebral metabolic rate in humans with F-18 2-fluoro-deoxyglucose: validation of method. *Ann. Neurol.,* **6,** 371–388.

Phelps, M.E., Mazziotta, J.C., Kuhl, D.E., Nuwer, M., Packwood, J., Metter, E.J., and Engel, J. (1981). Tomographic mapping of human cerebral metabolism, visual stimulation and deprivation. *Neurology,* **31,** 517–529.

Posner, M.I., Peterson, S.E., Fox, P.T., and Raichle, M.E. (1988). Localization of cognitive operations in the human brain. *Science,* **240,** 1627–1631.

Powers, W.J., Martin, W.R.W., Herscovitch, P., Raichle, M.E., and Grubb, A.L. (1984). Extracranial-intracranial bypass surgery: hemodynamic and metabolic results. *Neurology,* **34,** 1168–1174.

Reivich, M., Kuhl, D., Wolf, A., Greenberg, J., Phelps, M., Ido, T., Casella, V., Fowler, J., Hoffman, E., Alavi, A., Som, P., and Sokoloff, L. (1979). The (F^{18})-fluorodeoxyglucose method for the measurement of local cerebral glucose utilization in man. *Circ. Res.*, **44,** 127–137.

Reivich, M., Alavi, A., Wolf, A., Fowler, J., Russel, J., Arnett, C., MacGregor, R.R., Shiue, C.Y., Atkins, H., Anand, A., Dann, R., and Greenberg, J.H. (1985). Glucose metabolic rate kinetic model parameter determination in humans: the lumped constants and rate constants for (^{18}F) fluorodeoxyglucose and (^{11}C) deoxyglucose. *J. Cereb. Blood Flow Metab.*, **5,** 179–192.

Roland, P.E. (1984). Organization of motor control by the normal human brain. *Hum. Neurobiol.*, **2,** 205–216.

Sacks, W., Sacks, S., and Fletcher, A. (1983). A comparison of the cerebral uptake and metabolism of labeled glucose and deoxyglucose in vivo in rats. *Neurochem. Res.*, **8,** 661–685.

Salford, L.G., Duffy, T.E., and Plum, F. (1973). Altered cerebral metabolism and blood flow in response to physiological stimulation. *Stroke,* **4,** 351–362.

Sokoloff, L., Reivich, M., Kennedy, C., DesRosier, M.H., Patlak, C.S., Pettigrew, K.D., Sakurada, O., and Shinohara, H. (1977). The (C-14) deoxyglucose method for the measurement of local cerebral glucose utilization: theory, procedure and normal values in the conscious and anesthetized albino rat. *J. Neurochem.*, **28,** 897–916.

Stuss, D.T., and Benson, D.F. (1984). Neuropsychological studies of the frontal lobe. *Psychol. Bull.*, **95,** 3–28.

Syrota, A., Castaing, M., Rougemont, D., Berridge, M., Baron, J.C., Bousser, M.G., and Pocidalo, J.J. (1983). Tissue acid-base balance and oxygen metabolism in human cerebral infarction studied with positron emission tomography. *Ann. Neurol.*, **14,** 419–428.

Van Buren, J.M. (1975). The question of thalamic participation in speech mechanisms. *Brain Lang.*, **2,** 31–44.

Wise, R.J.S., Bernardi, S., Frackowiak, R.S.J., Legg, N.J., and Jones, T. (1983a). Serial observations on the pathophysiology of acute stroke, the transition from ischemia to infarction as reflected in regional oxygen extraction. *Brain,* **106,** 197–222.

Wise, R.J.S., Rhodes, C.G., Gibbs, J.M., Hatazawa, J., Palmer, T., Frackowiak, R.S.J., and Jones, T. (1983b). Disturbance of oxidative metabolism of glucose in recent human infarcts. *Ann. Neurol.*, **14,** 627–637.

Yamaguchi, F., Meyer, J.S., Sakai, F., and Yamamoto, M. (1980). Case reports of three dysphasic patients to illustrate rCBF responses during behavioral activation. *Brain Lang.*, **9,** 145–148.

Yarowsky, P., Kadekaro, M., and Sokoloff, L. (1983). Frequency-dependent activation of glucose utilization in the superior cervical ganglion by electrical stimulation of cervical sympathetic trunk. *Proc. Nat. Acad. Sci.*, **80,** 4179–4183.

5

Anatomic Imaging Methods for Neurobehavioral Studies

GREGORY G. BROWN AND ROBERT A. BORNSTEIN

From its beginning, the fundamental project of neuropsychology has been the mapping of human functions onto the three-dimensional structure of the brain. The central method of this project has been to correlate the location of a brain lesion with a behavioral description of the patient. Autopsies provided information about the location of a lesion in the classic tradition of Broca, Wernicke, Lichtheim, and Dejerine. The sectioning of the brain of a well studied patient was at times filled with drama and reached a high level of refinement in the hands of J.J. and Augusta Dejerine, who once sectioned the brain of a patient into 2000 slices (Caplan, 1987).

Radiologic imaging has largely replaced autopsy as the method of localizing a lesion in neuropsychological studies. In vivo imaging permits a description of the anatomy of a brain lesion at the time the patient is examined behaviorally and makes possible dynamic studies of brain-behavior correlations. Larger numbers of patients can be studied by in vivo imaging than come to autopsy, and anatomic descriptions of patients can be more consistently obtained, thus making the findings more representative. This chapter describes the two most common types of imaging used in neurobehavioral studies: computed tomography (CT) and magnetic resonance imaging (MRI). It provides an introduction to the principles of CT and MRI imaging, a description of the routine findings obtained with the two techniques in stroke, and a survey of methods for correlating the location and size of a lesion with neurobehavioral descriptions.

CT OF THE HEAD

Before the early 1970s, most neurodiagnostic methods offered few usable data for clinico-pathologic correlations of brain structure and function. Electroencephalography (EEG), angiography, and pneumoencephalography permitted only indirect inferences about lesion size or location. Skull radiographs were typically even less useful. Furthermore, angiography and pneumoencephalography entailed some degree of risk. The field of diagnostic brain imaging was radically transformed in 1973 when Hounsfield provided the first demonstration of reconstructive x-ray tomography in a living specimen. The applications of CT and of other methods for acquiring and analyzing imaging data have since expanded rapidly. As discussed later in this chapter, CT imaging in behavioral studies will likely be replaced in the future by MRI. However, the latter is not yet widely available, and most studies examining the neurobehavioral correlates of structural lesions have been based on CT technology.

Basic Principles of CT

The advance in diagnostic brain imaging represented by CT was made possible by linking computer technology to conventional x-ray imaging. In the years since the introduction of CT, several improvements have greatly increased the resolution of CT images. As with other x-ray procedures, CT imaging is based on the attenuation of x-rays as they pass through the body. With CT the calibrated x-ray beam is passed through the patient, and the degree of the attenuation varies with regard to the type of tissue. X-rays emerging from the patient are recorded by detectors. Several x-ray beams are passed in various directions through the subject, yielding attenuation data for a three-dimensional slice of the region being studied. Computer algorithms are used to resolve attenuation data from the slice into volume elements (voxels) that are then mapped onto a matrix of square picture elements (pixels). The CT image consists of this matrix of pixels. The degree of shading of each pixel's gray level represents the average linear attenuation coefficient of a small volume of the object under examination. Each coefficient is expressed as attenuation relative to water in Hounsfield units (HU). The value of a Hounsfield unit is given by the formula

$$\text{HU} = \frac{\mu(\text{tissue}) - \mu(\text{water})}{\mu(\text{water})} \times 1000$$

where μ represents the linear attenuation coefficient, and 1000 is a scaling factor. In general, air has an attenuation of -1000, water 0, and the densest bone $+1000$. These Hounsfield units represent the basic data acquired from CT imaging. The analogue image generated is based on the assignment of gray levels to a range of Hounsfield units. Dense structures that markedly attenuate x-rays fall at the bright end of the scale, while those with lowest attenuation fall toward the dark end. The actual range of the gray level scale is constrained to relatively few steps but may be manipulated within the range of acquired data. If the range of HU values were wide relative to the number of steps in the gray level scale, each tone in gray scale would represent a broad range of HU values, and diminished contrast discrimination would result. In addition to altering the range of numerical values to be sampled, CT data acquisition can also vary the thickness of the slice of the reconstructed image. Slice thickness depends on the collimation of the x-ray beam and can vary from 1.5 to 10.0 mm in most contemporary machines. Images may be acquired as overlapping or contiguous sections. Computer technology permits a variety of enhanced or refined

CT images. High resolution scans obtain data over a narrower field, which results in improved spatial resolution but also increases noise in the image. The data in CT are typically obtained and displayed in the axial (horizontal) plane. Current computer technology permits reformatting of the data to be displayed in other planes of view. Resolution in these images is never as good as in the plane of acquisition and depends on slice thickness during the initial acquisition of data.

A frequent augmentation to the CT procedure involves the use of intravenous contrast materials. Contrast media contain iodine, which can enhance some bright features of a CT image. With the injection of contrast medium into the blood, normal brain does not enhance because the contrast agent does not cross the blood-brain barrier, whereas pathologic tissue containing compromised blood-brain barrier does enhance. Contrast agents highlight increases in x-ray attenuation by approximately 25 HU for each 100 mg of iodine administered. Enhancement occurs in two stages, although the second, slower phase appears to be the best for differentiating between normal and pathologic brain tissue. Enhancement may persist for many hours or maybe days and appears unrelated to lesion vascularity (Stevens et al., 1988). Contrast enhancement is often needed when lesions are suspected in regions where CT artifacts are likely (e.g., posterior fossa and pituitary region) or when the lesion is isodense compared with surrounding brain tissue. Contrast-enhanced CT improves sensitivity in approximately 10% of arteriovenous malformations and in some cerebral infarctions between 1 and 3 weeks post-infarct (Stevens et al., 1988). Some clinical and experimental investigations have employed inhalation of stable xenon, which crosses the blood-brain barrier to selectively enhance brain tissue. The principal application of this technique is for evaluation of regional cerebral blood flow (see Chapter 3).

Basic CT Findings in Stroke Patients

Ischemic Cerebrovascular Disease

Approximately 80% of strokes are detectable by CT within 24 hours after infarction (Wall et al., 1981). Nevertheless, CT scans may be normal in as many as 25% of cases with well documented infarction (Kohlmeyer and Graser, 1978). Many of the missed cases of infarction are thought to be related to averaging of low and high density components of the lesion, resulting in an isodense appearance of the lesion (Alcala et al., 1978). Some studies (Inoue et al., 1980; Wall et al., 1981) have suggested that low density lesions could be identified 12 hours post-infarct in many patietns and as early as 3 to 6 hours post-infarct in some patients. Ischemic and hemorrhagic infarctions can be readily discriminated on nonenhanced CT images. Ischemic infarctions typically result in dark areas of low attenuation, whereas hemorrhagic infarctions produce bright areas of high attenuation (Figures 5–1 and 5–2). The low density areas associated with acute infarction correlate with increased water content. Early water changes are caused by cytotoxic edema, a form of intracellular edema caused by alterations of membrane permeability. Cytotoxic edema may begin to develop within seconds or minutes following hypoxia because of breakdown of the ATP-dependent sodium pump (Fishman, 1975). The appearance of cytotoxic edema (developing within the first 12 hours) is followed by vasogenic edema, caused by the breakdown of the blood-brain barrier. This second form of edema may further accentuate the

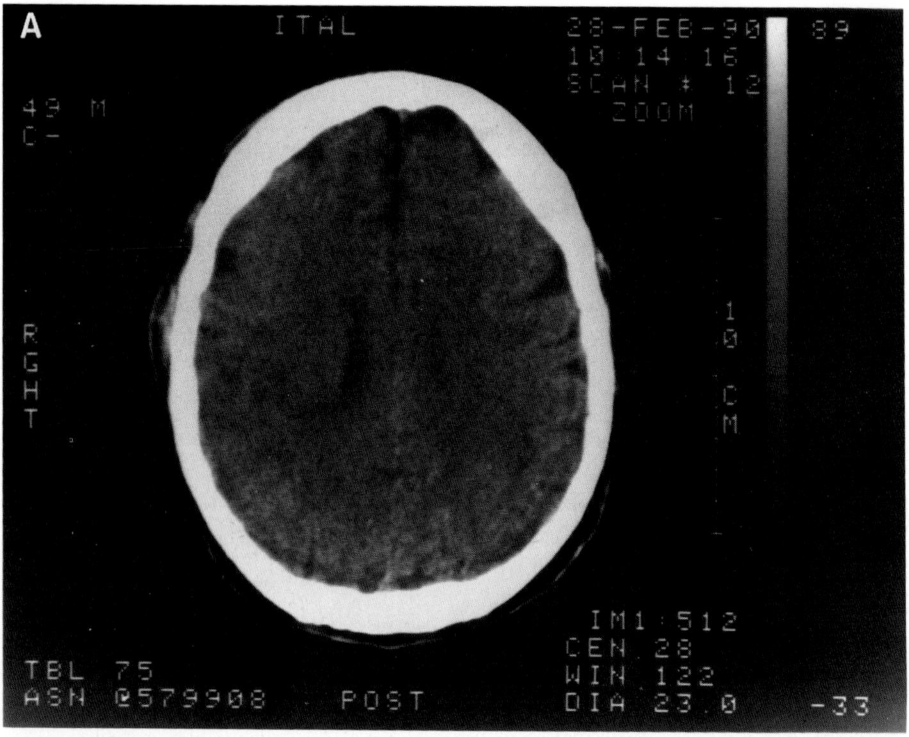

A

ITAL
28-FEB-90
10:14:16
SCAN # 12
ZOOM
89
49 M
C-
RIGHT
10 CM
IM1:512
CEN 28
WIN 122
DIA 23.0
-33
TBL 75
ASN 0579908
POST

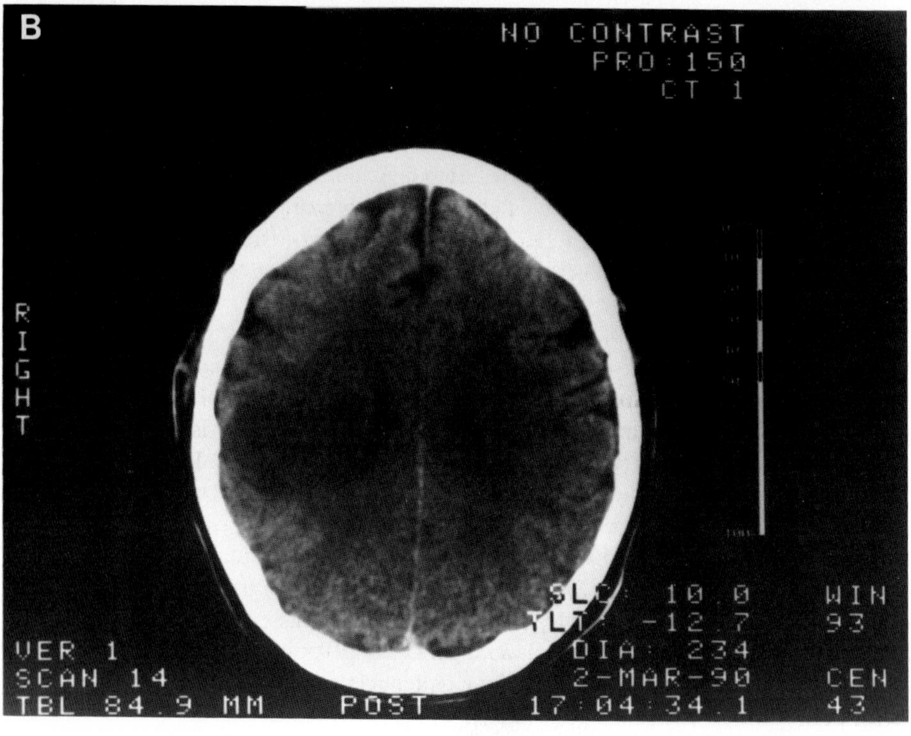

B

NO CONTRAST
PRO:150
CT 1
RIGHT
SLC: 10.0
TLT: -12.7
DIA: 234
2-MAR-90
17:04:34.1
WIN
93
CEN
43
VER 1
SCAN 14
TBL 84.9 MM
POST

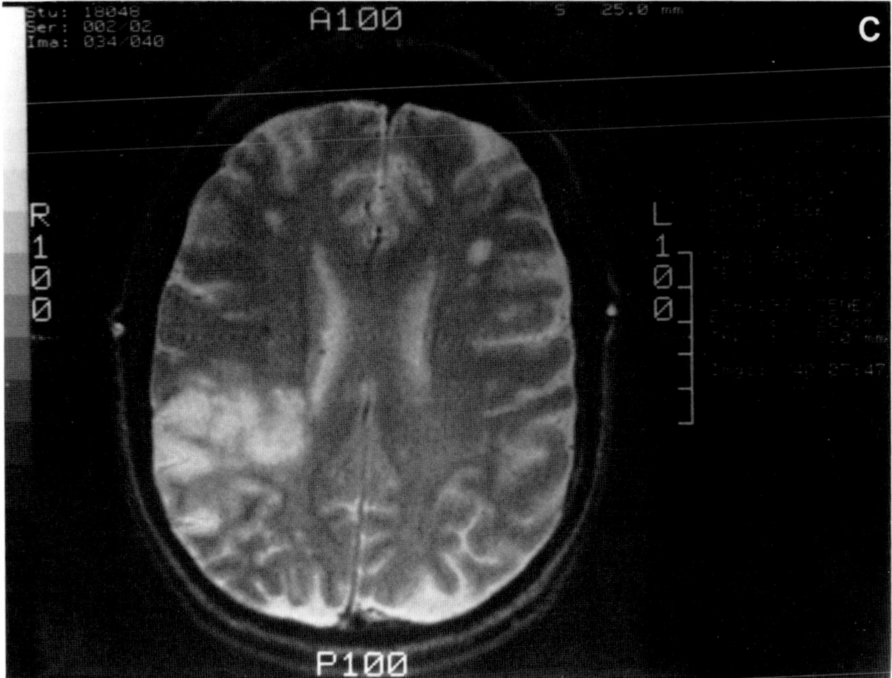

Figure 5–1 Computerized axial tomography scan and magnetic resonance imaging scan of a 49-year-old male with infarction in the territory of the right middle cerebral artery. (A) CT scan on the day of admission showing no clear delineation of the lesion. (B) CT scan performed 3 days following admission to hospital demonstrating low density in the distribution of the middle cerebral artery, consistent with ischemic infarction. (C) Magnetic resonance imaging scan on the same day as the second post-stroke day indicating large high signal area in the distribution of the right middle cerebral artery.

low attenuation attributable to cytotoxic edema. Swelling typically evolves over time and may be insufficient to produce shifts of midline structures until the second or third day post-infarction (Yamaguchi and Vemura, 1978; Inoue et al., 1980). This mass effect peaks on the third or fourth day and gradually resolves by the third week in survivors (Yamaguchi and Vemura, 1978).

The typical CT appearance in stroke changes as the lesion evolves (Russell, 1984). With acute infarctions (the first 5 days), low-density lesions corresponding to edema are the most frequent finding. Some lesions contain patchy areas of high attenuation related to hemorrhagic components. In fact, some lesions appear isodense owing to the averaging of low density edema and high density hemorrhage. In the acute stage contrast enhancement is typically unnecessary, although it may be helpful in the subacute (6 days to 3 weeks) or chronic (3 weeks or longer) stage. Approximately 10% of infarcts undetectable by unenhanced scans may be demonstrated with contrast enhancement (Wing et al., 1976). Patients studied during this subacute period often demonstrate enhancement, which is thought to be related to the evolution of the new capillaries in the area of infarction (Anderson et al., 1980; Inoue et al., 1980). During the subacute period the CT scan often reveals a lesion of lower density, with less mass effect than during the acute stage.

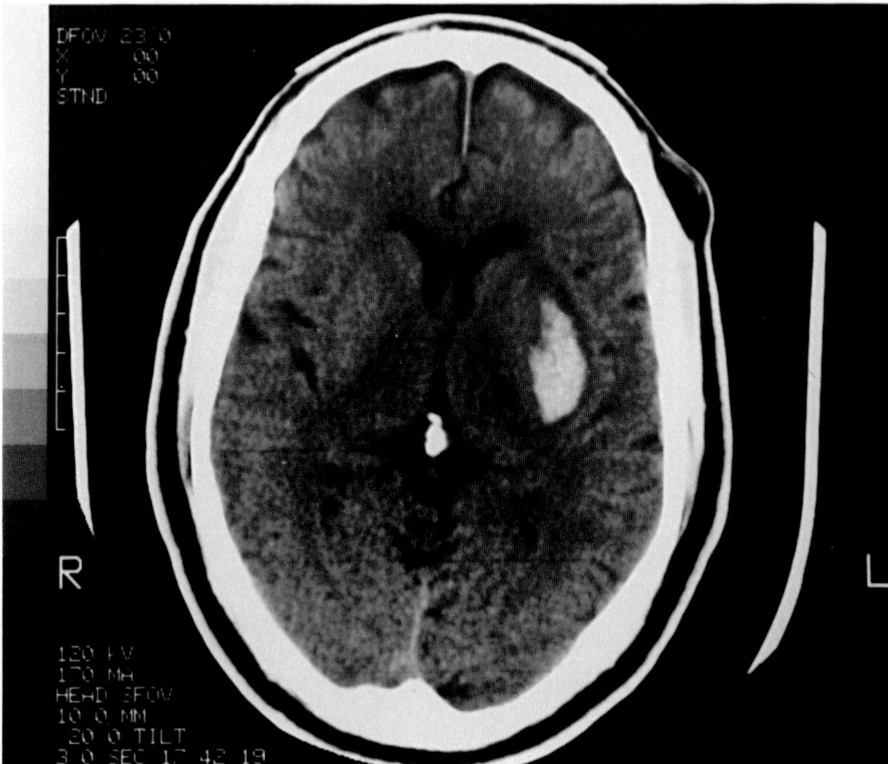

Figure 5–2 CT scan of a patient with a hemorrhagic stroke in the region of the basal ganglia.

In the chronic stage, the infarct appears as a well defined area of decreased attenuation with density similar to that of cerebrospinal fluid. In the later stages, there may be atrophy of cerebral gyri with resultant enlargement of subarachnoid spaces (Russell, 1984), which may appear as a prominence of the *sulci* or fissures, and there may be associated dilatation of the adjacent ventricular system.

Infarctions in the distribution of small penetrating vessels may produce lesions in the internal capsule or deep cortical gray masses. These lesions typically do not produce mass effect, and approximately 50% demonstrate enhancement during the first month post-infarction (Manelfe et al., 1981). Evolution of these lesions often leaves small cystic cavities referred to as "lacunes."

Intracerebral Hemorrhage

Within hours after hemorrhage, a hematoma appears as a bright, high-density region on CT. This bright region is typically surrounded by a faint, thin rim of dark, low-density signal (Dolinskas et al., 1977). As clotting occurs, the attenuation of x-rays by the hematoma increases until it peaks a few hours after its formation. The hemoglobin then begins to break down, and the signal darkens as a low density region develops, spreading from the periphery of the hematoma toward its center (Dolinskas et al., 1977). The evolution from a high to a low density region takes about 4 to 5 weeks and includes a period when the hemorrhage is as dense as surrounding brain tissue (Savoiardo, 1986). A hematoma often produces a mass effect, which can remain for months (Messina and Chernik, 1975). Ultimately, the hematoma evolves into a slit-like lesion of low density.

MRI OF THE HEAD

The principles of nuclear magnetic resonance (NMR) were established in 1946 by Bloch and coworkers at Stanford University (Bloch et al., 1946) and independently by Purcell and colleagues at the Radiation Laboratory, Massachusetts Institute of Technology (Purcell et al., 1946). After its discovery, NMR was used to measure the magnetic properties of various elements and their isotopes. One of the measurements made—the shift in resonance frequency of a particular nucleus as the nucleus was measured in different chemical environments—became a powerful analytic method in the fields of chemistry and biochemistry. In 1971 Damadian published a report suggesting that NMR might be useful in discriminating between malignant tumors and normal tissue. In 1973 Paul Lauterbur described a technique to produce an NMR image. Since the first images, magnetic resonance imaging (MRI) has been developed so that high resolution pictures of the normal and pathologic anatomy can be routinely obtained. In the following section, we first discuss the basic principles underlying MRI and then briefly review the application of MRI to the diagnosis of cerebrovascular disease.

Basic Principles of MRI

The NMR experiment fundamentally involves establishing a baseline condition in a system, activating the system, and obtaining measurements as the system returns to baseline (Table 5–1).

The means of establishing the baseline condition, the method of activating the system, and the measurements made depend on the magnetic properties of the nucleus of an atom. As with any magnetic phenomenon, the magnetic field produced by the spinning nucleus of an atom has a strength and an orientation along an axis that can be respresented by a vector quantity, the magnetic moment. Not all nuclei possess a magnetic moment. Of those nuclei that do, hydrogen, fluorine, sodium, and phosphorus have been most thoroughly studied in biologic systems (Gadian, 1982). Because the nucleus of hydrogen, i.e., the proton, is the most commonly imaged nucleus, we focus the remainder of the discussion on it.

Table 5–1 Basic Stages of an NMR Experiment

Stage	Manipulation	State of Nuclei
Baseline	Place nuclei in static magnetic field	Random precession
Activation	Introduce radiofrequency signal	Phase coherence
Return to baseline	Terminate radiofrequency signal and acquire NMR signal	Relaxation

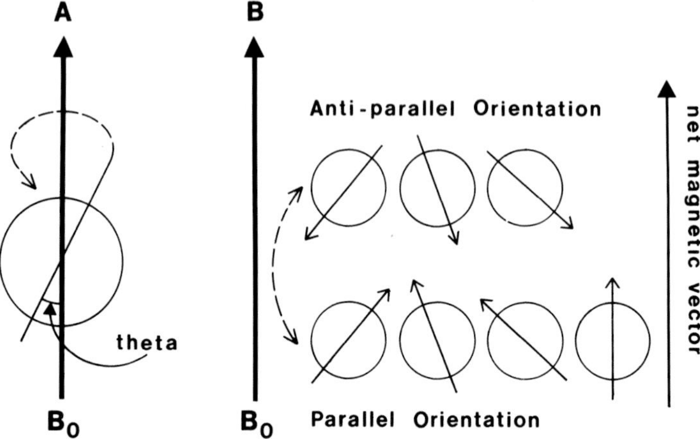

Figure 5–3 (A) Precession of a single proton tilted theta degrees from the axis of precession (B_o). (B) The result of a slight preponderance of protons precessing in a direction parallel to the static magnetic field (B_o) is represented by the net magnetic vector.

Baseline

When a proton is placed in a static magnetic field, the direction of its magnetic moment points either parallel or antiparallel to the axis of the static field (Figure 5–3B). Furthermore, the protons oriented parallel to the axis of the static field possess less energy than those oriented antiparallel (Brant-Zawadski, 1987). A close measurement of the alignment of the proton with the static magnetic field would show that the axis of spin of the proton is slightly tilted relative to the axis of the static magnetic field (Figure 5–3A). The angle of this tilt is conventionally called theta. As a result of this tilt, the proton precesses around the axis of the static magnetic field, much as a top, which is slightly off-center, precesses around an axis (Figure 5–3A). In the same magnetic field, nuclei of different atoms precess at different frequencies. The angular frequency of the precession (ω_o) is determined by the Larmor relation, $\omega_o = \gamma B_o$, where B_o is the strength of the static magnetic field, and γ is a physical constant, the magnetogyric ratio, which differs for different nuclei (Gadian, 1982).

In water there is a slightly greater number of protons precessing parallel around the axis of the static magnetic field than antiparallel (Brant-Zawadski, 1987). Furthermore, individual protons shift from one energy state to the other, depending on fluctuations of energy acting on each proton. At room temperature, there is roughly one additonal proton in the low energy state for every million protons in the high state. However, this slight preponderance of parallel-oriented protons means that the entire sample of water placed in the static magnetic field (i.e., the ensemble of nuclei) has a net magnetic moment, which results from the additive effects of the magnetic moments of the individual protons in the sample (Figure 5–3B).

The slight preponderance of nuclei oriented parallel to B_o can be represented as difference vectors that are also titled theta degrees from the main axis. The tips of the individual difference vectors are randomly distributed around B_o, forming the surface of a cone (Figure 5–4A). This cone represents the baseline condition of an NMR experiment and is not associated with any signal. That this baseline condition

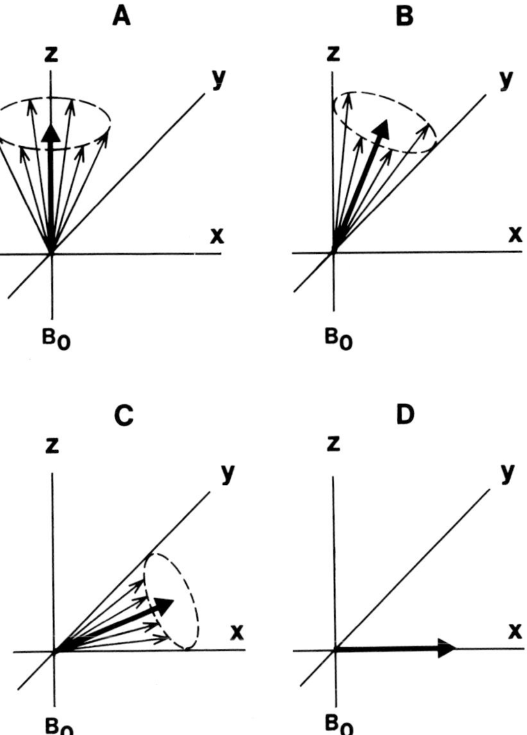

Figure 5–4 The increasing (A–D) tilt and phase coherence of difference vectors caused by applying a radiofrequency signal to the ensemble of nuclei.

has the potential to emit a signal depends on the energy difference between protons oriented in parallel and antiparallel directions.

Activation

The signal in an NMR experiment is generated by application of radiofrequency (rf) energy to the ensemble of protons. Prior to the application of rf energy, the ensemble is in "thermal equilibrium"; that is, the number of transitions that occur from the low to the high energy state is equal to the number of transitions from the high to the low energy state. To change this equilibrium, energy must be introduced into the ensemble. One method of introducing energy is to apply to the ensemble a common rf signal at the frequency determined by the Larmor relation and at right angles to the axis of the static magnetic field. As the ensemble of protons absorbs this energy, protons in the low energy state flip to the high energy state at a greater rate than the reverse transition. Consequently, one effect of applying the rf signal is to change the energy contained in the entire ensemble of protons. A second effect is that the tips of the magnetic vectors distributed around B_0 lose their random distribution around the central line of the baseline cone, producing coherence in the phase of rotation of these individual magnetic moments (Figure 5–4). As a result of these two effects, the orientation of the net magnetic vector begins to tilt away from the axis of the static magnetic field. As represented by Figure 5–5, this tendency to tilt combines with the

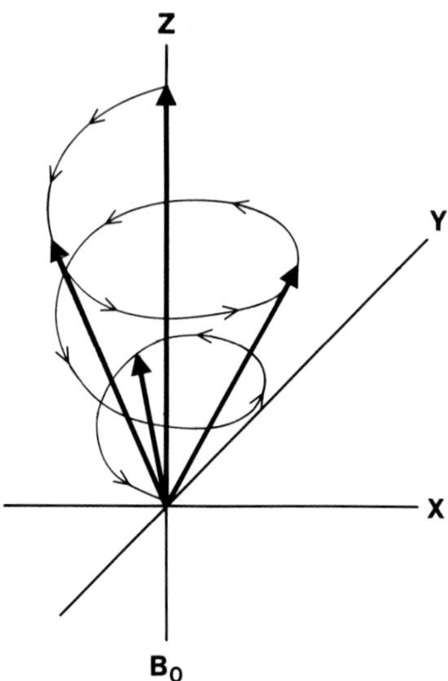

Figure 5–5 Spiraling of the net magnetic vector when radiofrequency energy is applied to the ensemble of nuclei.

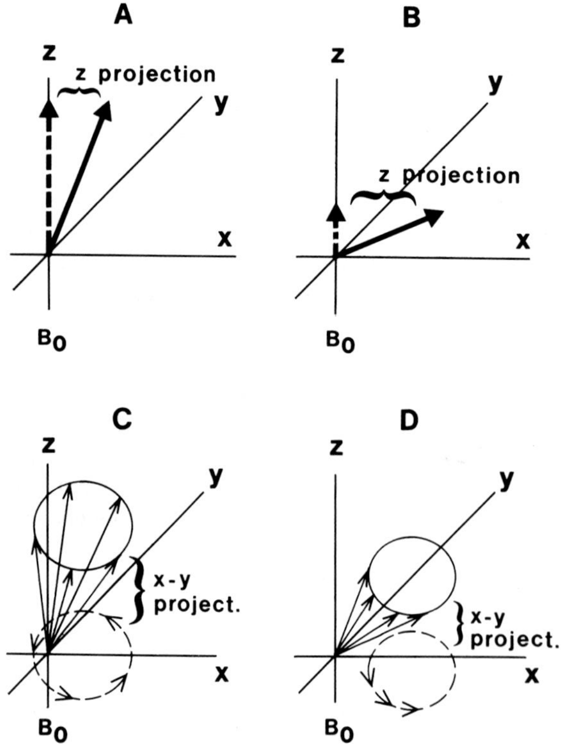

Figure 5–6 Longitudinal (A & B) and transverse (C & D) projections of the net magnetic vector.

precessional tendency of the net magnetic vector to cause it to spiral downward from its initial orientation (Brewer and Hahn, 1984). The extent to which this vector proceeds along the downward spiral is determined by the duration of the rf signal.

These two effects, spiraling and phase coherence, are shown in Figure 5–6. The Z-axis of that figure corresponds to the axis of the B_0 field. The X-Y plane corresponds to the plane of application of the rf signal. The downward spiral of the net magnetic vector and the increasing phase coherence can be represented by the projection of the former process onto the Z-axis and the projection of the latter onto the X-Y plane. These projections can be seen in Figure 5–6. Figures 5–6A–D suggest that the complicated changes induced by the rf signal can be understood by considering the longitudinal changes associated with the Z-projection of the net magnetic vector and by considering the transverse phase coherence represented by the projection of the net magnetic vector onto the X-Y plane.

Return to Baseline

When the rf signal is turned off, the ensemble of protons begin to return to the baseline state. This return to baseline involves a return to the previous energy level; the difference in energy is transmitted to the environment. The energy lost is emitted as an rf signal at frequencies near that of the rf signal originally used to pulse the ensemble; that is, the ensemble resonates to the rf signal. The signal in an NMR study is produced by only those nuclei whose rate of precession corresponds to the frequency of the rf signal used to pulse the sample. This resonance gives NMR its capability to study selected nuclei. For the simplest condition, the rf signal can be represented by the damping over time of the oscillation of a single frequency; this is the basic signal in a NMR experiment.

The return to baseline occurs over time. Two temporal parameters govern the duration of the signal, T_1 and T_2. Their meanings can be understood by considering what happens to the longitudinal and transverse projections of the net magnetic vector after the rf signal is turned off. At the termination of this signal, the projection of the net magnetic vector onto the Z-axis begins to grow until this signal returns to its baseline level. The time elapsed while the projection on the Z-axis returns to baseline is determined by a parameter intrinsic to the tissue studied, the longitudinal relaxation parameter (T_1). Simultaneously, the signal's coherence, as represented by the projection onto the X-Y p'ane, dissipates until the individual magnetic moments associated with the individual protons are once again precessing independently. The time taken to complete the loss of phase coherence is determined by a second intrinsic parameter, the transverse relaxation time (T_2). It is only the transverse portion of change in the ensemble that is detected in an NMR experiment, just as only a pulse of rf energy introduced at right angle to B_0 can induce the changes from baseline. Consequently, the signal observed in NMR studies fundamentally reflects the transverse relaxation time of the phenomenon under study. However a transverse signal can be detected only so long as a longitudinal projection of the magnetization vector has not returned to its baseline state. Consequently, factors that shorten T_1 limit the duration of the T_2 signal.

To obtain spatial information from an NMR experiment, an additional element must be introduced, a linear gradient of magnetic field that is static and varies in field strength across the physical dimensions of the sample studied. Figure 5–7 gives a

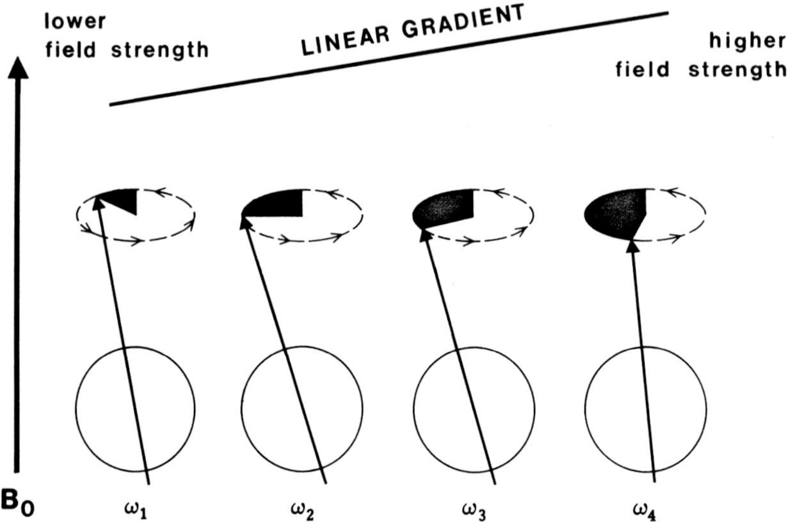

Figure 5–7 Increasing rate of precession of protons as the linear magnetic gradient increases. B_o = the static magnetic field; ω_i = the rate of precession of the ith proton.

representation of this concept. The frequency of precession of each proton along the linear gradient is determined by the field strength of the static magnet and the strength of the linear gradient at each point on the plane. Because the first effect is constant for a magnet with no fluctuations in the strength of its magnetic field, variations in frequency of precession occur as a function of the strength of the linear gradient at each point in the sample. Consequently, the range of frequencies detected across the gradient can be mapped to positions on the linear gradient and thereby encode spatial information. Applying gradients at different angles of orientation to the sample improves the ability to distinguish single points in the sample and makes possible the encoding of information about voxels.

The theory presented above implies that the intensity of the signal in an NMR experiment is determined by the density of the protons in the tissue and by T_1 and T_2. However, signal intensity is also determined by the degree to which the nuclei move (flow) during the NMR experiment and by the sequences of pulsed rf energy chosen by the operator. It is the control of these sequences of pulsed rf energy that generates contrast based on T_1, T_2, proton density, or flow.

To clarify how operator-determined pulse sequences can influence signal intensity, the commonly used spin-echo technique is described (Gadian, 1982). The technique involves applying the rf pulse sufficiently long to tilt the magnetization vector 90 degrees, placing it in the x-y plane. Linear magnetic field gradients are then applied to spatially tag nuclei. After a period of time (τ) elapses, a second rf signal is applied that flips the magnetization 180 degrees. During the τ milliseconds between the 90- and 180-degree pulses, the magnetization vector loses coherence as a result of T_2 relaxation, reducing the intensity of the signal. After the 180-degree pulse, the flipped magnetization almost paradoxically increases in coherence, and an echo of the effects of the 90-degree pulse reaches its peak coherence τ milliseconds (msec) after this second pulse (Brewer and Hahn, 1984). Typically, this sequence of pulses

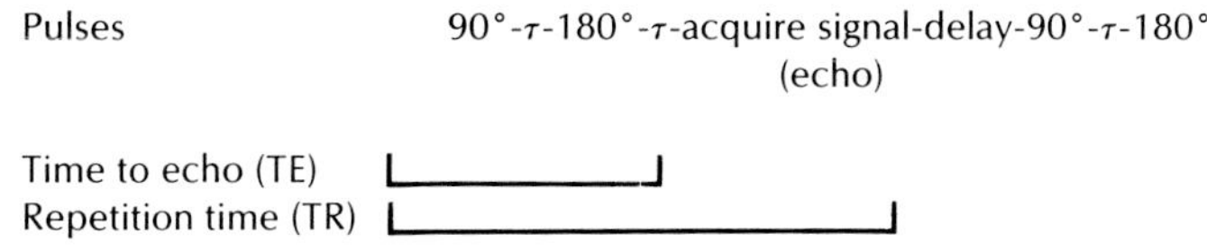

Figure 5–8 Steps in the spin-echo pulse sequence.

is repeated after a delay. Measurements of signal loss in this pulse sequence yield data from which inferences can be made about the duration of T_2 (Gadian, 1982). The time between consecutive repetitions of the 90-degree pulse (TR) and the time between the 90-degrees pulse and the peak coherence of the echo (2τ or TE) are parameters that can be chosen by an MRI operator (Figure 5–8). Short TRs (e.g., 600 msec) with short TEs (e.g., 24 msec) generate images with a T_1 weighting, whereas long TEs (e.g., 40 msec) with long TRs (e.g., 2000 msec) give images a T_2 weighting (Wehrli et al., 1984; Brant-Zawadski, 1987). Long TRs and short TEs are used to weight images by proton density. The T_1, T_2, and proton density of major central nervous system structures differ (Wehrli et al., 1984). These intrinsic parameters also vary from normal in stroke and other neurologic diseases (Bradley, 1987). The operator's ability to weight images by these intrinsic parameters and to use the MRI contrast agents being developed (McNamara, 1987) give radiologists unprecedented flexibility when imaging the anatomy of normal and pathological brain.

Basic MRI Findings in Stroke

When investigating the stroke patient, MRI is used to identify areas of ischemia or hemorrhage, to help in the detection of aneurysms and arteriovenous malformations and to rule out other focal diseases, such as tumors. Although MRI is useful for the evaluation of a patient with stroke, it is too expensive and nonspecific to be used to screen for stroke.

Ischemic Cerebrovascular Disease

Experimental and human studies agree that ischemic changes can be detected by MRI within the first few hours following the ictus (Sipponen et al., 1983; Unger et al., 1987). In the early stages of ischemia, an increase of both T_1 and T_2 occurs. As seen in Figure 5–9, these early ischemic effects are identified especially well as bright areas of high signal intensity seen on T_2-weighted images (Buonanno et al., 1986). Later in the ischemic process the infarct is better identified as a dark area of relatively low signal intensity seen on T_1-weighted images (Ramadan et al., 1989). The increased contrast of MRI allows for the identification of smaller regions of infarction, including lacunar infarcts, than does CT (Bradley, et al., 1984; Salgodo et al., 1986). Additionally, MRI may be sensitive to stroke in the intermediate stages when edema dissipates and before frank cavitation appears, a period when CT images of stroke often appear isodense with surrounding tissue (Ramadan et al., 1989). At this intermediate stage of stroke, MRI can frequently detect a rim of hyperintense signal on T_2 images surrounding a darker zone, representing the core of the infarct. Another advantge of MRI over CT is that infarcts can be better detected in the posterior fossa owing to the absence of bone artifacts (Buonanno et al., 1986).

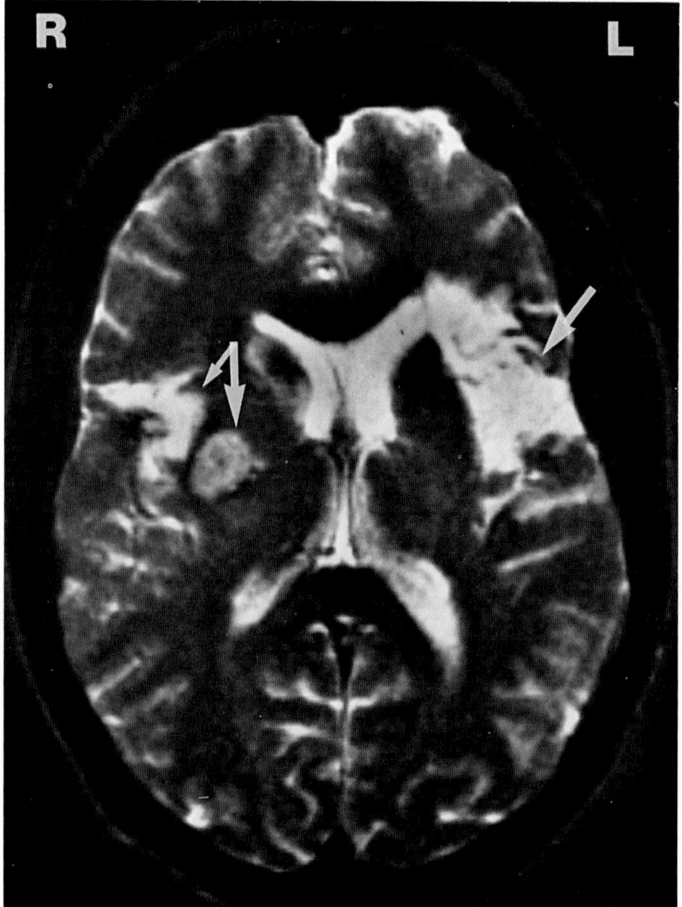

Figure 5–9 T_2-weighted MRI study of cerebral infarctions, indicated by arrows.

MRI improves the clinician's ability to determine the stage of a patient's infarction, elucidate the anatomy of smaller lesions, and detect lesions in the posterior fossa, where MRI images are uncomplicated by bone artifact. It is particularly useful in studying patients with transient ischemic attacks (TIAs). Abnormalities of CT are typically observed in patients with TIAs less than 20% of the time, whereas with MRI abnormalities have been observed in up to 80% of such patients (Salgado et al., 1986).

Intracerebral Hemorrhage

The effects of hemorrhage on MRI images varies as a function of chronicity of the hemorrhage and the T_1 or T_2 weighting of the image. Acutely, the hemoglobin in red blood cells is altered in a manner that produces lower signal intensities on T_2-weighted images. From the fourth to seventh days, a second alteration of hemoglobin produces increased signal intensities first on T_1-weighted images and later on T_2 images. During this subacute stage there are two zones observed on T_2 images: a dark medial zone, probably caused by hemosiderin, a protein that contains iron, and a

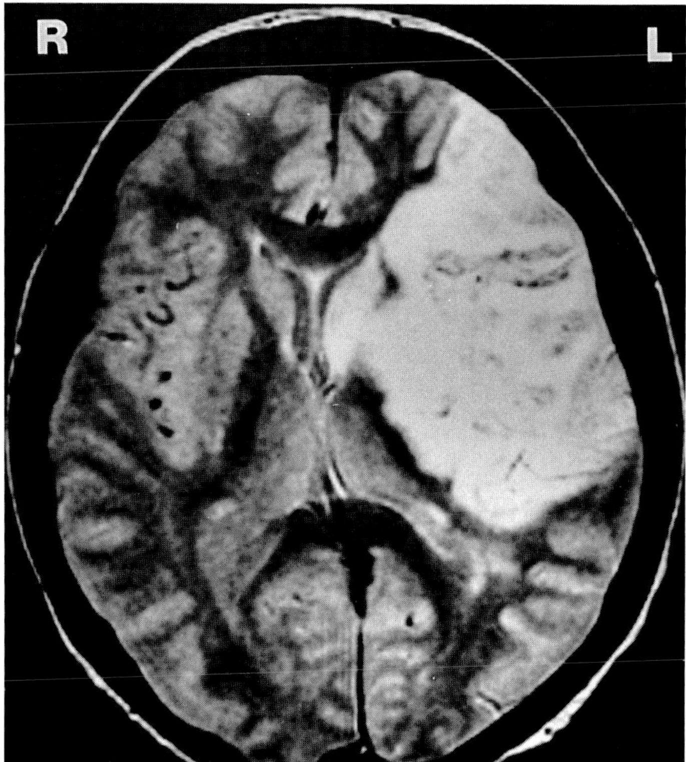

Figure 5–10 T_2-weighted MRI study of an intracerebral hemorrhage of the left frontal operculum with extensive surrounding vasogenic edema.

more peripheral bright zone of edema (Figure 5–10). In the chronic stage, a well delineated bright signal is seen from the whole blood clot on T_1-weighted images. On T_2-weighted images, there is likewise a bright zone. The increased signal intensity of a hematoma persists for as long as a year or more, until the hematoma is replaced by cerebrospinal fluid and the effects of T_1 prolongation appear. Therefore the image of an old clot more than 1 year of age appears as a dark signal on T_1 images and as a bright signal on T_2 images with a dark rim surrounding the cavity. This rim of hypointensity surrounding a bright region is useful for differentiating chronic ischemic infarction from chronic intracerebral hemorrhage.

Arteriovenous Malformations and Cerebral Aneurysms

The entagled dilated vessels of an arteriovenous malformation (AVM) can present as regions of inconsistent signal void, appearing mottled or mothworn in nature (Figure 5–11). The signal void appears as tagged protons flow rapidly through the AVM and out of the slice being imaged. This signal loss is exacerbated by flow turbulence within the AVM and by dephasing that results from the complexities of applying several linear gradients to the sample (Bradley, 1987). Furthermore, previous hemorrhage, cysts, or calcification may be evident on the MRI. Small aneurysms may be better detected by MRI than CT. In one study CT failed to identify aneurysms in 25

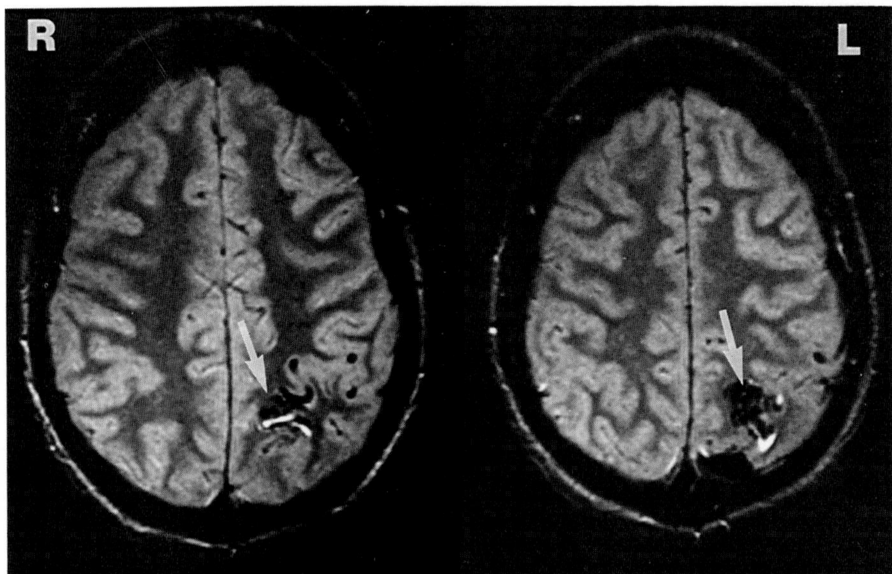

Figure 5–11 MRI study of an arteriovenous malformation in the left posterior parietal region. Note the speckled region of hypointense signal abutting regions of increased signal intensity.

of 30 cases, whereas in 14 of these cases MRI detected aneurysms (Jenkins et al., 1988). Although MRI may be more sensitive to the presence of aneurysms than CT, MRI is not considered to be a substitute for cerebral angiography when evaluating patients with potential aneurysms.

Thrombosed arteriovenous malformations, cavernous angiomas, capillary telangiectasia, and venous angiomas are better detected by MRI than CT. These abnormalities appear as mixed signal intensity in both T_1 and T_2 images (Ramadan et al., 1989).

Leukoaraiosis

Patchy, subcortical areas of high signal intensity, such as those seen in Figure 5–12, are often found on T_2-weighted images of elderly individuals (Awad et al., 1986). Corresponding regions of hypodensity have been reported on CT, although the extent of these changes is less than with MRI. Hachinski and colleagues (1987) have argued that an etiologically neutral term should be used to describe these radiologic changes, which they have called leukoaraiosis.

The presence of leukoaraiosis has been most strongly associated with age, hypertension, and ischemic stroke, although it is present in some patients with Alzheimer's disease (Steingart et al., 1987). Autopsy findings from a small, consecutive series of patients indicated that leukoaraiosis detected by postmortem MRI studies was associated with a variety of brain and vascular changes (Awad et al., 1986). They included gliosis, small areas of infarction, degeneration of myelinated axons, capillary telangiectasia, and a severe occurrence of at least one of the following three findings: arteriosclerosis, dilated perivascular spaces, and vascular ectasia. Awad and colleagues

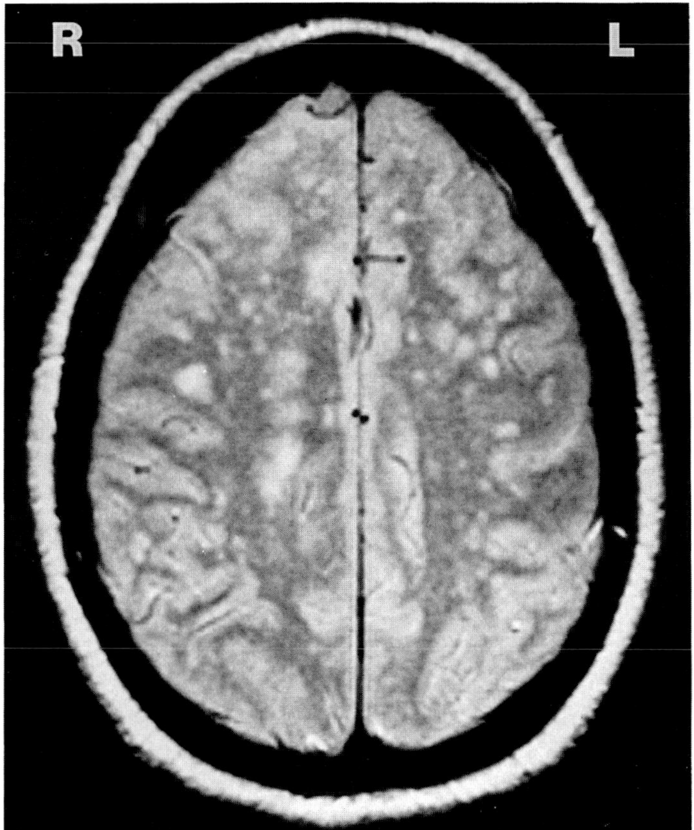

Figure 5–12 T_2-weighted MRI study showing subcortical white matter changes.

(1986a) theorized that "wear and tear" in brain parenchyma produces a network of perivascular tunnels filled with extracellular water. This state produced subcortical MRI changes not associated with any symptoms. As the "wear and tear" progresses, frank subcortical infarction develops, which also appears as subcortical white matter changes. Unfortunately, the pre- and postinfarction stages of leukoaraiosis are difficult to distinguish on MRI.

That leukoaraiosis can be seen in asymptomatic elderly individuals was confirmed by Hunt and colleagues (1989). They found no relation between performance on a comprehensive battery of neuropsychological tests and the degree of leukoaraiosis detected by MRI in a sample of 46 community-dwelling elderly individuals. All but one subject had no history of cerebrovascular disease. To our knowledge, no one has yet determined the correlation between extent of leukoaraiosis and neuropsychological impairment in patients with cerbrovascular disease. However, Steingart et al. (1987) found that the degree of leukoaraiosis observed on CT was associated with the degree of cognitive impairment in patients with mild to moderate Alzheimer's disease. Together the Hunt and Steingart studies suggest that the cause of leukoaraiosis might be as important as its extent in determining the behavioral significance of these commonly observed white matter changes.

Current research is extending NMR techniques beyond anatomic localization of ischemic or hemorrhagic disease. Advances have been made in developing magnetic resonance angiography (Ross et al., 1989), NMR blood flow techniques (Ewing et al., 1989), and NMR measurements of high energy phosphate metabolism (Petroff et al., 1984), phospholipid metabolism (Brown et al., 1989), pH (Petroff et al., 1985), and sodium (Ra et al., 1988). this one technology is potentially capable of a wide ranging description of the anatomic, physiologic, and metabolic aspects of cerebral vascular disease.

TOPOGRAPHIC AND VOLUMETRIC METHODS

The clinical radiologist visually interprets a radiographic image to determine the presence, size, and location of a lesion and its effects on brain structures outside the immediate area of the lesion. This information is communicated in written format, usually indicating the location of a lesion in terms of the lobes, ventricles, and major subcortical structures. Information about the size of the lesion is often communicated by using comparative terms (e.g., small, large, giant) that convey rank order information about the size of the lesion. When measurements are made they generally reflect the cross section rather than the volume of a lesion. When more information is needed, as often happens with surgical intervention, the original image is inspected by the person needing the information.

Clinical methods of communicating the results of imaging scans are adequate for the medical management of large numbers of clinical patients, but they have limitations for neurobehavioral studies. The location of a lesion is often not given precisely enough; judgments about lesion size are subjective and insufficient for many quantitative analyses. A survey of methods for making the results of imaging studies less subjective and more quantitative follows. This survey has led to a series of questions, presented in Table 5–2, that are useful to keep in mind when reading studies that correlate imaging and neurobehavioral findings.

Table 5–2 Issues in the Quantifying Anatomic Lesions in Imaging Studies

1. From what orientations is the brain imaged?
2. What brain atlas is used in the study?
3. What is the size of the pixel matrix?
4. How thick are the slices studied?
5. Are consecutive slices separated by nonimaged tissue? If so, by what distance are the slices separated?
6. What is the total number of slices studied?
7. What portion of the total brain is studied?
8. If a brain atlas or templates are used, how is the outline of the lesion transferred to the atlas or template?
9. What is the reliability of the measurements made?
10. How are interindividual variations in brain volume, shape, and gyral anatomy handled?
11. How is the density or completeness of a lesion within a region taken into account?

Image Characteristics

The number of slices obtained and their thickness, as well as the pixel size of the matrix underlying the image, influence the amount of information that a CT or MRI study can convey about the size and location of a lesion. Although these factors are not the only ones that determine the visual information available in CT or MRI scans, they vary across neurobehavioral studies and complicate comparisons of their findings (Kertesz et al., 1979; Naeser et al., 1981; Knopman et al., 1983). Ideally, voxels from many contiguous, thin slices would be mapped to a high-dimensional matrix of pixels. However, the constraints on radiation dosage with CT and on total imaging time with MRI force trade-offs among the size of the pixel matrix, slice thickness, and number of slices. Even though these trade-offs are always present, few authors discuss the trade-offs involved when choosing the particular values used in their studies.

Lesion Location

Early descriptions of the location of lesions on CT were hampered by the absence of an anatomic atlas that displayed the brain sectioned at planes used for CT slices. Several atlases now exist that present brain sections cut 15 to 20 degrees above the orbitomeatal line. Matsui and Hirano's (1978) atlas presents slices at 12 angles. Damasio (1983) has developed a guide to CT slices that identifies Brodmann's architectonic areas and major vascular territories. These atlases present brain slices only for specific angles, thickness, and spacing. Before beginning a research project, investigatiors must choose the atlas they are going to use and then obtain CT slices that correspond to those in the atlas of choice.

Descriptions of the location of a stroke must take into account the variability of normal cerebral anatomy. The location of brain sulci, which demarcate the major regions of the lateral cortex, can vary substantially (Cunningham, 1892; Connolly, 1950). When sulci are obliterated by a cerebral infarct or hemorrhage, the researcher is faced with a difficult problem in localization. Often the anatomy of the homologous region of the contralateral hemisphere is examined for landmarks to make decisions about the location of the lesion. However, significant asymmetries in sucal anatomy exist. The location of the posterior branch of the sylvian sulcus of the left hemisphere presents a particular problem. It separates the inferior parietal lobe from the temporal gyri, distinguishing two regions that might contribute differently to language functioning. However, portions of this sulcus are often longer in the left hemisphere and have a different slope than in the right hemisphere (Cunningham, 1892; Connelly, 1950). Furthermore, individual differences in the degree of these asymmetries exist (Ruebens, 1977).

Another method to identify anatomic landmarks obscured by infarction or hemorrhage involves viewing the landmark from different perspectives. Also adjacent landmarks, viewed from several perspectives, can be used to infer the most likely location of an obscured landmark. Knopman and colleagues (1983) have used this approach with CT, where they inferred the location of the posterior sylvian fissure from both axial and coronal slices. The total amount of radiation to which a patient can be exposed, the rigidity involved in the fixed placement of detectors, and patient compliance limit the range of perspectives obtainable in a single patient by CT. MRI is inherently more flexible, with the imaging of any cerebral plane possible. Given the fast imaging techniques developed for MRI (Frahm et al., 1990; Haase, 1990; Ordidge et al., 1989) an interactive approach to lesion localization is possible.

To effectively localize partly obscured anatomic landmarks, more information is needed about the intrahemispheric relations among structures, especially as a function of individual differences in cerebral asymmetries. It might be possible to develop a general index of asymmetry that is strongly related to local asymmetries or to develop regression equations to predict a specific anatomic asymmetry from other asymmetries.

Lesion Size

Areas and volumes of lesions, either unweighted or weighted by the severity of the tissue destruction, have been used to measure lesion size. As currently performed by most investigators, these measures involve a human operator outlining the boundary of a lesion on some type of template, which represents a slice of the brain seen on CT or MRI. Areas of the lesion can then be calculated and combined into measurements of volumes. Whatever is known about the sources of error involved in drawing the original boundaries has influenced few neurobehavioral studies. Experience of the human judge, the similarity between the templates and imaging slices, the visual contrast of the lesion, the regularity of the lesion's boundary, and the lesion's proximity to ventricles or skull likely contribute to the precision of the outline. However, we have not found any systematic study of the effects of these factors on interobserver agreement about the boundaries and sizes of infarctions. When studied, the ratings of different observers have been found to be significantly correlated for presence, number, size, site, and severity of infarct (Knopman & Rubens, 1986; Lee et al., 1987). However, the sizes of these correlations are rarely reported. When a statistic reflecting the degree of agreement is reported, appropriate measures of interobserver agreement are not always presented (Shrout & Fleiss, 1979).

Because strokes and hemorrhages are three-dimensional structures, measurements of their volumes seem to be the most appropriate metric of size. However, not all researchers have been able to obtain contiguous slices of images through the infarction or hemorrhage. When contiguous slices are obtained, they can be as much as 1 cm thick (Naeser et al., 1981). Assumptions about the regularity of the lesion between and within slices must be made, and they introduce some error in volume calculations that are not present in the area measures. Consequently, some investigators have chosen to use area measurements to indicate lesion size. In particular, Robinson and colleagues (1986) measured infarct size as a ratio of the largest area of the lesion on any CT slice divided by the largest area of total brain seen on a CT slice passing through the lateral ventricles. This ratio correlated 0.94 with measurement of lesion volume in 20 randomly selected scans of patients with strokes. This method assumes that the surface of the three-dimensional stroke is relatively smooth and that the volume is primarily determined by the cross section of the lesion as its widest extent. These assumptions seem at least as problematic as those needed to calculate volumes. To choose between volume and area measures of infarct size, data about the degree of interobserver agreement for the two measures are needed.

Because an infarct might only partially damage a specific region of interest, some investigators have tried to develop benchmarks of the extent of damage within a region. These approaches have involved techniques based on human judgment, attenuation coefficients, or eigenimage filtering.

Knopman and colleagues (1983) used human judges to determine the completeness of damage to a specific region. They divided each hemisphere into 40 regions, which were then rated by a neuroradiologist as having no lesions, a questionable lesion, a definite lesion less than one-half of the region damaged, damage to more than one-half of the region, and complete damage (Knopman & Rubens, 1986). The volume of the lesion was calculated by software provided by Siemens Corporation for regions that had ratings of a definite lesion, regardless of completeness of the damage (Knopman et al., 1983). The rating scale was used to assess the relation between severity of a neurologic deficit and completeness of the stroke within critical regions. For example, the severity of a patient's hemiparesis was found to be associated with the completeness of the infarction within the corona radiata (Knopman & Rubens, 1986). Although this approach assesses the volume and completeness of damage within a region, the volume measure is only weakly weighted by completeness of the damage.

Naeser and colleagues (1981) discussed a method based on CT attenuation numbers that attempts to strongly weight lesion volume by the extent of damage to a region. The method utilizes the attentuation matrix that is mapped to the visually presented gray levels. It involves a semiautomated approach based on the Automated Framing Program (AFP). This program is a variant of the one developed by Jernigan and coworkers (1979) to study the size of ventricles. The AFP identifies an area of infarction within a region framed by a user. This identification is accomplished by comparing the CT numbers within the framed region with values from the presumably normal, homologous region of the other hemisphere. The mean and standard deviation of the CT numbers associated with the pixels in the homologous region of the uninvolved hemisphere are calculated. The mean CT number of the homologous region serves as a standard. Subsequently, *t*-tests are used to compare this standard with the mean CT numbers of successive four pixel parcels in the region framed by the user. Probability values are used to identify four pixel parcels that appear to deviate from the standard. Ideally, these deviant four-pixel parcels would be contiguous and would identify an area of abnormality. The area of the abnormality can be calculated in pixels, and descriptive statistics based on the CT numbers associated with the pixels within the region can be calculated. Naeser and colleagues (1981) interpreted the CT numbers as representing varying combinations of infarcted and noninfarcted tissue within a four-pixel region. Right minus left hemispheric differences correlated −.63 with the auditory comprehension subtest from the Boston Diagnostic Aphasia Examination. The variations of CT numbers in regions identified by AFP as abnormal are apparently related to the severity of behavioral impairment following stroke. It is not known if this variation simply reflects different combinations of normal and infarcted tissue. The evolution of an infarction covers a spectrum of phenomena including edema, ischemic demyelination, death of the nerve cell body, alterations of the blood-brain barrier, astrocytic infiltration, and development of a frank cystic cavity. The contribution of each of these changes to alterations of CT numbers remains an unresolved issue.

Eigenimage filtering is a technique currently being developed to isolate features of interest within an image while suppressing other interfering features (Windham et al., 1988). The technique uses a linear filter that produces a composite image obtained from a weighted summation of images from the same anatomic site. By selecting infarcted tissue as the desirable feature and normal gray matter, white matter, and cerebrospinal fluid as interfering features, a volume of infarction, weighted by the severity of tissue destruction, can be calculated.

In its application to MRI, eigenimage filtering takes advantage of the fact that the intensity of the signal depends on the NMR parameters intrinsic to the tissue (T_1, T_2, proton density) and on parameters selected by the operator (e.g., TR, TE). By controlling the operator-selectable parameters, a sequence of images of a specific anatomic site can be obtained in which the pixel intensities for different tissue types vary characteristically throughout the image sequence. For example, the intensity of each pixel might be determined at five points in time, after termination of an rf signal, for a 256×256 matrix. The resulting three-dimensional matrix (two dimensions in space and one in time) would contain a large amount of correlated information. As with any correlated data set, the three-dimensional matrix would have an underlying eigenvalue structure. Much as the factor analysis of a battery of behavioral tests can identify separate factors responsible for the variation of scores on a single test in the battery, so eigenimage filtering can separate features of an image at a subpixel level of analysis. The analogy between eigenimage filtering and traditional factor analysis breaks down when considering the general goal of the analysis: Factor analysis is used to identify the fundamental dimensions underlying the covariance structure of a set of measures. Eigenimage filtering, on the other hand, is used to highlight information regarding some features of the data while suppressing others.

Eigenimage filtering has been applied to the problem of distinguishing edema from tumor (Windham et al., 1988), and its applications to stroke are currently being studied. This method has the potential to separately estimate volumes of gray matter, white matter, cerebrospinal fluid, edema, and signal changes related to cerebral infarction. Verification in animal models using meticulous histologic correlation is required before this approach can be widely used in neurobehavioral studies.

FUTURE DEVELOPMENTS

Most of the CT and MRI technology discussed above has been developed since the early 1970s. We can expect a continuation of this rapid growth in the development of imaging tools. The first steps in developing magnetic resonance angiography have been taken (Ross et al., 1989) and will likely lead to techniques to jointly image the parenchymal and vascular anatomy of the brain. Techniques have also been developed to map metabolic data from PET onto MR images (Evans et al., 1988). Metabolic information obtained from NMR spectroscopy could be mapped to MR images even more directly than positron emission tomography (PET) data. These methods will lead to better localization of metabolic information. Rapid imaging techniques being developed for MRI (Frahm et al., 1990; Hasse, 1990; Ordidge et al., 1989) coupled with the multiperspective capability of MRI could make three-dimensional imaging of the brain routinely available. Three-dimensional images would improve the localization of infarcts or hemorrhages, especially when the stroke obscures some anatomic landmarks. Variations in head size and shape limit the use of standard atlases when identifying anatomic landmarks in the brain. Techniques must be developed to transform an image from a standard atlas to make it more nearly conform to the variations in major skull and cerebral landmarks seen in individual patients. The complications caused by individual differences in cerebral anatomy when attempting to localize a focal brain lesion remain a major problem for studies of brain-behavior relations.

Keeping astride future developments in brain imaging will require a significant commitment of time and effort on the part of scientists and clinicians who are primarily interested in the behavioral effects of cerebrovascular disease. However, this commitment of time will likely lead to new insights into the functional organization of the brain and to new information about the breakdown of this organization following stroke.

REFERENCES

Alcala, H., Gado, M., and Torack, R.M. (1978). The effect of size, histologic elements, and water content on the visualization of cerebral infarcts: a computerized cranial tomographic study. *Arch. Neurol.,* **35,** 1–7.

Anderson, O.C., Coss, D.T., Jacobson, R.L. and Meyer, M.W. (1980). Tissue pertechnetate and iodinated contrast material in ischemic stroke. *Stroke,* **11,** 617–621.

Awad, I.A., Johnson, P.C., Spetzler, R.F., and Hodak, J.A., (1986a).Incidental subcortical lesions identified on magnetic resonance imaging in the elderly. II. Postmortem pathological correlations. *Stroke,* **17,** 1090–1097.

Awad, I.A., Spetzler, R.F., Hodak, J.A., Awad, C.A., and Carey, R. (1986b). Incidental subcortical lesions identified on magnetic resonance imaging in the elderly. I. Correlation with age and cerebrovascular risk factors. *Stroke,* **17,** 1084–1089.

Bloch, F., Hansen, W.W., and Packard, M. (1946). Nuclear induction. *Phys. Rev.,* **69,** 127.

Bradley, W.G., Jr., Waluch, V., Yadley, R.A., and Wycoff, R.R. (1984). Comparison of CT and MR in 400 patients with suspected disease of the brain and cervical spinal cord. *Radiology,* **152,** 695–702.

Bradley, W.G., Jr. (1987). Magnetic resonance appearance of flowing blood and cerebrospinal fluid. In: M. Brant-Zawadzki and D. Norman, eds., *Magnetic Resonance Imaging of the Central Nervous System,* pp. 83–96. New York: Raven Press.

Brant-Zawadzki, M. (1987). Magnetic resonance imaging principles: the bare necessities. In: M. Brant-Zawadzki and D. Norman, eds., *Magnetic Resonance Imaging of the Central Nervous System,* pp. 1–12. New York: Raven Press.

Brewer, R.G., and Hahn, E.L. (1984). Atomic memory. *Sci. Am.,* **251**(6), 50–57.

Brown, G.G., Levine, S.R., Gorell, J.M., Pettegrew, J.W., Gdowski, J.W., Bueri, J.A., Helpern, J.A., and Welch, K.M.A. (1989). In vivo ^{31}P NMR profiles of Alzheimer's disease and multiple subcortical infarct dementia. *Neurology,* **39,** 1423–1427.

Buonanno, F.S., Fossel, E.T., and Kistler, J.P. (1986). Nuclear magnetic resonance in stroke. In: H.J.M. Barrett, J.P. Mohr, B.M. Stein, and F.M. Yatsu, eds., *Stroke: Pathophysiology, Diagnosis, and Management,* Vol. 1, pp. 165–180. New York: Churchill Livingstone.

Caplan, D. (1987). *Neurolinguistics and Linguistic Aphasiology: An Introduction.* New York: Cambridge University Press.

Connolly, C.J. (1950). *External Morphology of the Primate Brain.* Springfield, Charles C. Thomas.

Cunningham, D.F. (1892). *Contribution to the Surface Anatomy of the Cerebral Hemispheres.* Dublin: Royal Irish Academy.

Damadian, R. (1971). Tumor detection by nuclear magnetic resonance. *Science,* **171,** 1151–1153.

Damasio, H. (1983). A computed tomographic guide to the identification of cerebral vascular territories. *Arch. Neurol.,* **40,** 138–142.

Dolinskas, C.A., Bilaniuk, L.T., Zimmerman, R.A., and Kuhl, D.E. (1977). Computed tomography of intracerebral hematomas. I. Transmission CT observations on hematoma resolution. *Am. J. Roentgenol.,* **129,** 681–688.

Evans, A.C., Beil, C., Marrett, S., Thompson, C.J., and Hakim, A. (1988). Anatomical-functional correlation using an adjustable MRI-based region of interest atlas with positron emission tomography. *J. Cereb. Blood Flow Metab.,* **8,** 513–530.

Ewing, J.R., Branch, C.A., Fagan, S., Helpern, J.A., and Welch, K.M.A. (1989). A multi-component measurement of CBF using FC-23 and 19-F NMR detection. *J. Cereb. Blood Flow Metab.,* **9**(suppl 1), S101.

Fishman, R.A. (1975). Brain edema. *N. Engl. J. Med.,* **293,** 706–711.

Frahm, J., Merboldt, K-D., Bruhn, H., Gyngell, M.L., Hanicke, W., and Chien, D. (1990). 0.3 Second FLASH MRI of the human heart. *Magn. Reson, Med.,* **13,** 150–157.

Gadian, D. (1982). *Nuclear Magnetic Resonance and Its Applications to Living Systems.* Oxford: Clarendon Press.

Haase, A. (1990). Snapshot FLASH MRI: application to T_1, T_2, and chemical-shift imaging. *Magn. Reson. Med.,* **13,** 77–89.

Hachinski, V.C., Potter, P., and Merskey, H. (1987). Leukoaraiosis. *Arch. Neurol.,* **44,** 21–23.

Hounsfield, G.N. (1973). Computerized transverse axial scanning (tomography). *Br. J. Radiol.,* **46,** 1016–1022.

Hunt, A.L., Orrison, W.W., Yeo, R.A., Haaland, K-Y., Ryhne, R.L., Garry, P.J., and Rosenberg, G.A. (1989). Clinical significance of MRI white matter lesions in the elderly. *Neurology,* **39,** 1470–1474.

Inoue, Y., Takemoto, K., Miyamoto, T., Yoshikawa, N., Taniguchi, S., Saiwai, S., Nishimura, Y., and Komatsu, T. (1980). Sequential computed tomography scans in acute cerebral infarction. *Radiology,* **135,** 655–662.

Jenkins, A., Hadley, D.M., Teasdall, G.M., Condon, F., Macpherson, P., and Patterson, J. (1988). MR imaging of acute subarachnoid hemorrhage. *J. Neurosurg.,* **68,** 731–736.

Jernigan, T.L., Zatz, L.M., and Naeser, M.A. (1979). Semiautomated methods for quantitating CSF volume on cranial computed tomography. *Radiology,* **132,** 463–466.

Kertesz, A., Harlock, W., and Coates, R. (1979). Computer tomographic localization, lesion size, and prognosis in aphasia and nonverbal impairment. *Brain Lang.,* **8,** 34–50.

Knopman, D.S., and Rubens, A.B. (1986). The validity of computed tomographic scan findings for localization of cerebral functions: the relationship between computed tomography and hemiparesis. *Arch. Neurol.,* **43,** 328–332.

Knopman, D.S., Selnes, O.A., Niccum, N., Rubens, A.B., Yock, D., and Larson, D. (1983). A longitudinal study of speech fluency in aphasia: CT correlates of recovery and persistent nonfluency. *Neurology,* **33,** 1170–1178.

Kohlmeyer, K., and Graser, G. (1978). Comparative study of computed tomography and carotid angiography in stroke patients. *Neuroradiology,* **16,** 162–163.

Lauterbur, P.C. (1973). Image formation by induced local interactions:examples employing nuclear magnetic resonance. *Nature,* **242,** 190–191.

Lee, D., Fox, A., Vinuela, F., Pelz, D., Lau, C., Donald, A., and Merskey, H. (1987). Interobserver variation in computed tomography of the brain. *Arch. Neurol.,* **44,** 30–31.

Manelfe, C., Clanet, M., Gigaud, M., Bonafe, A., Guiraud, B., and Rascol, A. (1981). Internal capsule: normal anatomy and ischemic changes demonstrated by computed tomography. *Am. J. Neuroradiol.,* **2,** 149–155.

McNamara, M.T. (1987). Paramagnetic contrast media for magnetic resonance imaging of the central nervous system. In: M. Brant-Zawadzki and D. Norman, eds., *Magnetic Resonance Imaging of the Central Nervous System,* pp. 97–106.. New York: Raven Press.

Matsui, T., and Hirano, A. (1978). *An Atlas of the Human Brain for Computerized Tomography.* New York: Igaku-Shoin.

Messina, A.V., and Chernik, N.L. (1975). Computed tomography: the "resolving" intracerebral hemorrhage. *Radiology,* **118,** 609–613.

Naeser, M.A., Hayward, R.W., Laughlin, S.A., and Zatz, L.M. (1981). Quantitative CT scan studies in aphasia. I. Infarct size and CT numbers. *Brain Lang.,* **12,** 140–164.

Ordidge, R.J., Howseman, A., Coxon, R., Turner, R., Chapman, B., Glover, P., Stehling, M., and Mansfield, P. (1989). Snapshot imaging at 0.5T using echo-planar techniques. *Magn. Reson. Med.,* **10,** 227–240.

Petroff, O.A.C., Prichard, J.W., Behar, W.L., Alger, J.R., and Shulman, R.G. (1984). In vivo phosphorus nuclear magnetic resonance spectroscopy in status epilepticus. *Ann. Neurol.,* **16,** 169–177.

Petroff, O.A.C., Prichard, J.W., Behar, K.L., Alger, J.R., den Hollander, J.A., and Shulman, R.G. (1985). Cerebral intracellular pH by ^{31}P nuclear magnetic resonance spectroscopy. *Neurology,* **35,** 781–788.

Purcell, E.M., Torrey, H.C., and Pound, R.V. (1946). Resonance absorption by nuclear magnetic moments in a solid. *Phys. Rev.,* **69,** 37–38.

Ra, J.B., Hilal, S.K., Oh, C.H., and Mun, I.K. (1988). In vivo magnetic resonance imaging of sodium in the human body. *Magn. Reson. Med.,* **7,** 11–22.

Ramadan, N.M., Deveshwar, R., and Levine, S.R. (1989). Magnetic resonance and clinical cerebrovascular disease: an update. *Curr. Concepts Cerebrovasc. Dis. Stroke,* **24,** 13–18.

Robinson, R.G., Bolla-Wilson, K., Kaplan, E., Lipsey, J.R., and Price, T.R. (1986). Depression influences intellectual impairment in stroke patients. *Br. J. Psychiatry,* **148,** 541–547.

Ross, J.S., Masaryk, T.J., Modic, M.T., Harik, S.I., Wiznitzer, M., and Selman, W.R. (1989). Magnetic resonance angiography of the extracranial carotid arteries and intracranial vessels: a review. *Neurology,* **39,** 1369–1376.

Ruebens, A.B. (1977). Lateralization in the nervous system. In: S. Harnad, R.W. Doty, L. Goldstein, J. Jaynes, and G. Krauthamer, eds., *Lateralization in the Nervous System,* pp. 503–516. New York: Academic Press.

Russell, W.F. (1984). The CT scan in extracranial vascular disease. In: R.R. Smith, ed., *Stroke and the Extracranial Vessels.* pp. 99–110. New York: Raven Press.

Salgado, E.D., Weinstein, M., Furlan, A.J., Madic, M.T., Beck, G.J., Estes, M., Awad, I., and Little, J.R. (1986). Proton magnetic resonance imaging in ischemic cerebrovascular disease. *Ann. Neurol.,* **20,** 502–507.

Savoiardo, M. (1986). CT scanning. In: H.J.M. Barnett, B.M. Stein, J.P. Mohr, and F.M. Yatsu, eds., *Stroke: Pathophysiology, Diagnosis, and Management,* Vol. 1, pp. 189–219. New York: Churchill Livingstone.

Shrout, P.E., and Fleiss, J.L. (1979). Intraclass correlations: uses in assessing rater reliability. *Psychol. Bull.,* **86,** 420–428.

Sipponen, J.L., Kaste, M., Sepponen, R.E., Kuurne, T., Suorantz, H., and Sivula, A. (1983). Nuclear magnetic resonance imaging in reversible cerebral ischemia. *Lancet,* **1,** 294–295.

Steingart, A., Hachinski, V.C., Lau, C., Fox, A.J., Fox, H., Lee, D., Inzitari, D., and Merskey,

H. (1987). Cognitive and neurologic findings in demented patients with diffuse white matter lucencies on computed tomographic scan (leuko-araoisis). *Arch. Neurol.,* **44,** 36–39.

Stevens, J.M., Valentine, A.R., and Kendall, B.E. (1988). *Computed Cranial and Spinal Imaging.* Baltimore: Williams & Wilkins.

Unger, E.D., Gado, M.H., Fulling, K-F., and Littlefield, J.L. (1987). Acute cerebral infarctions in monkeys: an experimental study using MR imaging. *Radiology,* **162,** 789–795.

Wall, S.D., Brant-Zawadzki, M., Jeffrey, R.B., and Barnes, B. (1981). High frequency CT findings within 24 hours after cerebral infarction. *Am. J. Neuroradiol.,* **2,** 553–557.

Wehrli, F.W., MacFall, J.R., Shutts, D., Breger, R., and Herfkens, R.J. (1984). Mechanisms of contrast in NMR imaging. *J. Comput. Assist. Tomogr.,* **8,** 369–380.

Windham, J.P., Abd-Allah, M.M., Reimann, D.A., Froelich, J.W., and Haggar, A.M. (1988). Eigenimage filtering in MR imaging. *J. Comput. Assist. Tomogr.,* **12,** 1–9.

Wing, S.D., Norman, D., Pollock, J.A., and Newton, T.H. (1976). Contrast enhancement of cerebral infarcts in computed tomography. *Radiology,* **121,** 89–92.

Yamaguchi, K., and Vemura, K. (1978). An angiographic study of brain swelling in cerebral infarction. *Neuroradiology,* **16,**, 150–151.

II
Clinical Neuropsychology of Stroke

6

Overview of Clinical Issues in Stroke

SAMUEL WIEBE-VELAZQUEZ AND VLADIMIR HACHINSKI

Stroke is the leading cause of focal neuropsychological impairment in adults. The abrupt onset and possibly devastating course are best conveyed by the lay term "stroke," in preference to labels such as "cerebrovascular accident," which usually are neither cerebrovascular in origin nor accidental. Stroke—the sudden occurrence of paralysis and loss of consciousness or sensation—has been recognized since the times of Hippocrates (Clarke, 1963). Its relation to occlusive cerebrovascular disease of the carotid and vertebral arteries was established in 1658 by Wepfer (Gurdjian and Gurdjian, 1979), and by the midnineteenth century the concepts of cerebral embolism and thrombosis were substantiated by Virchow (Schiller, 1970).

Notwithstanding the disorder's antiquity, it is only during the second half of the twentieth century that we are witnessing increasing awareness and understanding of stroke. Advances have included the identification of risk factors (notably hypertension, atherosclerosis, and rheumatic heart disease), information about epidemiology and current trends, the advent of enlightening diagnostic tools such as angiography and computed tomography (CT), and the introduction of preventive and therapeutic strategies. All of these developments have contributed to the progressive decline in stroke mortality that has been observed over the last three decades (Barnett, 1982; Hachinski, 1984; Whisnant, 1984) (Figure 6–1).

As understanding of the problem is gained, previous stroke nosologies become inadequate, either because they are too brief, vague, and overlapping (e.g., the International Classification of Diseases) or too exhaustive and impractical, e.g., those elaborated by various experts. Thus it is time for a classification that has applicability at the bedside and takes into account the anatomic location, nature, cause, and tem-

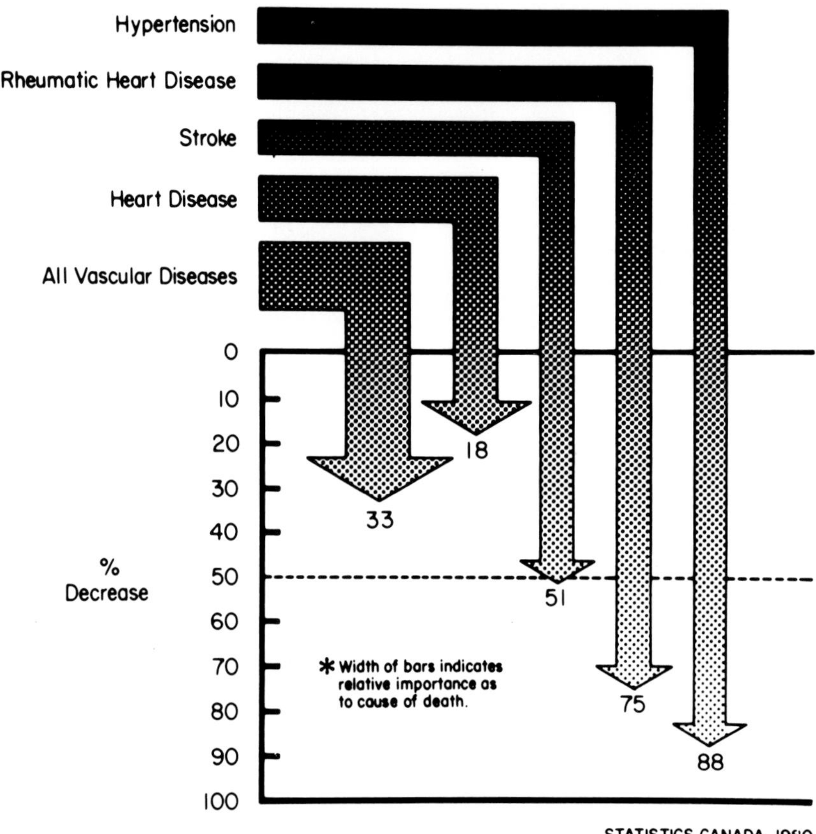

Figure 6–1 Decrease in mortality rates for hypertension, heart disease, and stroke in individuals aged 65 and under in Canada from 1953 to 1978. (Reproduced with permission from Barnett, 1982.)

poral evolution, as well as management categories of stroke. The major management categories include TIA and minor stroke, major stroke, deteriorating stroke, and young stroke (Table 6–1). These categories are based on the observation that patients in the various groups usually have a different type, pathophysiology, and prognosis of stroke and hence call for different diagnostic, therapeutic, and prophylactic approaches (Hachinski and Norris, 1985).

EPIDEMIOLOGY

Diagnostic accuracy is the essential prerequisite for the development of epidemiologic data on neurologic diseases. A number of factors influence diagnostic accuracy including the skill of the diagnostician, the nomenclature in use, the frequency of the disease in the population studied, and the availability and reliability of diagnostic tests (Kurtzke, 1986). Clinically silent strokes may occur in the basal ganglia, white matter, and frontal lobes. Nonhemiplegic strokes (up to 30% of all strokes) have a

Table 6–1 Suggested Classification of Stroke

- *Category*
  - Presumed stroke
  - Presumed TIA
  - Other
- *Anatomic classification*
  - By axial location
    - Supratentorial
      - Lobar (specify)
      - Centrencephalic (specify)
    - Infratentorial
      - Cerebellar (specify)
      - Brain stem (specify)
  - By vascular territory
    - Carotid (specify)
    - Vertebrobasilar (specify)
- *Etiologic classification*
  - By result
    - Cerebral infarct
      - Arterial
      - Arteriolar (lacunar)
      - Venous
    - Cerebral hemorrhage
      - Intraparenchymal
      - Subarachnoid
- *Etiologic classification* (*cont.*)
  - By cause
    - Ischemia
      - Extracranial vascular disease
      - Embolism
      - Other
    - Hemorrhage
      - Hypertension
      - Amyloid angiopathy
      - Vascular malformation
      - Other
- *Management classification*
  - TIA and minor stroke
  - Major stroke
  - Deteriorating stroke
  - Young stroke

Source: Hachinski and Norris (1985).

higher chance of not being detected (Hatano, 1976). The significance of diagnostic skill is hence emphasized.

After diagnosis, the next important item is the frequency of stroke. It entails risks of selection bias and nonrepresentativeness of the population under study in reports of series of cases. On the other hand, in studies based on death rate, the accuracy of classification is affected by changing fashions in death certification and imprecision in diagnosis (Corwin et al., 1982). Finally, pathologic series are unrepresentative for epidemiologic purposes (Wylie, 1972). Nonetheless, certain points can be made from epidemiologic studies.

1. There is a reciprocal relation between the incidence of cerebrovascular and cardiovascular disease that has an impact on reports of incidence rates (Ostfeld, 1980).
2. As with other neurologic diseases, a distinction between social and racial factors is not made easily. There is a significant geographic and social variation in stroke incidence throughout the world, which in certain instances could be accounted for by differences in the quality of reporting among countries. Nevertheless, there are also differences in incidence within the same country, e.g. in the United States it is higher in Blacks than in Whites and higher in the southeastern states than in midwestern states (Kuller, 1978).
3. The incidence of stroke rises with age; consequently, relatively minor increases in the mean age of the population result in relatively large increases in stroke incidence (Fries, 1980).

4. In North America, for every 1000 population, six individuals are expected to have had a stroke; and each year two new strokes and one stroke death per 1000 population would be expected. Four of five new strokes are thrombo-embolic, one of eight is a cerebral hemorrhage, and one of twelve is a subarachnoid hemorrhage (Kurtzke, 1980).
5. Stroke is still the third commonest cause of death in North America and Europe, and in some countries (Japan and China) it continues to be the most important cause of death (Lambo, 1979; Wu, 1979; Kurtzke, 1980).

STRATEGY FOR STROKE

Having considered the epidemiologic magnitude of stroke, how should we approach the problem? First, stroke patients are not to be considered terminal or irreversible cases. A nihilistic therapeutic attitude born from ignorance hinders the search for effective therapy. Many negative attitudes toward the management of stroke patients revolve around the widespread, though inaccurate, conception that the clinical effects of stroke are due to local brain death and result in irreversible neurologic deficits. Indeed, studies of stroke outcome disprove this idea (Whisnant et al., 1971; Norris et al., 1984), and we know that ischemic stroke produces a broad array of potentially reversible events that antedate brain death (Hachinski and Norris, 1985).

Stroke is a medical emergency necessitating hospitalization for diagnostic, but not necessarily treatment, purposes and because it is the best way to optimize patient care, foster research on cerebrovascular disorders, and promote education in all aspects of stroke. However, factors such as scarcity of hospital beds, finances, cultural determinants, and belief that hospitalization does not change prognosis have an influence in reducing the number of patients who are hospitalized. Second, the use of a standardized functional scale for assessing stroke patients is desirable for a number of reasons. It provides the basis for comparison among studies, helps to detect deterioration, and allows clinicians to monitor the course of the patient.

MORBIDITY AND MORTALITY OF STROKE

Death during the first few days after stroke usually occurs as a consequence of primary neurologic causes and later, in the following stages, from systemic causes (Figure 6–2). Unfortunately, little can be done in the way of specific therapy for the brain in stroke patients (Kennedy et al., 1970), except to prevent further damage. Morbidity primarily caused by brain damage is not likely to be affected by medical intervention, and several determinants of subsequent neurologic impairment have been identified, e.g., severity of the initial lesion, older age, impairment of consciousness on admission, persistent forced conjugate gaze, and the presence of hemispheric lesions (Carpenter and Reed, 1972; Drake et al., 1973; Haerer and Woosley, 1975; Oxbury et al., 1975; Norris et al., 1984).

On the other hand, morbidity secondary to complications, e.g., pneumonia, urinary tract infections, decubital ulcers, and myocardial infarction, are amenable to prevention and treatment. Thus the short-term outcome depends to a large extent on continuous and adequate care. Medium- and long-term prognosis of functional

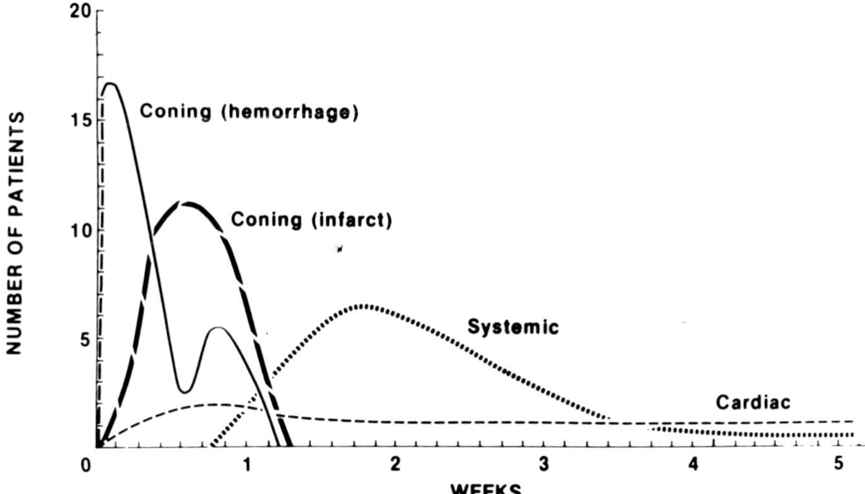

Figure 6–2 Cause of death in 180 consecutive patients following supratentorial stroke. (Reproduced with permission from Silver et al., 1984.)

recovery is directly related to the severity and reversibility of the brain damage. Specialized care in stroke units should therefore be offered to patients with minimal neurologic lesions and threatened strokes.

STRUCTURE AND FUNCTION OF THE CEREBRAL VASCULATURE

Arteries

The brain is supplied by the carotid and basilar arteries. The medial and basal portions of the brain and brain stem (the centrencephalon) are supplied by short penetrating arteries that sustain relatively high gradients of pressure over a short segment. As a result, this region becomes the major site of small lacunar infarcts and hypertensive hemorrhages (Figure 6–3). Cerebral arteries have thinner walls than similar sized arteries elsewhere in the body and are prone to rupture and bleed into the brain.

The human cerebral vasculature is also particularly prone to atherosclerosis, an age-dependent phenomenon that affects, in chronologic sequence, the aorta, coronary arteries, and cervical and cerebral arteries. It causes gradual, progressive stenosis that usually allows collateral flow to develop.

Blood-Brain Barrier

The blood-brain barrier is a complex structure that protects the brain by preventing systemic substances from entering the central nervous system. Tight junctions among endothelial cells in the brain capillaries make them highly impermeable. The blood-brain barrier is notably resistant to ischemic damage, which ultimately causes vasogenic cerebral edema. Understanding the pathogenesis of ischemic injury is of primary clinical importance, as acute morbidity and mortality in stroke are the result of cerebral edema.

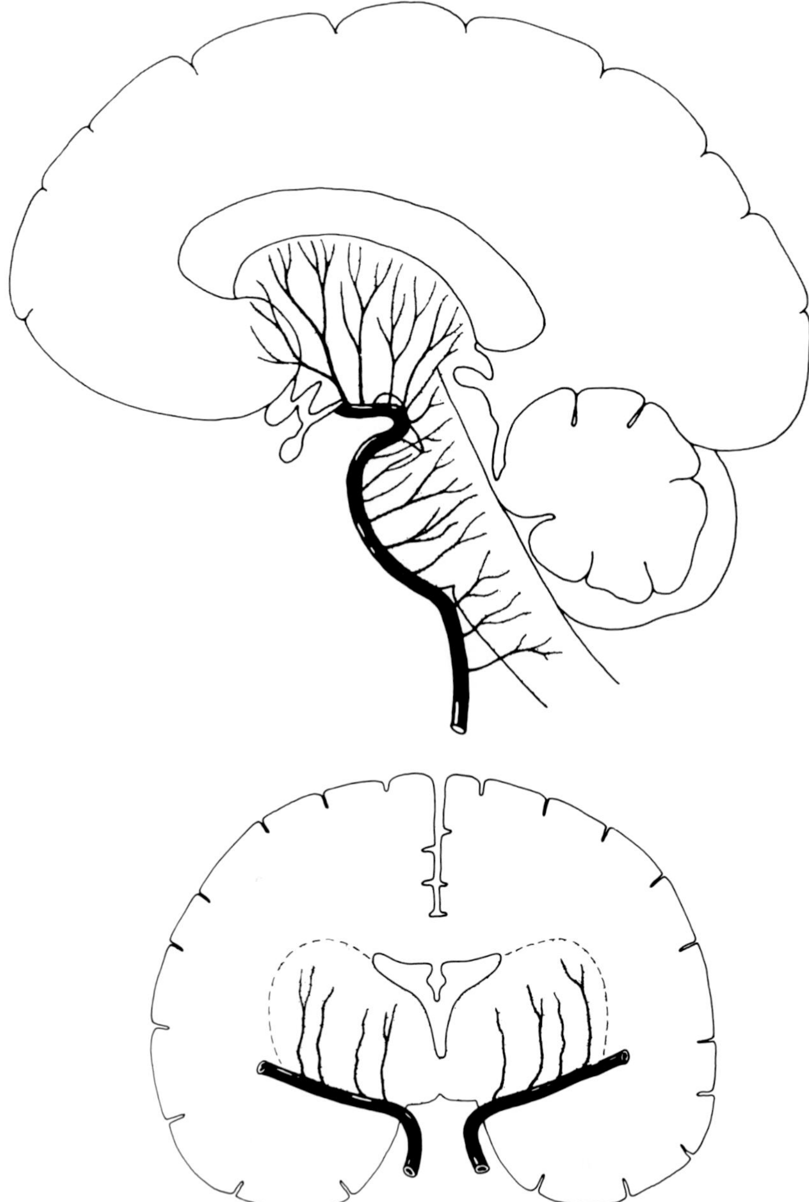

Figure 6–3 Vascular centrencephalon, the major site of lacunar infarcts and hypertensive hemorrhages: sagittal (top), coronal (bottom), and horizontal (top of next page) sections of the brain. (Reproduced with permission from Hachinski and Norris, 1985.)

Cerebral Blood Flow and Metabolism

The brain is richly perfused, having one of the highest blood supplies per gram of tissue in the body. Its exquisite sensitivity to ischemia is revealed when complete stoppage of blood flow causes unconciousness almost immediately and irreversible

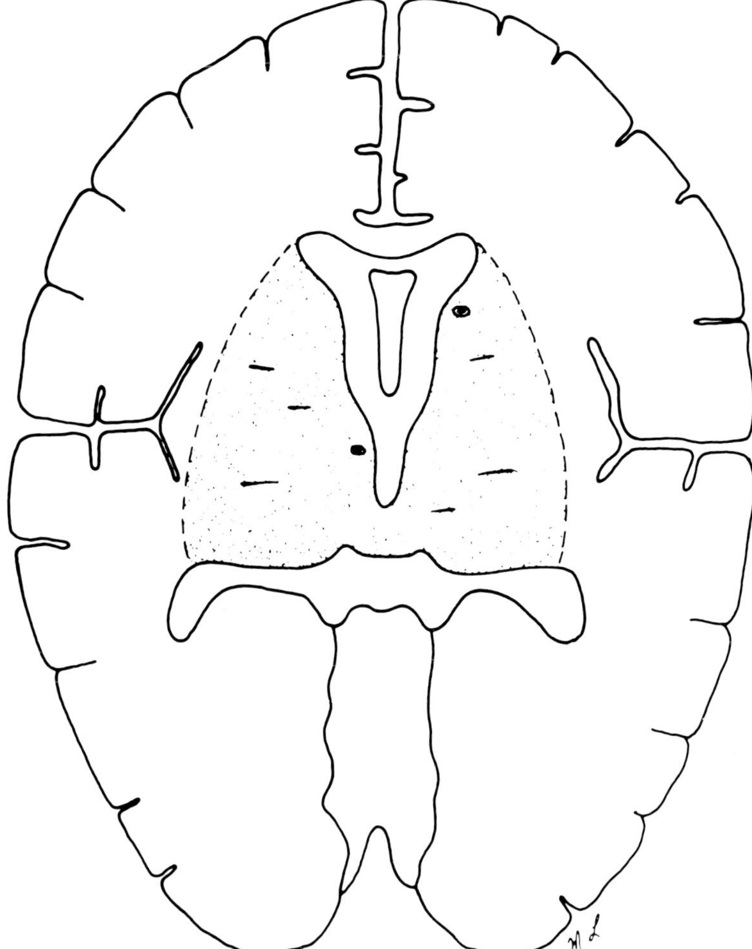

Figure 6–3 *(continued)*

brain damage after 5 minutes. Glucose and oxygen are the brain's main sources of energy, although some ketone bodies can be metabolized during hypoglycemia. Energy reserves are minimal in the brain, and it depends on a constant provision of oxygen and glucose—hence its particular vulnerability to impaired perfusion.

Autoregulation

The brain is capable of efficiently adjusting its own blood flow, which allows it to be in constant homeostasis and yet in constant change focally. In general, autoregulation can maintain blood perfusion within a normal narrow range despite relatively wide changes in systemic blood pressure (Figure 6–4). However, it is sensitive to CO_2, and slight CO_2 increases are followed by relatively large increments in cerebral blood flow. Accordingly, it has been shown by positron emission tomography (PET) and xenon 133 (^{133}Xe) studies that various mental activities involving language and

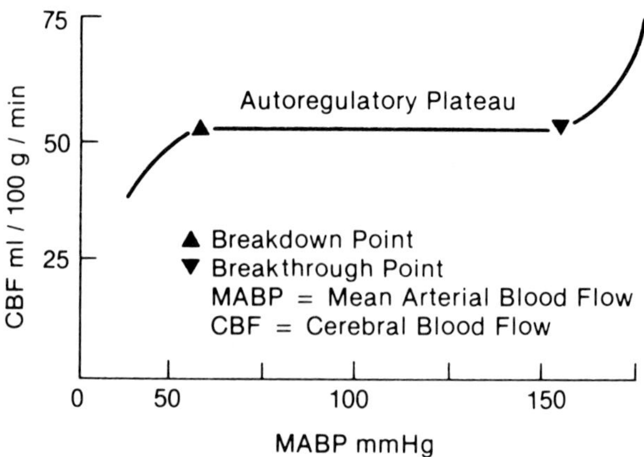

Figure 6–4 Cerebral autoregulation. Cerebral blood flow remains constant between the mean arterial blood pressures of approximately 50 to 150 torr. (Reproduced with permission from Hachinski, 1984.)

motor and visual functions are accompanied by corresponding local changes and redistribution of cerebral blood flow and metabolism (Lassen et al., 1978; Phelps et al., 1982).

CLINICAL PICTURE OF STROKE

The diagnosis of stroke depends on the history and examination, which should guide judiciously the radiologic and laboratory investigations so they complement the diagnostic evaluation. The clinical picture usually decides the cerebral location of the stroke, and location in turn suggests etiology (Figure 6–5). The history offers valuable information about the type and cause of the lesion. Characterization of the temporal profile and the initial symptoms are of paramount importance in diagnosis, as they frequently provide the best clues to localization and etiology. By way of illustration, severe headache of abrupt onset suggests subarachnoid hemorrhage but is unusual in cerebral infarction. Loss of consciousness evolving rapidly after onset occurs more frequently in cerebral hemorrhage of brain stem stroke, and seizures are more common in cerebral embolism and hemorrhage.

A practical attitude concerning the interpretation of information is to first analysze unequivocal data of the history and examination. Less clear-cut findings can reinforce a working diagnosis but if overemphasized may confuse or mislead.

MAJOR TYPES OF STROKE

The hallmarks of stroke diagnosis are accurate cerebral localization and definition of underlying pathology. Current diagnostic procedures can localize lesions with great precision. Diagnostic investigation of stroke now has practical application, as it is strongly directed toward the cause of the lesion and its susceptibility to therapy. For example, it is more important to know if an embolic event has a cardiac origin and can be treated than to know the exact site of cerebral infarction. Thus diagnosis deter-

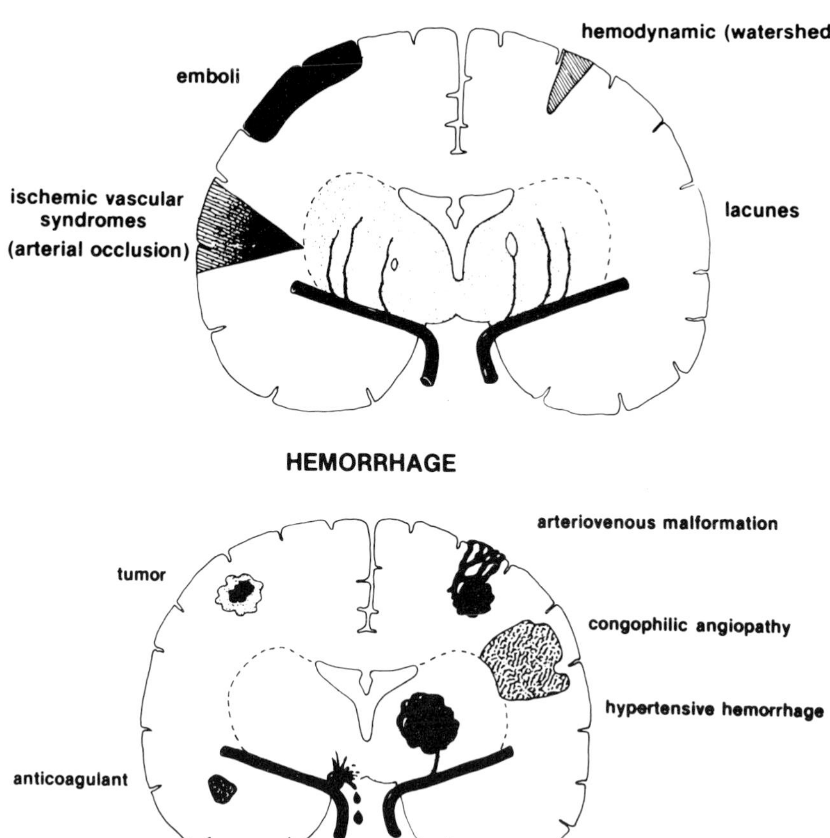

Figure 6–5 Typical locations of cerebral infarction (top) and hemorrhage (bottom). Stroke location suggests the etiology. (Reproduced with permission from Hachinski and Norris, 1985.)

mines therapy. The temporal description of cerebrovascular events are of more value in determining therapy than the countless vascular syndromes arising from the variants of vascular supply.

Major Stroke

The neurologic deficit in patients with major stroke is usually stable and extensive. Early rehabilitation is warranted if intellect and personality are not severely impaired. It may decrease the number of complications and have social and psychological benefits. Management should include general measures referred to later in this chapter, anticoagulation if it is of embolic cardiac origin, and treatment of risk factors that may be present. Investigation should also be directed to the possible cause of stroke, e.g., heart disease or hypertension. The final outcome is largely determined by the severity of the lesion.

TIAs and Minor Stroke

Patients with TIAs have no lasting deficit; yet they are at high risk of stroke and should be thoroughly investigated. The diagnosis is made by the history, as the TIAs are seldom witnessed, and physical examination is negative (Calanchini et al., 1977). The term "presumed TIA or minor stroke" would probably be more suitable in the initial setting. It is generally agreed that TIAs last no more than 24 hours, and studies have confirmed the notion that most TIAs last minutes and resolve within 1 hour. In fact, TIAs lasting 4 hours or more are really strokes (Levy, 1988; Werdelin and Juhler, 1988). The possiblity of finding an abnormality on CT scanning grows as the duration of the TIA increases, and several studies have found CT scan abnormalities in up to 50% of TIA patients (Bogousslavsky and Regli, 1984; Calandre et al., 1984; Mirsen & Hachinski, 1988; Turnbull and Bannister, 1985; Weisberg and Lacorte, 1985; Werdelin and Juhler, 1988).

The most frequent presentation of carotid TIAs have been reported to be monocular blindness, contralateral motor or sensory impairment, and speech disturbances, whereas vertebrobasilar TIAs most commonly present with bilateral visual blurring, diplopia, ataxia, and dizziness (Futty et al., 1977). Uncommon features include seizures, loss of consciousness, drop attacks, and transient global amnesia. The differential diagnosis is broad and includes postictal states, complicated migraine, cerebral tumor and aneurysm, chronic subdural hematoma, hypoglycemia, hysteria, and multiple sclerosis (Table 6–2). The most important point to be remembered in this condition is the great risk of stroke and the potential for prevention.

Deteriorating Stroke

This category includes patients whose condition deteriorates during the first week. Prospective studies show that it occurs in approximately 30% of stroke patients (Car-

Table 6–2 Initial Complaint and Final Diagnosis in 123 Patients Found Not to Have TIA[a]

Initial Complaint	Final Diagnosis	No.
Fainting	Postural hypotension	18
	Syncope	16
Dizziness	Vertigo	7
	Other (including cardiac arrhythmias)	16
Loss of consciousness	Seizures	18
Anxiety	Neurosis	14
Headache	Migraine and tension	5
Visual symptoms	Papillitis	2
	Retinal artery occlusion	2
Confusion	Other organic confusional states	7
Other	Tumor, iatrogenic, and others	18

Source: Calanchini et al. (1977).

[a]A total of 95 patients with completed stroke were excluded.

Table 6–3 Causes of Deterioration in Stroke

Cerebral factors	Systemic factors
Infarction	Cardiac
Cerebral edema	Heart failure
Hemorrhagic infarction	Cardiac arrhythmias
Recurrent embolism	Pulmonary
Progressive thrombosis	Pneumonia
(Postictal states)	Pulmonary embolism
Hemorrhage	Metabolic
Cerebral edema	Renal/hepatic failure
Rebleeding	Syndrome of inappropriate ADH
Acute hydrocephalus	Septicemia
(Postictal states)	Psychological
	Drugs

Source: Hachinski and Norris (1985).

ter, 1960; Jones and Millikan, 1976; Hachinski and Norris, 1981). Primary cerebral causes such as edema, hemorrhage, and recurrent embolism are responsible for 69% of these cases, and systemic factors (cardiopulmonary, metabolic, drugs) account for the remaining 31% (Hachinski and Norris, 1981) (Table 6–3). Documentation of a causal relation is frequently not possible, so we can only stress a strong association between events.

Secondary hemorrhage is more common with embolic infarction, where anticoagulants are most indicated. However, the risk of hemorrhage due to anticoagulation in embolic stroke has been probably overemphasized in the past and should not preclude the use of such drugs when indicated (Furlan et al., 1982; Yatsu and Mohr, 1982). With ischemic stroke, the relation between clinical deterioration and progressive brain swelling is controversial. With hemorrhagic stroke, deterioration is probably more commonly due to cerebral edema than to rebleeding (Ransohoff et al., 1971). Early cognition of deterioration is sine qua non to successful therapy—hence the importance of close clinical vigilance of stroke patients. Urgent CT scanning can differentiate between infarction and hemorrhage and can identify massive edema, thereby guiding therapy.

Stroke in the Young

Young stroke patients (16–45 years of age) suffer from reversible lesions more often than elderly patients, and thorough investigation is necessary in all cases. The approximate proportion of young patients suffering stroke is 3 to 4% in the United States, Walker et al., 1981, but the age structure of the population clearly has an influence on these figures; i.e., a greater proportion of young individuals results in a greater proportion of young stroke patients (Dalal, 1979). The causes of stroke in this age group are different from those in older patients, atherosclerosis being uncommon. The most common causes of ischemic stroke are embolism of cardiac origin, migraine, trauma, arteritis, and coagulopathies. Hemorrhagic stroke results from arteriovenous malformations and aneurysms (Figure 6–6; Table 6–4).

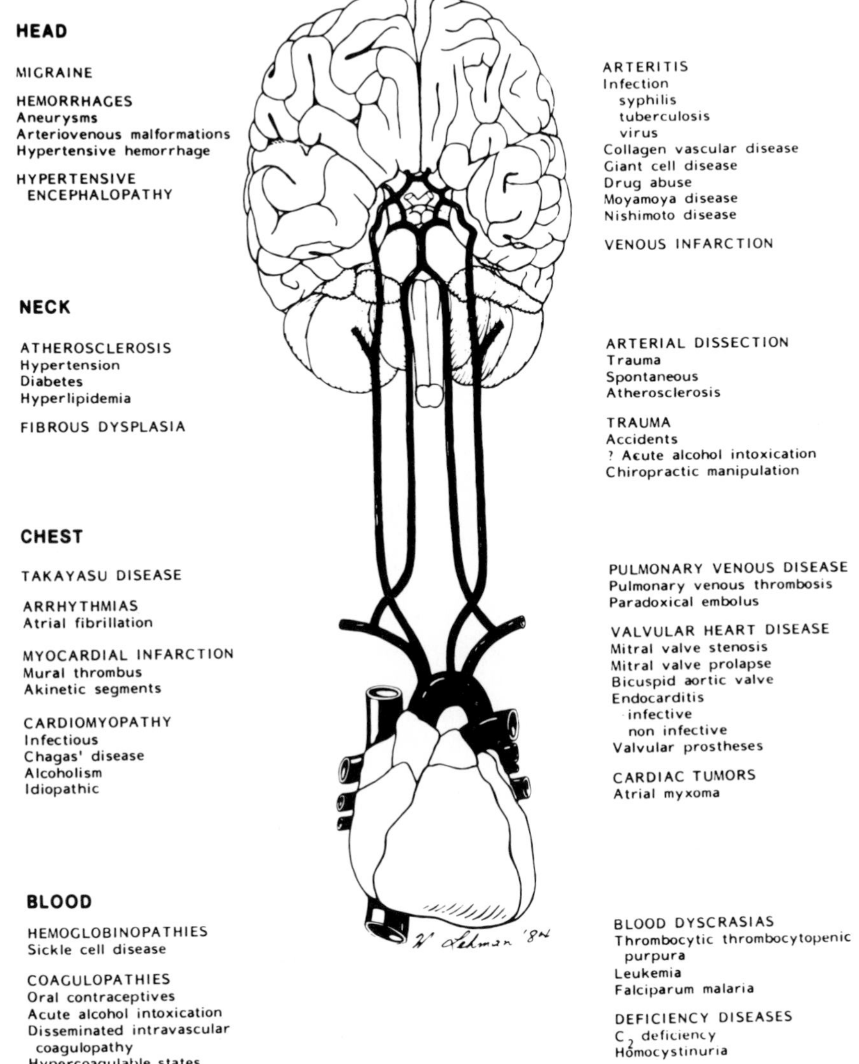

Figure 6–6 Causes of stroke in the young. (Reproduced with permission from Hachinski and Norris, 1985.)

HEART–BRAIN INTERACTIONS

The cardiovascular and cerebrovascular systems are interrelated closely and in a complex way. Brain and heart are sensitive to ischemia, and vascular disease is the commonest affliction of both. As a result of improved diagnostic tools and prospective epidemiologic studies, we know that hypertension, chronic atrial fibrillation, and diabetes are notable risk factors for stroke (Kannel, 1971; Kannel et al., 1983; Wolf et al., 1978). Stroke patients are more likely to die from heart disease than from subsequent stroke. Conversely, stroke causes cardiac arrhythmias, inverted T waves,

Table 6–4 Risk Factors for Stroke in the Young

1. Cardiac disease
   a. Valvular heart disease, especially mitral valve prolapse
   b. Cardiomyopathies
   c. Atrial myxoma
2. Hypertension
3. Migraine
4. Hyperlipidemia
5. Oral contraceptives
6. Cigarette smoking
7. Trauma
8. Drug abuse
9. Alcohol
10. Neurosyphilis

Source: Hachinski and Norris (1985).

and prolonged QT interval on electrocardiogram (ECG), as well as neurogenic pulmonary edema, which are probably causally related to increased catecholamine activity. This heart–brain interdependence clearly has major therapeutic implications.

VASCULAR DEMENTIA

The term "cerebral arteriosclerosis" has been used to imply dementia caused by slow, continuous deprivation of the brain of its nutrients. Two major points have been clarified. First, the commonest cause of stroke is not vascular but degenerative, predominantly Alzheimer's disease. Postmortem studies have found that approximately 20% of all demented patients have vascular dementia, although vascular factors may contribute to the clinical features in a larger proportion (Tomlinson et al., 1970; Tomlinson and Henderson, 1976; Wells, 1978).

Second, when vascular disease causes dementia, it results from repetitive embolic cerebral infarcts, which produce a multiinfarct dementia (Harchinski et al., 1974). Most such emboli arise from the heart and extracranial vessels, and the most important conditions predisposing to their occurrence are atherosclerosis, hypertension, cardiac disease, and diabetes. Adequate treatment of these conditions is the best way to prevent strokes and multiinfarct dementia.

To make the diagnosis of vascular dementia one must first search for other causes of intellectual impairment. Notable among them in older age groups is depression, which impairs cognitive functions that can improve with treatment. Wells (1979) found that certain features suggest a depressive origin, i.e., an abrupt onset, a previous history of psychiatric disease, and complaints of memory loss by the patient himself instead of his family. On the other hand, stroke causes depression that may impair cognitive functions in the absence of multiinfarct dementia.

An ischemia score (Hachinski et al., 1975; Wade and Hachinski, 1986, 1987) (Table 6–5) that has been validated in clinico-pathologic studies (Rosen et al., 1980) is helpful for distinguishing Alzheimer's disease from multiinfarct dementia. A score of 4 or less suggests Alzheimer's disease and a score of 7 or more multiinfarct demen-

Table 6–5 Ischemic Scores[a]

Feature	Score
Abrupt onset	2
Stepwise deterioration	1
Fluctuating course	1
Nocturnal confusion	1
Relative preservation of personality	1
Depression	1
Somatic complaints	1
Emotional incontinence	1
History of hypertension	1
History of strokes	2
Evidence of associated atherosclerosis	1
Focal neurologic symptoms	2
Focal neurologic signs	2

Source: Hachinski et al. (1975).

[a]Patients attaining 7 points or more are likely to have either multiinfarct dementia or a vascular component to their mental impairment.

tia. However, the two may coexist (mixed dementia), and the ischemic score does not discriminate well between pure multiinfarct dementia and mixed dementia (Wade et al., 1987).

The correlation of cerebral lesions on CT scan and dementia has been evaluated by Loeb and colleagues (1988). No significant correlation was found between the volume of the lesions and dementia except in patients with unilateral lesions and in those with bilateral cortical and subcortical lesions. Brain atrophy was significantly related to multiinfarct dementia.

LEUKOARAIOSIS

The eponym "Binswanger's disease" has been used to refer to neuropathologically nonspecific changes in the hemispheric white matter of elderly patients with chronic hypertension. Relatively large numbers of patients with white matter lesions on CT scan and MRI have been classified as Binswanger's disease. However, the nature and significance of these abnormalities remain unclear, and agreement on the correlation between these lesions and intellectual impairment has not been reached (George et al., 1986a,b; Steingart, 1987a,b). Until sufficient understanding is obtained, we propose use of the descriptive term "leukoaraiosis" in these cases, meaning a diminution of the density of the white matter, in preference to eponyms which can be misleading (Hachinski et al., 1987).

TREATMENT

Treatment for the established stroke is limited, attitudes toward therapy ranging from ignorant nihilism to misguided polypharmacology. The careful practice of a number of general measures is warranted in stroke patients.

1. Maintaining blood pressure within safe limits to avoid hypoperfusion and hypertension
2. Keeping a patent and clean airway
3. Avoiding drugs that impair alertness
4. Assessing the metabolic profile and the water and electrolyte balance
5. Detecting and treating infections that befall the bedridden
6. Preventing deep venous thrombosis and pulmonary thromboembolism by the judicious use of low dose heparin

Specific Therapy for Ischemic Stroke

Therapy of proved benefit includes osmotic agents and anticoagulants. Osmotic agents (e.g., mannitol, glycerol) should be used cautiously and as a temporary decompressive measure preceding surgery. The risk/benefit ratio of anticoagulation must be assessed in each patient with cardiac embolic sources. We think that the risk of recurrent strokes from cardiac embolism is greater than that of hemorrhage due to anticoagulant drugs, and these agents should be used when indicated.

There are a number of therapeutic measures of unproved usefulness, notably vasodilators and steroids. Vasodilators may actually cause "cerebral steal" and further damage (Hoedt-Rasmussen et al., 1967), and steroids have been shown to increase morbidity without beneficially altering the outcome (Dyken and White, 1956; Bauer and Tellez, 1973; Norris, 1976; Norris and Hachinski, 1985).

Specific Therapy for Hemorrhagic Stroke

Surgery has a role in decompressing lobar cerebral and cerebellar hemorrhages that cause increased intracranial pressure and threaten brain stem compression. Surgery for deep or devastating lesions may change the prognosis from death to a living death.

PROGNOSIS

A number of factors that adversely affect functional recovery and survival have been identified (Table 6–6). Approximately one-fifth of patients die during the first month after stroke. The longer the patient lives, the more likely he is to sustain a fatal myocardial infarction, the commonest cause of death in stroke patients (Whisnant, 1983).

In general, the best prognosis can be expected in the patient who is less than 65 years old, who has no previous history of cardiovascular or cerebrovascular disease, and who suffers a minor stroke. The single most important determinant of prognosis is the severity of stroke, regardless of its etiology and location.

PREVENTION

Prevention is the mainstay of medical intervention in stroke. It can be carried out at several stages in the natural history of the disease (Table 6–7), and it can be extended to the patient's relatives who are at risk (Hachinski, 1983). Prevention is directed

Table 6–6 Factors That Negatively Influence the Prognosis of Stroke

Neurologic Factors
- Site of lesion
  - Within the brain
    - Hemisphere vs. brainstem
    - Right hemisphere vs. left hemisphere
  - Vascular location
    - Intracranial carotid
      - vs. Middle cerebral artery stenoses and occlusions
      - vs. Cervical carotid occlusion
    - Basilar vs. vertebral artery lesions
- Nature of lesion
  - Hemorrhage vs. infarct
  - Hemispheric vs. centrencephalic infarct
  - Centrencephalic vs. hemispheric hemorrhage
- Severity of lesion
  - Decreased level of consciousness
  - Forced gaze deviation
  - Dense hemiplegia
  - Loss of movement in distal limbs
  - Dense hemisensory impairment
  - Slow recovery rate
  - CT—hypodense lesion
  - Isotope brain scan—increased uptake
- Number of lesions
  - Recurrent stroke

General factors
- Age
- Cardiac disease
- Polycythemia
- Hyperglycemia
- Hyperthermia
- Hypertension?

Complicating factors
- Cardiac complications
- Infections
  - Pneumonia
  - Urinary tract infection
  - Septicemia
- Deep venous thrombosis and pulmonary embolism
- Depression
- Seizures
- Recurrent stroke
- Multiinfarct dementia

Source: Hachinski and Norris (1985).

toward the risk factors (Table 6–8). Hypertension is the most important of these factors, and strict control is mandatory. Also important are heart disease, diabetes, TIAs, polycythemia, and smoking (Kannel, 1976).

The only drugs that have been shown to be of benefit in stroke prophylaxis are aspirin as an antiplatelet agent, in doses of 1300 mg per day, and anticoagulants in emboli of cardiac origin. Ticlopidine hydrochloride, another platelet inhibitor, effec-

Table 6–7 Therapeutic Opportunities in the Prevention of Stroke

Asymptomatic phase
- Treatment of risk of factors
- Management of asymptomatic bruits and stenoses

Warning phase
- Diagnosis and management of TIAs and minor strokes

Recurrent phase
- Management to prevent further strokes

Source: Hachinski and Norris (1985).

Table 6–8 Risk Factors for Stroke

Hypertension (diastolic and systolic)
Cardiac disease
- Ischemic/hypertensive
  - Coronary heart disease
  - Myocardial infarction
    - Acute endocardial damage → thrombi
    - Chronic: akinetic segments → thrombi
  - Congestive heart failure
  - Left ventricular hypertrophy
    - On ECG
    - On chest radiograph
- Valvular
  - Rheumatic heart disease
  - Prolapsing mitral valve
  - Endocarditis
    - Infectious
    - Marantic
  - Aortic stenosis
  - Prosthetic heart valves
  - ? Calcified mitral annulus
- Arrhythmias
  - Atrial fibrillation
  - Sick sinus syndrome

Diabetes
Erythrocytosis
Cigarette smoking
Other
- Physical inactivity
- Hyperlipidemia
- Heredity
- Environmental factors

Source: Hachinski and Norris (1985).

tively prevents recurrent stroke, myocardial infarction, and vascular death (Gent et al., 1988), but it is not yet available in North America.

Extracranial to intracranial bypass surgery has limited if any value in the prevention of stroke, and carotid endarterectomy has a good rationale but an unproved record. The best course for patients, physicians, and society at large is to refer suitable candidates to one of several studies being carried out (North American Symptomatic Carotid Endarterectomy Study Group, 1987).

REFERENCES

Barnett, H.J.M. (1982). Platelet antiaggregants in stroke prevention: a review of rational and results. In: H.J.M. Barnett, J. Hirsch, and J.F. Mustard, eds., *Acetylsalicylic Acid: New Uses for an Old Drug,* p. 175. New York: Raven Press.

Bauer, R.B., and Tellez, H. (1973). Dexamethasone as a treatment in cerebrovascular disease. 2. A controlled study in acute cerebral infarction.*Stroke,* **4,** 547–555.

Bogousslavsky, J., and Regli, F. (1984). Cerebral infarction with transient signs (CITS): do TIAs correspond to small deep infarcts in internal carotid artery occlusion? *Stroke,* **15,** 536–539.

Calanchini, P.R., Swanson, P.D., Gotshall, R.A., et al. (1977). Cooperative study of hospital frequency and character of transient ischemic attacks. IV. The reliability of diagnosis. *J.A.M.A.,* **238,** 2029–2033.

Calandre, L, Gomara, S., Bermejo, F., et al. (1984). Clinical CT correlations in TIA, RIND and strokes with minimum residuum. *Stroke,* **15,** 663–666.

Carpenter, R.R., and Reed, D.E. (1972). The outcome for patients with cerebrovascular disease in university and community hospitals. *Stroke,* **3,** 747–758.

Carter, A.B. (1960). Ingravescent cerebral infarction. *Q. J. Med.,* **29,** 611–625.

Clarke, E. (1963). Apoplexy in the Hippocratic writings. *Bull. Hist. Med.,* **37,** 301–314.

Corwin, L.I., Wolf, P.A., Kannel, W.B., and McNamara, P.M. (1982). Accuracy of death certification of stroke: the Framingham Study. *Stroke,* **13,** 818–821.

Dalal, P.M. (1979). Strokes in the young in west central India. *Adv. Neurol.,* **25,** 339.

Drake, W.E., Hamilton, M.J., Carlsson, M., et al. (1973). Acute stroke management and patient outcome: the value of neurovascular care units (NCU).*Stroke,* **4,** 933–945.

Dyken, M., and White, P.T. (1956). Evaluation of cortisone in the treatment of cerebral infarction. *J.A.M.A,* **132,** 1531.

Fries, J.F. (1980). Aging, natural death and the compression of morbidity. *N. Eng. J. Med.,* **303,** 130–135.

Furlan, A.J., Cavalier, S.J., and Hobbs, R.E. (1982). Hemorrhage and anticoagulation after nonseptic embolic brain infarction. *Neurology,* **32,** 280–282.

Futty, D.E., Conneally, M., Dyken, M., et al. (1977). Cooperative study of hospital frequency and character of transient ischemic attacks v. symptom analysis. *J.A.M.A,* **238,** 2386–2390.

Gent, M., Blakely, J.A., Easton, J.D., et al. (1988). The Canadian American Ticlopidine Study (CATS) in thromboembolic stroke. *Stroke,* **19,** 1203–1210.

George, A.E., De Leon, M.J., Gentes, C.T., et al. (1986a). Leukoencephalopathy in normal and pathologic aging. I. CT of brain lucencies. *Am. J. Neuroradiol.,* **7,** 561–566.

George, A.E., De Leon, M.J., Kalnin, A., et al. (1986b). Leukoencephalopathy in normal and pathologic aging. II. MRI of brain lucencies. *Am. J. Neuroradiol.,* **7,** 567–570.

Gurdjian, E.S., and Gurdjian, E.S. (1979). History of occlusive cerebrovascular disease. I. From Wepfer to Moniz. *Arch. Neurol.,* **36,** 340–343.

Hachinski, V.C. (1983). Prognostic indicants in cerebrovascular disease. In: M. Reivich and H.I. Hurtig, eds., *Cerebral Vascular Diseases,* pp. 41–50. New York: Raven Press.

Hachinski, V.C. (1984). Decreased incidence and mortality of stroke. *Stroke,* **15,** 376–378.

Hachinski, V.C., and Norris, J.W. (1981). The deteriorating stroke. In: J.S. Meyer, H. Lechner, M. Reivich, et al., eds., *Cerebral Vascular Disease, Vol. 3,* pp.315–318. Amsterdam: Excerpta Medica.

Hachinski, V.C., and Norris, J.W. (1985). *The Acute Stroke*. Philadelphia: Davis.

Hachinski, V.C., Lassen, N.A., and Marshall, J. (1974). Multi-infarct dementia a cause of mental deterioration in the elderly. *Lancet*, **2**, 207–209.

Hachinski, V.C., Iliff, L.D., Phil, M., Zilhka, E., et al. (1975). Cerebral blood flow in dementia. *Arch. Neurology*, **32**, 634–637.

Hachinski, V.C., Potter, P., and Merskey, H. (1987). Leukoaraiosis. *Arch. Neurol.*, **44**, 21–23.

Haerer, A.F., and Woosley, P.C. (1975). Prognosis and quality of survival in a hospitalized stroke population from the south. *Stroke*, **6**, 543–548.

Hatano, S. (1976). Experience from a multicenter stroke register: a preliminary report. *Bull. W.H.O.*, **54**, 541–553.

Hoedt-Rasmussen, K., Skinhoj, E., Paulson, O., et al. (1967). Regional cerebral blood flow in acute apoplexy: the "luxury perfusion" syndrome of brain tissue. *Arch. Neurol.*, **17**, 271–281.

Jones, H.R., and Millikan, C.H. (1976). Temporal profile (clinical course) of acute carotid system cerebral infarction. *Stroke*, **7**, 64–71.

Kannel, W.B. (1971). Current status of the epidemiology of brain infarction associated with occlusive arterial disease. *Stroke*, **2**, 295–318.

Kannel, W.B. (1976). Epidemiology of cerebrovascular disease. In: R.W. Ross Russell, ed., *Cerebral Arterial Disease*, p. 1. Edinburgh: Churchill-Livingstone.

Kannel, W.B., Wolf, P.A., and Verter, J. (1983). Manifestations of coronary disease predisposing to stroke: the Framingham Study. *J.A.M.A*, **250**, 2942–2946.

Kennedy, F.B., Pozen, T.J., Gabelman, E.H., et al. (1970). Stroke intensive care—an appraisal. *Am. Heart J.*, **80**, 188–196.

Kuller, L.H. (1978). Epidemiology of stroke. *Adv. Neurol.*, **19**, 281.

Kurtzke, J.F. (1980), Epidemiology of cerebrovascular disease. In: R.G. Siekert, ed., *Cerebrovascular Survey Report*, p. 135, Bethesda: National Institute of Neurological and Communicative Disorders and Stroke.

Kurtzke, J.F. (1986). Epidemiology. In: H.J.M. Barnett, J.P. Mohr, B.M. Stein, and F.M. Yatsu, eds., *Stroke: Pathophysiology, Diagnosis and Management*. p. 3. New York: Churchill Livingstone.

Lambo, T.A. (1979). Stroke—a worldwide health problem. *Adv. Neurol.*, **25**, 1–3.

Lassen, N.A., Ingvar, D.H., and Skinhoj, E. (1978). Brain function and blood flow. *Sci. Am.*, **239**, 62–71.

Levy, D.E. (1988). How transient are transient ischemic attacks? *Neurology*, **38**, 674–677.

Loeb, C., Gandolf, C., and Bino, G. (1988). Intellectual impairment and cerebral lesions in multiple cerebral infarcts: a clinical-computed tomography study. *Stroke*, **19**, 560–565.

Mirsen, T.R., and Hachinski, V.C. (1988). Transient ischemic attacks and stroke. *Can. Med. Assoc, J.*, **138**, 1099–1105.

Norris, J.W. (1976). Steroid therapy in acute cerebral infarction. *Arch. Neurol.*, **33**, 69–71.

Norris, J.W., and Hachinski, V.C. (1985). High dose steroid treatment in cerebral infarction. *Br. Med. J.*, **292**, 21–23.

Norris, J.W., Chambers, B.R., Shurvell, B.L., and Hachinski, V.C. (1984). Outcome of brainstem strokes. In: R. Berguer and R.B. Bauer, eds., *Vertebrobasilar Arterial Occlusive Arterial Disease*, pp. 37–44. New York: Raven Press.

North American Symptomatic Carotid Endarterectomy Study Group. (1987). Carotid endarterectomy: three critical evaluations. *Stroke*, **18**, 987–989.

Ostfeld, A.M. (1980). A review of stroke epidemiology. *Epidemiol. Rev.*, **2**, 136–152.

Oxbury, J.M., Greenhall, R.C.D., and Grainger, K.M.R. (1975). Predicting the outcome of stroke: acute stage after cerebral infarction. *Br. Med. J.*, **3**, 125–127.

Phelps, M.E., Mazziotta, J.C., and Huang, S-C. (1982). Study of cerebral function with positron computed tomography. *J. Cereb. Blood Flow Metab.*, **2**, 113–162.

Ransohoff, J., Derby, B., and Kricheff, I. (1971). Spontaneous intracerebral hemorrhage. *Clin. Neurosurg.*, **18,** 247–266.

Rosen, W.G., Terry, R.D., Fuld, P.A., et al. (1980). Pathological verification of ischemic score in differentiation of dementias. *Ann. Neurol.*, **7,** 486–488.

Schiller, F. (1970). Concepts of stroke before and after Virchow. *Med. Hist.*, **14,** 115–131.

Silver, F.L., Norris, J.W., Lewis, A.J., et al. (1984). Early mortality following stroke: a prospective view. *Stroke,* **15,** 492–496.

Steingart, A., Hachinski, V. C., Lau, C., et al., (1987a). Cognitive and neurological findings in subjects with diffuse white matter lucencies on computed tomographic scan (leuko-araiosis). *Arch. Neurol.*, **44,** 32–35.

Steingart, A., Hachinski, V.C., Lau, C., et al. (1987a). Cognitive and neurological findings in demented patients with diffuse white matter lucencies on computed tomographic scan (leuko-araiosis). *Arch. Neurol.*, **44,** 36–39.

Tomlinson, B.E., and Henderson, G. (1976). Some quantitative cerebral findings in normal and demented old people. In: R. D. Terry and S. Gershon, eds., *Neurobiology of Aging, Vol. 3,* New York: Raven Press.

Tomlinson, B.E., Blessed, G., and Roth, M. (1970). Observations on the brains of demented old people. *J. Neurol. Sci.*, **11,** 205–242.

Turnbull, I.W., and Bannister, C.M. (1985). CT observations on the natural history of asymptomatic cerebral infarction following transient ischemic attacks. *Neurol. Res.*, **7,** 190–193.

Wade, J., and Hachinski, V.C. (1986). Revised ischemic score for diagnosis multi-infarct dementia. *J. Clin. Psychiatry,* **47,** 437.

Wade, J.P.H., and Hachinski, V.C. (1987). Multi-infarct dementia. In: B.M. Pitt, ed., *Dementia (Medicine in Old Age),* pp. 209–228. London: Churchill Livingstone.

Wade, J.P.H., Mirsen, T.R., Hachinski, V.C., et al. (1987). The clinical diagnosis of Alzheimer's disease. *Arch. Neurol.*, **44,** 24–29.

Walker, A.E., Robins, M., and Weinfeld, F.D. (1981). Clinical findings. *Stroke,* **12**(suppl 1), 13–31.

Weisberg, L.A., and Lacorte, W.S. (1985). Computerized tomographic abnormalities in patients with transient episodes of focal neurological dysfunction. *Comput. Radiol.*, **9,** 247–254.

Wells, C.E. (1978). Role of stroke in dementia. *Stroke,* **9,** 1–3.

Wells, C.E. (1979). Pseudodementia. *Am. J. Psychiatry,* **136,** 895–900.

Werdelin, L., and Juhler, M. (1988). The course of transient ischemic attacks. *Neurology,* **38,** 677–680.

Whisnant, J.P. (1983). The role of the neurologist in the decline of stroke. *Ann. Neurol.*, **14,** 1–7.

Whisnant, J.P. (1984). The decline of stroke. *Stroke,* **15,** 160–168.

Whisnant, J.P., Fitzgibbons, J.P., Kurland, L.T., et al. (1971). Natural history of stroke in Rochester, Minnesota, 1945 through 1954. *Stroke,* **2,** 11–22.

Wolf, P.A., Dawber, T.R., Thomas, H.E., and Kannel, W.B. (1978). Epidemiologic assessment of chronic atrial fibrillation and risk of stroke: the Framingham Study. *Neurology,* **28,** 973–977.

Wu, Y.K. (1979). Epidemiology and community control of hypertension, stroke and coronary heart disease in China. *Chin. Med. J.*, **92,** 665 [English].

Wylie, C.M. (1972). Epidemiology of cerebrovascular disease. In: P.J. Vinken and G.W. Bruyn, eds., *Handbook of Clinical Neurology, Vol. 11,* P. 183. Amsterdam: North Holland.

Yatsu, F.M. and Mohr, J.P. (1982). Anticoagulation therapy for cardiogenic emboli to the brain. *Neurology,* **32,** 274–275.

7
Cerebrovascular Dementia

JEFFREY L. CUMMINGS AND MICHAEL E. MAHLER

Vascular disease accounts for a major portion of the neurologic morbidity of the elderly and may occur in younger individuals as well. Often the volume, number, or location of the cerebrovascular lesions is sufficient to impair intellectual activities and produce a dementia syndrome (Tomlinson et al., 1970; Benson et al., 1982; Volpe and Petito, 1985). This chapter provides an overview of the vascular dementias. The prevalence, clinical characteristics, neuroimaging, pathology, and treatment of the dementia syndromes produced by cerebrovascular injury are discussed.

Terminology regarding vascular dementia is evolving, and a consensus has not been reached regarding the appropriate names for the vascular dementia syndromes. Multiinfarct dementia (MID) is the most commonly used term; but dementia may occur with hemorrhagic as well as ischemic injuries, and in some cases a single infarction is sufficient to produce a dementia syndrome. Therefore this term may be appropriate for a subset of the vascular dementias but is not broadly inclusive. In this chapter, the term cerebrovascular dementia (CVD) is used to refer to dementing syndromes as a group, whereas MID is used for the specific subgroup of vascular dementias related to multiple ischemic injuries.

PREVALENCE

Few studies have attempted to determine the prevalence of CVD. Difficulties with valid sampling of a large population, detection of dementia within the sampled group and determination that the cause of the dementia was a vascular process represent formidable methodological challenges.

Studies of stroke in the United States indicate a prevalence of approximately 794 per 100,000 individuals. Below age 45, the prevalence was 66 per 100,000; between ages 46 and 65, the prevalence rose to 998 per 100,000; and over age 65 the prevalence was 5063 per 100,000 (Wolf et al., 1984). The number of stroke patients who develop CVD is unknown. Hershey and colleagues (1987) found that 23.5% of stroke patients had CVD and an additional 23.5% had evidence of intellectual impairment without completely fulfilling diagnostic criteria for the syndrome.

In one of the earliest studies to attempt to quantify the prevalence of CVD, Akesson (1969) used hospital and nursing home records to obtain the names of demented patients in the community. A prevalence of CVD of 210 per 100,000 individuals was suggested. Broe et al. (1976) assayed a random community sample of individuals over age 65 and found the prevalence of CVD to be 1856 per 100,000. Sulkava and colleagues (1985), using a Finnish sample, determined the overall prevalence of CVD to be 2700 per 100,000, higher than that found in the United States and Great Britain. The age-specific prevalence was found to be 1900 per 100,000 in 65- to 74-year-olds, 4300 per 100,000 in the 75- to 84-year-old group, and 2500 per 100,000 in those age 85 and above. Thus a prevalence of CVD in the elderly of 1800 to 2700 per 100,000 is indicated by these studies. The variability in the existing studies suggests that the true community prevalence has yet to be determined, that it varies from country to country, and that it may be changing as the prevalence of stroke changes.

Investigations of the prevalence of vascular disease among autopsied dementia patients have also been reported. Tomlinson et al. (1968, 1970) studied the brains of 50 patients with severe chronic dementia and 28 nondemented elderly subjects. Only 20% of the brains of dementia patients and 28% of the controls were free of ischemic injuries. Infarctions exceeding 20 ml in volume were significantly more common in the demented group (40% versus 21% in the controls). Histologic study suggested that one-half of the 50 patients had Alzheimer's disease (AD) as the principle cause of the dementia, 17% had CVD, and 16% percent had mixed CVD–AD. Todorov and colleagues (1975) found that of 682 patients with dementia studied pathologically 19% had CVD and 37% had combined CVD–AD. Autopsy studies do not lend themselves to demographic extrapolation but do suggest that among patients with fatal dementing illnesses CVD accounts for 15 to 20% of cases and contributes to another 15 to 35%.

Together, the different approaches to the demography of CVD indicate that it accounts for 20% or more of dementia syndromes and contributes to an additional 15 to 20%. About 25 to 50% of stroke patients eventually develop CVD.

CLINICAL CHARACTERISTICS

Clinical History

Hachinski and colleagues (1975) developed an Ischemia Scale to call attention to the historical and examination findings typical of CVD (Table 7–1). Most studies have confirmed that these scale items are cardinal clinical symptoms. An abrupt onset and stepwise deterioration have been observed in CVD in several studies (Hachinski et al., 1975; Rosen et al., 1980; Gustafson and Nilsson, 1982). These typical historical

Table 7–1. Clinical Features and Relative Importance Assigned to Each Element in the Ischemia Scale

Characteristics	Assigned Weight
Historical features	
Abrupt onset	2
Stepwise deterioration	1
Fluctuating course	2
Nocturnal confusion	1
History of hypertension	1
History of strokes	2
Focal neurological symptoms	2
Examination findings	
Relative personality preservation	1
Depression	1
Somatic complaints	1
Emotional incontinence	1
Evidence of associated atherosclerosis	1
Focal neurological signs	2
Total possible score 18; score of 7 or higher is consistent with CVD.	

Source: Hachinski et al. (1975).

features are not present in all cases, however, and CVD patients may have courses characterized by insidious deterioration, partial intellectual recovery, or periods of stability (Hershey et al., 1987).

Hypertension is the most common risk factor for CVD, and a history of hypertension is found in 80% of CVD patients (Hachinski et al., 1975; Ladurner et al., 1982a; St. Clair and Whalley, 1983; Bucht et al., 1984; Tresch et al., 1985). Other cardiovascular abnormalities are also common. Patients manifest an increased frequency of retinal vascular abnormalities, heart murmurs, angina, heart failure, and electrocardiographic (ECG) abnormalities (St. Clair and Whalley, 1983; Bucht et al., 1984; Tresch et al., 1985). The likelihood that a dementia syndrome is vascular in origin is also increased if there is evidence of a past myocardial infarction (Hontela and Schwartz, 1979).

A history of focal neurologic symptoms, e.g., transient ischemic attacks (TIAs), or of completed strokes is also common in CVD (Hachinski et al., 1975; Rosen et al., 1980; Loeb and Gandolfo, 1983; Kotsoris et al., 1987). In the study by Ladurner et al. (1982a) most CVD patients exhibited symptoms involving the dominant hemisphere (24 of 37) or occurring bilaterally (9 of 37). Localized right hemisphere symptoms occurred in only 11% of patients (4 of 37).

Neurologic Examination

Focal abnormalities on the neurologic examination reflect localized brain injury and support a diagnosis of CVD (Hachinski et al., 1975; Rosen et al., 1980; Loeb and Gondolfo, 1983; Bucht et al., 1984). Bucht et al. (1984) found that 70% of CVD patients had focal signs, and Ladurner and coworkers (1982a) found that 63% had focal abnormalities and 8% had symmetric disturbances. Sluss and colleagues (1982) found the following frequencies of neurologic findings among 13 CVD patients: abnormal gait 92%, facial asymmetry 69%, visual disturbances 62%, aphasia or dysarthria 54%, limb weakness 46%. Psychomotor slowing, muscular rigidity, incontinence, and gait changes have been emphasized as particularly common accompaniments of CVD (Bruetsch and Williams, 1954; Ishii et al., 1986; Hershey et al., 1987; Kotsories et al., 1987; Roman, 1987). Occasionally, CVD mimics the neurologic syndromes of Parkinson's disease or progressive supranuclear palsy (de Reuck et al., 1980; Dubinsky and Jankovic, 1987). It is notable that up to 30% of CVD patients have normal neurologic examinations (Bucht et al., 1984; Ladurner et al., 1982a).

Cognitive Aspects

There have been few studies of the neuropsychological features of CVD. Perez et al. (1975) found that when the performance of patients with MID, vertebrobasilar insufficiency with dementia, and Alzheimer's disease were compared on standard neuropsychological tests, the latter were the most impaired, the vertebrobasilar group was least impaired, and the MID sample exhibited an intermediate dementia severity. Using the Wechsler Adult Intelligence Scale, Perez and colleagues (1976) also demonstrated that MID patients were relatively more impaired on the performance subscales than Alzheimer's disease patients.

Language alterations in CVD have been more rigorously investigated. Ladurner et al. (1982a) noted that, among 37 CVD patients, 18 had an identifiable aphasia syndrome. Hier and colleagues (1985) compared CVD and Alzheimer's disease patients and found that the former had more of a "Brocoid" type output with shortened phrase length, restricted lexical variability, and simplified syntax. Bayles and Tomoeda (1983) and Powell and colleagues (1988) demonstrated that CVD patients have naming impairments that are less severe than those of comparably demented Alzheimer's disease patients. The language changes in CVD correlate with the overall dementia severity and with the amount of tissue loss as reflected in ventricular enlargement on computed tomography (CT) (Aharon-Peretz and Cummings, 1988; Powell et al., 1988 Cummings, 1989).

Specific CVD syndromes with more unique patterns of neuropsychological deficits are described below (Subtypes of Vascular Dementia).

Neuropsychiatric Aspects

Psychosis and depression are the two principal neuropsychiatric disorders reported with CVD. Delusions occur in up to 50% of CVD patients at some point in the course of their illness (Cummings et al., 1987; Leuchter and Spar, 1985). The patients entertain false beliefs involving threats of personal harm, theft of belongings, or marital infidelity. Occasional cases of Capgras syndrome (believing that one's spouse or other important person has been replaced by an identical-appearing imposter) have been described (Cummings et al., 1987). There is little correlation between the occurrence of delusions and the severity of dementia.

Depression is also common in CVD. Cummings and coworkers (1987) found that 25% of CVD patients had major depressive episodes and 60% exhibited depressive symptoms, whereas 17% of patients with Alzheimer's disease had symptoms and none experienced a major mood disorder. Bucht et al. (1984) also found depression to be common in CVD, occurring in 32% of patients. Depression is a component of the Ischemia Scale, and its presence supports the diagnosis of CVD (Hachinski et al., 1975; Gustafson and Nilsson, 1982). The components of the depression syndrome accompanying CVD are identical to those of idiopathic major depression.

ELECTROENCEPHALOGRAPHY

Electroencephalographic (EEG) abnormalities are present in most CVD patients (Table 7–2). Results of existing studies have varied considerably regarding the type of abnormality observed. Approximately 25% of patients have normal EEGs, and 75% have generalized slowing, focal abnormalities, or both (Roberts et al., 1978; Harrison et al., 1979; Striano et al., 1981; Bucht et al., 1984).

NEUROIMAGING

Imaging studies of CVD have involved primarily x-ray CT. More recently, new technologies such as magnetic resonance imaging (MRI), positron emission tomography (PET), and single photon emission computed tomography (SPECT) have also been employed.

X-Ray Computed Tomography

The CT abnormalities in CVD include discrete infarcts, white matter low density areas, and diffuse atrophy (Ladurner et al., 1982a,b; Erkinjuntti et al., 1984, 1987). Ladurner and colleagues (1982a) reported that among 40 patients with CVD 2 had normal CT scans, 9 had atrophy as the only visible abnormality, 16 had unilateral infarcts (equally distributed between the hemispheres), and 13 had bilateral infarcts. Ladurner et al. (1982b) also reported CT findings from 204 patients with ischemic strokes, 84 of whom were demented. Only one of the 84 had a normal scan, whereas 76 demonstrated infarcts and 73 had atrophy. In 39 the infarcts were multiple and bilateral, in 7 multiple and unilateral, and in 30 single. Atrophy and multiple, bilateral infarcts occurred more frequently in demented than nondemented stroke patients.

The high frequency of visible infarcts reported by Ladurner and colleagues contrasts with a study by Roberts et al. (1978), who found no CT evidence of infarct in 62% of CVD patients. Methodologic differences could account for the discrepancy of results: Ladurner et al. looked for demented subjects among identified stroke

Table 7–2 Results of Investigations Reporting EEG Abnormalities in CVD

Study	No.	Normal	Generalized Slowing	Focal Abnormalities
Roberts et al. (1978)	57	11 (19%)	22 (39%)	24 (42%)
Harrison et al. (1979)	21	NR	NR	8 (38%)
Striano et al. (1981)	30	NR	18 (60%)	12 (40%)
Bucht et al. (1984)	20	4 (20%)	3 (15%)	13 (65%)

NR = not reported.

patients, whereas Roberts and colleagues looked for infarctions in those identified first on the basis of cognitive impairment.

The size of ischemic lesions varies according to the type and etiology of CVD. Small deep lesions, lacunar infarctions, are characteristic of the most common type of CVD. According to Fisher (1965) only 17% of lacunar infarctions are larger than 1 cm in diameter. This point has particular relevance to early studies using CT scans with limited spatial resolution, as infarctions smaller than 2 cm in diameter are not visible on most CT scans (Kinkel, 1988).

Atrophy or periventricular areas of white matter low attenuation occur but are not specific for CVD. Whereas 88.6% of patients with definite CVD and 41.3% of patients with probable CVD demonstrated CT lesions consistent with infarcts, only 1.5% of Alzheimer's disease patients had a discrete lesion (Erkinjuntti et al., 1987). At the same time, white matter low attenuation occurred in 72.1%, 50.0%, and 19.1% of these groups, respectively. The CT scans of 10 to 15% of the normal elderly and 30 to 40% of Alzheimer's disease patients show these white matter changes (London et al., 1986; Inzitari et al., 1987; Steingart et al., 1987a,b).

Magnetic Resonance Imaging

Magnetic resonance imaging appears to be more sensitive than CT for defining the existence and extent of cerebrovascular ischemic lesions (Figure 7–1) (DeWitt et al., 1985; Salgado et al., 1986; Kertesz et al., 1987), although CT is superior for detecting acute intracerebral hemorrhage (Kertesz et al., 1987). MRI sequences that yield a mixture of T_1- and T_2-weighted images demonstrate ischemic infarctions in the subcortical and periventricular white matter particularly well (Kistler et al., 1984; Salgado et al., 1986). Preliminary studies of small numbers of CVD patients (Besson et al., 1983, 1985; Erkinjuntti et al., 1984) suggest that focal hypodense areas on T_1 images, increased white matter proton density, and increased T_2 signals are characteristic.

Although the sensitivity of MRI is high in ischemic infarcts, 10 to 20% of strokes may be missed by MRI, with sensitivity declining with elapsed time after the event (Kertesz et al., 1987). Cortical infarctions are least well seen (Salgado et al., 1986).

The specificity of MRI findings must be defined in relation to differentiation of CVD from other types of dementia, determining criteria that distinguish between pathologic lesions and changes seen in normal elderly, and correlating observed lesions with the symptoms of dementia. Erkinjuntti et al. (1987) examined 29 CVD patients and 22 Alzheimer's disease patients with both MRI and CT. Of the 29 CVD patients, 19 (65.5%) demonstrated infarctions by MRI, whereas 18 (62.1%) of the CT scans showed infarction. No Alzheimer's disease patients had infarcts detected by either technique. All of the CVD patients showed periventricular white matter changes on the MRI, whereas 8 of the 22 DAT patients did also. CT detected similar changes in 26 (89.7%) of the CVD patients but in only one of the Alzheimer's group. The sensitivity of MRI was 100% when either infarcts or white matter changes were seen versus 96.6% for CT. Both methods were highly specific when infarcts were seen, but only the CT was specific when white matter changes were evaluated.

Hershey et al. (1987) compared demented and nondemented patients with ischemic cerebrovascular disease using MRI. All eight demented patients had white mat-

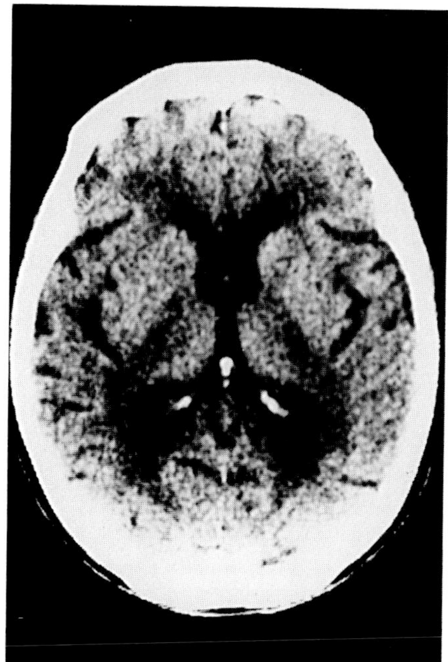

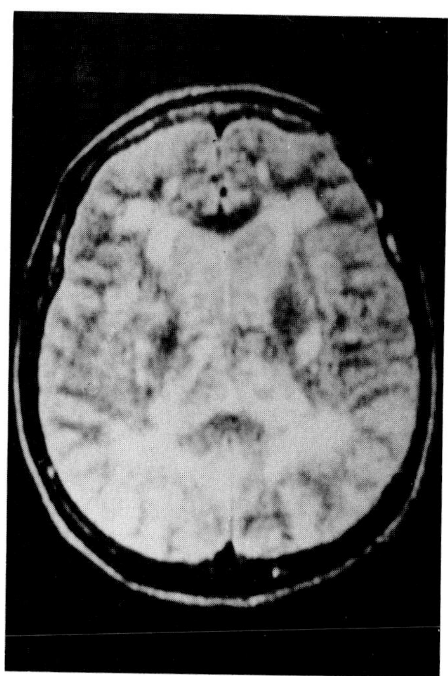

Figure 7–1 CT scan (right) and MRI (left) of a patient with Binswanger's disease. The CT shows excessive periventricular lucencies, and the MRI reveals pathologic high signal lesions in the same regions.

ter lesions in the cortex, basal ganglia, or periventricular white matter. The latter site was involved most commonly. However, these changes were seen in five of eight patients with equivocal evidence of CVD and 11 of 18 nondemented patients. One-half of the demented patients had enlarged central cerebrospinal fluid spaces, compared to only 6% of the nondemented group. Cortical cerebrospinal fluid spaces were enlarged in one-half of each group.

The high signal lesions seen in white matter on MRI and the low density areas seen on CT of most CVD patients also occur in some elderly patients without clinical evidence of stroke or overt dementia (Goto et al., 1981; Bradley et al., 1984; Brant-Zawadzki et al., 1985; Zimmerman et al., 1985; London et al., 1986; Inzitari et al., 1987; Steingart et al., 1987a,b). The periventricular changes correlate with the presence of cerebrovascular risk factors (Gerard and Weisberg, 1986; Sarpel et al., 1987); and pathologically the MRI findings reflect imcomplete infarctions (Englund et al., 1987; Kirkpatrick and Hayman, 1987). Thus mild ischemic lesions may occur in those without dementia and those with nonvascular dementia syndromes; the severity of the white matter changes may prove useful for differentiating among these clinical groups (Aharon-Peretz et al., 1988).

Cerebral Blood Flow and Metabolic Imaging Techniques

Whereas CT and MRI result in images of brain structure, other techniques are available to produce images corresponding to cerebral blood flow (CBF) and metabolism (see Chapters 3 and 4).

In a seminal study Hachinski and colleagues (1975) classified a group of patients into those with primary degenerative dementia and those with MID. They found that CBF, measured by the ^{133}Xe inhalation technique, was reduced in the MID group but not in the primary degenerative dementia group. There was an inverse relation between the degree of dementia and the CBF in the MID group.

Despite the promising findings of Hachinski and colleagues, determining mean CBF does not help in the diagnosis of CVD because it can be reduced in a variety of diseases, including Alzheimer's disease (Rogers et al., 1986; Deutsch and Tweedy, 1987). However, patchy changes with reductions of regional flow (rCBF) occur in CVD prior to the onset of dementia symptoms, whereas in Alzheimer's disease CBF is reduced following dementia onset (Rogers et al., 1986).

SPECT utilizes either an iodine-123-labeled iodoamphetamine tracer (IMP) or a technetium-99-labeled hexamethylpropylene amineoxine (HMPAO) to create a tomographic image of cerebral perfusion and rCBF. In CVD, SPECT shows a pattern of multiple, asymmetric flow defects involving both white and gray matter or gray matter alone (Cohen et al., 1986). In Alzheimer's disease, SPECT shows a predominantly symmetric reduction of perfusion in the temporoparietal regions (Jagust et al., 1987; Johnson et al., 1987). With improved resolution and more widespread availability, SPECT may become an important tool for the diagnosis of CVD.

Like SPECT, PET creates tomographic images utilizing energetic emissions from specially prepared isotopes. When labeled oxygen is used as a positron emitter, regional cerebral oxygen utilization is measured. The use of 18-fluorodeoxyglucose (FDG) allows the measurement of regional glucose metabolism.

There have been only a few studies of PET with CVD patients. Frackowiak and coworkers (1981) measured CBF, oxygen utilization, and oxygen extraction in normals, CVD patients, and Alzheimer's disease patients. The CBF and oxygen utilization were reduced in both patient groups, with parietotemporal defects in the Alzheimer's disease group and more variable, but predominantly parietal, defects in the CVD group. Regional changes of CBF and oxygen utilization were coupled in the CVD patients, leading to the conclusion that there was no chronic ischemia as a cause of dementia symptoms.

Benson et al. (1983) reported on a small number of CVD patients studied with the FDG-PET method. Multiple asymmetric regions of glucose hypometabolism were seen. This pattern contrasted with the bilaterally symmetric frontal and parietal hypometabolism reported in Alzheimer's disease by these and other investigators (Benson et al., 1983; Foster et al., 1983, 1984). PET is a promising research technique for understanding the pathophysiology of CVD, but it is not sufficiently widely available to support clinical diagnosis.

SUBTYPES OF VASCULAR DEMENTIA

There are several syndromes within CVD corresponding to the pattern of cerebral injury, the size of the blood vessel involved, and the etiology of the vascular disorder (Cummings and Benson, 1983). The clinical features and pathology of the principal subsyndromes are summarized in Table 7–3.

Table 7–3 Subtypes of Cerebrovascular Dementia

Syndrome	Pathologic Anatomy
Lacunar state	Lacunar infarctions in the basal ganglia, internal capsule, and related deep hemispheric structures
Binswanger's disease	Ischemic lesions in hemisphere white matter with sparing of u-fibers (lacunar state often coexists)
Thalamic dementia	Paramedian thalamic and rostral midbrain infarctions
Border zone syndrome	Infarction of cortical and subcortical border zone regions produced by bilateral carotid occlusion or systemic hypotension
Angular gyrus syndrome	Infarction of the left angular gyrus region (inferior parietal lobule).
Microangiopathy	Innumerable small infarctions of the cerebral cortex

Lacunar State

Lacunes are small infarctions located preferentially in the deep hemispheric regions, brain stem, and cerebellum; they result from occlusion of penetrating branches of the major cerebral arteries. Vascular occlusion in lacunar state usually results from hyaline changes of the vessel wall produced by long-standing hypertension. Recognized clinical syndromes produced by single lacunar infarctions include pure sensory strokes, pure motor strokes, ataxic hemiparesis, dysarthria-clumsy hand syndrome, and Wallenberg's lateral medullary syndrome (Fisher, 1982). When multiple lacunes occur, the syndrome is known as a lacunar state, and dementia is commonly present.

Ishii et al. (1986) reported that among 30 patients with a minimum of six lacunes and no complicating cortical infarcts or other pathology, all had abulia-aspontaneity, 80% had dysarthria, 73% were incontinent, 67% had mood disturbances, 63% had lower limb spasticity, and 57% had gait abnormalities. Dubinsky and Jankovic (1987) reported that 79% of patients with lacunar state imitating progressive supranuclear palsy had dementia syndromes. Critchley (1929), Alvarez (1946), Bruetsch and Williams (1954), and Hughes and colleagues (1954) emphasized the occurrence of bradyphrenia, cognitive deterioration, and mood alterations in patients with lacunar state.

The locations of lacunes associated with dementia include the striatum (caudate and putamen), internal capsule, thalamus, subthalamic nucleus, and rostral brain stem (Critchley, 1929; Rothschild, 1942; Alvarez, 1946; Hughes et al., 1954; de Reuck et al., 1980, 1982; Ishii et al., 1986).

Computed tomography reveals lacunar infarcts in 40 to 70% of patients with appropriate clinical syndrome (Roberts et al., 1978; Donnan et al., 1982), and MRI demonstrates small punctuate lesions in the deep gray or white matter (Hershey et al., 1987).

Binswanger's Disease

Binswanger's disease (also known as subcortical arteriosclerotic encephalopathy, SAE) is a gradually progressive syndrome resulting from ischemic injury to the deep white matter of the cerebral hemispheres. It is associated with occlusion of the lumens of the deep penetrating arterioles (Olszewski, 1962; Babikan and Ropper, 1987; Roman, 1987). Clinically, the patients manifest a dementia syndrome, asymmetric weakness, pyramidal tract signs, and pseudobulbar palsy. Extrapyramidal system dysfunction occurs in some patients but is less common than pyramidal tract abnormalities (Caplan and Schoene, 1978; Loizou et al., 1981).

Pathologically, Binswanger's disease is characterized by demyelination of the hemispheric white matter, sparing the short arcuate fibers. There is loss of myelin and oligodendroglia as well as the presence of astrogliosis. The penetrating white matter vessels show fibrohyaline thickening. The ventricular system is enlarged, and lacunes are frequently present in the deep gray matter structures (Roman, 1987).

Computed tomography reveals symmetric lucent regions in the periventricular regions, and MRI reveals high signal areas on T_2-weighted images in the periventricular areas, extending irregularly into the white matter of the corona radiata (Figure 7–1) (Rosenberg et al., 1979; Roman, 1987). These findings may occur to at least a limited extent in other disorders and cannot be regarded as pathognomonic of Binswanger's disease.

Thalamic Dementia

Thalamic dementia is a CVD syndrome resulting from bilateral occlusion of the thalamosubthalamic paramedian artery with bilateral infarction of anterior medial thalamus. Clinically, the patients have an initial period of stupor or coma and ocular motility deficits. This phase is followed by partial recovery with a subcortical dementia syndrome, including visuospatial, memory, and personality changes. Language alterations (initial muteness followed by anomia and paraphasia) are present if the left thalamus is the predominant site of infarction (Guberman and Stuss, 1983; Graff-Radford et al., 1984). Abnormal movements such as tremor or asterixis may emerge during the recovery period (Castaigne et al., 1981).

Pathologically, there is infarction bilaterally of the median, central, intralaminar, and parafascicular nuclei. In most cases the red nuclei, fasciculus retroflexus, median reticular nuclei, substantia nigra, superior cerebellar peduncle, and medial cerebral peduncle are also encompassed within the infarcted region (Castaigne et al., 1981). The infarcts can usually be visualized by CT (Guberman and Stuss, 1983; Graff-Radford et al., 1984).

Large Vessel Syndromes

Lacunar state, Binswanger's disease, and thalamic dementia result from occlusion of small penetrating arterioles. Large vessel occlusion may also produce CVD. Two recognized large vessel syndromes are (1) dementia with bilateral carotid artery occlusion producing border zone infarctions; and (2) angular gyrus syndrome.

In the border zone syndrome, there is ischemic injury to the cortex in the regions between the primary distributions of the anterior, middle, and posterior cerebral arteries. Superficial border zone infarctions involve primarily the lateral convexities of the hemisphere, and deep border zone lesions occupy the corner of the lateral ventricles in the hemispheric white matter. Border zone lesions may occur with occlusion of the carotid arteries or systemic hypotension. The resulting syndrome is characterized by a mixed transcortical aphasia combined with visuospatial, memory, and personality abnormalities.

Angular gyrus syndrome results from a branch occlusion of the left middle cerebral artery with infarction of the inferior parietal lobule. The resulting clinical syndrome includes anomia, Gerstmann's syndrome (agraphia, right-left disorientation, finger agnosia, acalculia), alexia, and verbal amnesia, and may be mistaken for Alzheimer's disease (Benson et al., 1982). The patient may have a normal neurologic examination, or there may be subtle right-sided abnormalities. Posterior left-hemispheric dysfunction may be revealed by EEG, CT, MRI, or PET.

In general, the large vessel syndromes are comprised of disturbances consistent with dysfunction of cerebral cortex, whereas the small vessel disorders produce more subcortical dysfunction.

Microangiopathy

A rare cause of CVD results from progressive diffuse occlusion of the small arterial vessels supplying the cerebral cortex as well as other body regions (Torvik et al., 1971). Clinically, the patients exhibit progressive aphasia, memory loss, and cortical blindness, as well as advancing motor and sensory dysfunction. Autopsy studies reveal multiple infarctions of the cerebral cortex and other organs.

ETIOLOGIES AND RISK FACTORS

Thrombotic Disorders

It is currently assumed that the risk factors for CVD are the same as those for thrombotic stroke. Hypertension is the principal determinant. Other factors that increase the likelihood of stroke and CVD include diabetes, hyperlipidemia, and cigarette smoking (Rogers et al., 1983; Abbot et al., 1987; Meyer et al., 1987). The risk of stroke is also elevated in men and in nonwhites (Schoenberg et al., 1986).

Table 7–4 summarizes the thrombotic and nonthrombotic disorders that may produce dementia syndromes and are considered in the differential diagnosis of CVD. Among the rare causes of thrombosis are amyloidosis, fibromuscular dysplasia, Fabry disease, homocystinuria, Moyamoya disease, pseudoxanthoma elasticum, radiation-induced vasculopathy, and neoplastic angioendotheliosis (Cummings and Benson, 1983).

Nonthrombotic Disorders

Embolic disorders produce multiple branch artery occlusions. Fibrin–platelet emboli may arise from cardiac valve diseases or carotid artery changes. Other substances can

Table 7–4 Etiologies of Cerebrovascular Dementia

Thrombosis
Atherosclerosis
Arteriosclerosis
Diabetic vasculopathy
Amyloidosis
Fibromuscular dysplasia
Fabry disease
Homocystinuria
Moyamoya disease
Pseudoxanthoma elasticum
Radiation-induced injury
Neoplastic angioendotheliosis
Emboli
Cardiac origin
Large vessel origin
Hemorrhage
Direct brain injury
Posthemorrhagic hydrocephalus
Hemosiderosis (with recurrent hemorrhage)
Aneurysm
Obstructive hydrocephalus
Cerebral hemorrhage
Inflammatory (infectious and noninfectious)
Cerebritis
Thrombotic occlusion
"Pipe stem" basilar artery
Obstructive hydrocephalus
Hypotension
Border zone (gray or white matter) infarction
Medial temporal lobe ischemia

also enter the vascular system, such as tumor cells, air, fat, bacteria, parasites, ova, or injected foreign bodies.

Cerebral hemorrhage can cause direct brain injury at the hemorrhagic site, produce posthemorrhagic obstructive hydrocephalus, or result in central nervous system hemosiderosis if hemorrhage is recurrent. Arteriovenous malformations may steal cerebral blood flow from adjacent tissues or they may rupture and bleed into surrounding tissues. Likewise, cerebral aneurysms may cause obstructuve hydrocephalus or, if they rupture, produce hemorrhage-related CVD (see Chapter 10).

Infectious and noninfectious inflammatory disease may produce diffuse cerebritis or may cause an inflammatory vasculitis with multiple branch occlusions. Calcified "pipe stem" basilar arteries intrude into the floor of the third ventricle, occluding the cerebral aqueduct and causing obstructive hydrocephalus. Hypotension leads to cerebral ischemia and can produce several types of CVD. there may be injury in the cortical border zone or the damage may occur in the deep border zone in the white matter at the corner of the lateral ventricles. Hypotension can also produce a bilateral medial temporal lobe ischemia syndrome with CVD (Volpe and Petito, 1985).

TREATMENT

Two types of treatment are pursued in CVD: (1) therapy of the underlying etiologic disorders and risk factors; and (2) treatment of secondary behavioral disturbances and physical complications (Cummings, 1987). Improved control of hypertension (to the upper limits of normal) results in improved cognition in hypertensive CVD patients, and abstinence from cigarette smoking enhances intellectual performance in normotensive CVD patients (Meyer et al., 1986). Aspirin therapy (in dosages of 325–1300 mg/day) decreases the risk of stroke and presumably slows the progression of CVD (Dyken, 1979). Antibiotics, anticoagulants, or steroids are indicated only in specific disease-related circumstances.

Treatable complications of CVD include psychosis, depression, pseudobulbar palsy, spasticity, and seizures. Depression accompanying stroke syndromes may be treated with antidepressants that produce limited side effects, such as nortriptyline or trazodone (Reding et al., 1983; Lipsey et al., 1984). Psychosis leading to agitation or bizarre behavior may be successfully treated with conservative doses of high potency (i.e., fluphenazine hydrochloride, haloperidol) or low potency (i.e., thioridazine) agents (Cummings, 1988). Aggressive or impulsive behavior may improve with small doses of major tranquilizers, lithium, carbamazepine, or propranolol hydrochloride (Elliott, 1977; Yudofsky et al., 1984). Pseudobulbar palsy may respond to conventional doses of levodopa or amantadine hydrochloride or to low-dosage tricyclic antidepressant therapy (amitriptyline 50–75 mg/day, doxepin 100 mg/day) (Wolf et al., 1979; Schiffer et al., 1983; Udaka et al., 1984). Dantrolene sodium (up to 100 mg q.i.d.) may relieve spasticity and improve gait and coordination; seizures should be treated with phenytoin or carbamazepine (dosages to be determined by serum anticonvulsant levels). Occupational, physical, and speech therapy may help optimize the patient's functional abilities.

Patients with CVD frequently have coexisting cardiac or renal diseases that require careful monitoring and surveillance. When CVD becomes severely disabling, the patient's hydration, nutrition, and skin integrity must be ensured. Optimization of general health maximizes cerebral function, and minimization of drug use avoids potential toxic complications.

CONCLUDING COMMENTS

Although we know much about cerebrovascular dementia, several fundamental questions remain unanswered. One that has stimulated considerable debate involves the precise criteria necessary for a diagnosis of CVD (Brust, 1988; O'Brien, 1988). Published criteria vary on the type, location, and amount of ischemic change required to support the pathologic diagnosis of MID and other types of CVD (Tomlinson et al., 1970; Molsa et al., 1985; Erkinjuntti et al., 1988; Tierney et al., 1988). Clinical diagnosis is heavily dependent on the criteria embodied in the Hachinski Ischemia Score (Hachinski et al., 1975), but some authors have questioned the validity of this instrument (Liston and LaRue, 1983).

The contribution of CVD to the cognitive and cerebral changes seen during aging and in Alzheimer's disease is also an unresolved issue. Awad and colleagues (1986) have suggested that the white matter anomalies seen on imaging studies of nondemented elderly individuals might contribute to the neuropsychological changes observed with normal aging. Similarly, Steingart et al. (1987a) have reported that deep white matter anomalies seen on CT and MRI are associated with low psychometric scores. Englund and colleagues (1987, 1988) suggested that deep white matter changes commonly found in Alzheimer's disease reflect a cerebrovascular disorder. Furthermore, the presence of deep white matter changes on imaging studies predicted greater cognitive impairment among mildly to moderately impaired Alzheimer's disease patients (Steingart et al., 1987b).

The pathophysiologic mechanisms of CVD have yet to be determined. In the angular gyrus syndrome (Benson et al., 1982) the relation between the clinical symptoms and the underlying lesion is clear, but in many cases of CVD the lesions occur in subcortical gray matter and deep white matter pathways (Fisher, 1965, 1982; Tomlinson et al., 1970) making correlations between the lesions and loss of function more obscure. Fisher (1965, 1982) and Tomlinson and colleagues (1970) suggested that dementia is associated with a large total volume of infarcted tissue (more than 100 ml). Brust (1983) concluded that the locations of the lesions were most important, and that the mere presence of an infarct did not prove that the infarct led to the dementia syndrome. Hachinski et al. (1975) proposed that CBF was inadequate to the metabolic needs of the brain in CVD. Glucose PET studies of CVD have demonstrated multiple, focal, asymmetric areas of hypometabolism as well as global reductions in glucose metabolic rates (Benson et al., 1983), indicating an important relation between the infarcted areas and the dementia. Which, if any, of these factors is primarily responsible for the cognitive decline remains an open question. It is probable that multiple pathophysiologic mechanisms exist to account for the various subtypes of CVD.

These fundamental questions have made CVD an active topic of research. Current investigations will lead to new ideas that will not only clarify the nature of CVD but will influence general theories of dementia, aging, and the neurologic basis of intellectual function.

ACKNOWLEDGMENTS

This project was supported by the Veterans Administration and by a VA Merit Review Grant. The manuscript was prepared by Ms. Norene Hiekel.

REFERENCES

Abbot, R.D., Donahue, R.P., MacMahon, S.W., Reed, D.M., and Yano, K. (1987). Diabetes and the risk of stroke. *J.A.M.A.*, **257,** 949–952.

Aharon-Peretz, J., and Cummings, J. L., and Hill, M.A., (1988). Vascular dementia and dementia of the Alzheimer type: cognition, ventricular size and leuko-araiosis. *Arch. Neurol.*, **45,** 719–721.

Akesson, H.D. (1969). A population of senile and arteriosclerotic psychosis. *Hum. Hered.* **19,** 546–566.

Alvarez, W.C. (1946). Cerebral arteriosclerosis with small, commonly unrecognized apoplexies. *Geriatrics,* **1,** 189–216.

Awad, I.A., Spetzler, R.F., Hodak, J.A., Awad, C.A., and Carey, R. (1986). Incidental subcortical lesions identified on magnetic resonance imaging in the elderly. I. Correlation with age and cerebrovascular risk factors. *Stroke,* **17,** 1084–1089.

Babikan, V., and Ropper, A.H. (1987). Binswanger's disease: a review. *Stroke,* **18,** 2–12.

Bayles, K.A., and Tomoeda, C.K. (1983). Confrontation naming in dementia. *Brain Lang.,* **19,** 98–114.

Benson, D.F., Cummings, J.L., and Tsai, S.Y. (1982). Angular gyrus syndrome simulating Alzheimer's disease. *Arch. Neurol.* **39,** 616–620.

Benson, D.F., Kuhl, D.E., Hawkins, R.A., Phelps, M.E., Cummings, J.L., and Tsai, S.Y. (1983). The fluorodeoxyglucose F-18 scan in Alzheimer's disease and multi-infarct dementia. *Arch. Neurol.,* **40,** 711–714.

Besson, J.A.O., Corrigan, F.M., Foreman, E.I., Ashcroft, G.W., Eastwood, L.M., and Smith, F.W. (1983). Differentiating senile dementia of the Alzheimer type and multi-infarct dementia by proton NMR imaging. *Lancet,* **2,** 789.

Besson, J.A.O., Corrigan, F.M., Foreman, E.I., Eastwood, L.M., Smith, F.W., and Ashcroft, G.W. (1985). Nuclear magnetic resonance (NMR). II. Imaging in dementia. *Br. J. Psychiatry,* **146,** 31–35.

Bradley, W.G., Waluch, V., Brant-Zawadzki, M., Yadley, R.A., and Wycoff, R.W. (1984). Patchy, periventricular white matter lesions in the elderly: a common observation during NMR imaging. *Noninvas. Med. Imag.,* **1,** 35–41.

Brant-Zawadski, M., Fein, G., Van Dyke, C., Kiernan, R., Davenport, L., and de Groot, J. (1985). MR imaging of the aging brain: patchy white matter lesions and dementia. *Am. J. Neuroradiol.,* **6,** 657–682.

Broe, G.A., Akhtar, A.J., Andrews, G.R., Caird, F.I., Gilmore, A.J., and McLennan, W.J. (1976). Neurological disorders in the elderly at home. *J Neurol. Neurosurg. Psychiatry,* **39,** 362–366.

Bruetsch, W.L., and Williams, C.L. (1954) Arteriosclerotic muscular rigidity with special reference to gait disturbances. *Am. J. Psychiatry,* **111,** 332–336.

Brust, J.C.M. (1983). Vascular dementia-still over diagnosed. *Stroke,* **14,** 298–300.

Brust, J.C.M. (1988). Vascular dementia is overdiagnosed. *Arch. Neurol.,* **45,** 799–800.

Bucht, G., Adolfson, R., and Winblad, B. (1984). Dementia of the Alzhemier type and multi-infarct dementia: a clinical description and diagnostic problems. *J. Am. Geriatr. Soc.,* **32,** 491–497.

Caplan, L.R., and Schoene, W.C. (1978). Clinical features of subcortical arteriosclerotic encephalopathy (Binswanger disease). *Neurology,* **25,** 1206–1215.

Castaigne, P., Lhermitte, F., Buge, A., Escourolle, R., Hauw, J. J., and Lyon-Caen O. (1981). Paramedian thalamic and midbrain infarcts: clinical and neuropathological study. *Ann. Neurol.,* **10,** 127–148.

Cohen, M.B., Graham, L.S., Kale, R., Metter, E.J., Fitten, J., Kulkarni, M.K., Sevrin, R., Yamada, L., Chang, C.C., Woodruff, N., and Kling, A.S. (1986). Diagnosis of Alzheimer's disease and multiple infarct dementia by tomographic imaging of iodine-123 IMP. *J. Nucl. Med.,* **27,** 769–774.

Critchley, M. (1929). Arteriosclerotic parkinsonism. *Brain,* **52,** 23–83.

Cummings, J.L. (1987). Multi-infarct dementia: diagnosis and management. *Psychosomatics,* **28,** 117–126

Cummings, J.L. (1988). Organic psychosis. *Psychosomatics,* **29,** 16–26.

Cummings, J.L. (1989). Vascular dementia and dementia of Alzheimer-type cognition [letter]. *Arch. Neurol.,* **46,** 1046–1047.

Cummings, J.L., and Benson, D.F. (1983). *Dementia: A Clinical Approach.* Boston: Butterworths.

Cummings, J.L., Miller, B., Hill, M.A., and Neshkes, R. (1987). Neuropsychiatric aspects of multi-infarct dementia and dementia of the Alzheimer type. *Arch. Neurol.*, **44,** 389–393.

De Reuck, J., Sieben, G., de Coster, W., and van der Eecken, H. (1980). Parkinsonism in patients with cerebral infarcts. *Clin. Neurol. Neurosurg.*, **82,** 177–185.

De Reuck, J., Sieben, G., de Coster, W., and van der Eecken, H. (1982). Dementia and confusional state in patients with cerebral infarcts. *Eur. Neurol.*, **21,** 94–97.

Deutsch, G., and Tweedy, J.R. (1987). Cerebral blood flow in severity-matched Alzheimer and multi-infarct patients. *Neurology,* **37,** 431–438.

DeWitt, L.D., Grek, A.J., Buonanno, F.S., Levine, D.N., and Kistler, J.P. (1985). MRI and the study of aphasia. *Neurology,* **35,** 861–865.

Donnan, G.A., Tress, B.A., and Bladin, P.F. (1982). A prospective study of lacunar infarction using computerized tomography. *Neurology,* **32,** 49–56.

Dubinsky, R.M., and Jankovic, J. (1987). Progressive supranuclear palsy and a multi-infarct state. *Neurology,* **37,** 570–576.

Dyken, M.L. (1979). Assessment of the role of antiplatelet aggregating agents in transient ischemic attacks, stroke and death. *Stroke,* **10,** 602–604.

Elliott, F.A. (1977). Propranolol for the control of belligerent behavior following acute brain damage. *Ann. Neurol.*, **1,** 489–491.

Englund, E., Brun, A., and Persson, B. (1987). Correlations between histopathologic white matter changes and proton MR relaxation times in dementia. *Alzheimer Dis. Relat. Disord.*, **1,** 156–170.

Englund, E., Brun, A., and Alling, C. (1988). White matter changes in dementia of Alzheimer's type: biochemical and neuropathological correlations. *Brain,* **111,** 1425–1439.

Erkinjuntti, T., Ketonen, L., Sulkava, R., and Sipponen, R.E. (1984). Cerebral NMR and CT imaging in dementia. *J. Comput. Assist. Tomogr.*, **8,** 614–618.

Erkinjuntti, T., Ketonen, L., Sulkava, R., Sipponen, J., Vuorialho, M., and Iivanainen, M. (1987). Do white matter changes on MRI and CT differentiate vascular dementia from Alzheimer's disease? *J. Neurol. Neurosurg. Psychiatry,* **50,** 37–42.

Erkinjuntti, T., Haltia, M., Palo, J., Sulkava, R., and Paetau, A. (1988). Accuracy of the clinical diagnoses of vascular dementia: a prospective clinical and post-mortem neuropathological study. *J. Neurol. Neurosurg. Psychiatry,* **51,** 1037–1044.

Fisher, C.M. (1965). Lacunes, small deep cerebral infarcts. *Neurology,* **15,** 774–784.

Fisher, C.M. (1982). Lacunar strokes and infarcts: a review. *Neurology,* **32,** 871–876.

Foster, N.L., Chase, T.N., Fedio, P., Patronas, N.J., Brooks, R.A., and DiChiro, G. (1983). Alzheimer's disease: focal cortical changes shown by positron emission tomography. *Neurology,* **33,** 961–965.

Foster, N.L., Chase, T.N., Mansi, L., Brooks, R., Fedio, P., Patronas, N.J., and Di Chiro, G. (1984). Cortical abnormalities in Alzheimer's disease. *Ann. Neurol.*, **16,** 649–654.

Frackowiak, R.S.J., Pozzilli, C., Legg, N.J., du Boulay, G.H., Marshall, J., Lenzi, G.L., and Jones, T. (1981). Regional cerebral oxygen supply and utilization in dementia. *Brain,* **104,** 753–778.

Gerard, G., and Weisberg, L.A. (1986). MRI periventricular lesions in adults. *Neurology,* **36,** 998–1001.

Goto, K., Nobuyoshi, T., and Fukasawa, H. (1981). Diffuse white-matter disease in the geriatric population. *Radiology,* **141,** 687–695.

Graff-Radford, N.R., Eslinger, P.J., Damasio, A.R., and Yamada, T. (1984). Nonhemorrhagic infarction of the thalamus: behavioral, anatomic, and physiologic correlates. *Neurology,* **34,** 14–23.

Guberman, A., and Stuss, D. (1983). The syndrome of bilateral paramedian thalamic infarction. *Neurology,* **33,** 540–546.

Gustafson, L., and Nilsson, L. (1982). Differential diagnosis of presenile dementia on clinical grounds. *Acta Psychiatr. Scand.*, **65,** 194–209.

Hachinski, V.C., Iliff, L.D., Zilhka, L., Du Boulay, G.H., McAllister, V.L., Marshall, J., Russell, R.W.R., and Symon, L. (1975). Cerebral blood flow in dementia. *Arch. Neurol.*, **32,** 632–637.

Harrison, M.J.G., Thomas, D.J., Du Boulay, G.H., and Marshall, J. (1979). Multi-infarct dementia. *J Neurol. Sci.*, **40,** 97–103.

Hershey, L.A., Modic, M.T., Greenaugh, G., and Jaffe, D.F. (1987) Magnetic resonance imaging in vascular dementia. *Neurology,* **37,** 29–36.

Hier, D.B., Hagenlocker, K., and Shindler, A.G. (1985). Language disintegration in dementia: effects of etiology and severity. *Brain Lang.*, **25,** 117–133.

Hontela, S., and Schwartz, G. (1979). Myocardial infarction in the differential diagnosis of dementias in the elderly. *J. Am. Geriatr. Soc.*, **27,** 104–106.

Hughes, W., Dodgson, M.C.H., and MacLennan, D.C. (1954). Chronic cerebral hypertensive disease. *Lancet,* **2,** 770–774.

Inzitari, D., Diaz, F., Fox, A., Hachinski, V.C., Steingart, A., Lau, C., Donald, A., Wade, J., Mulic, H., and Merskey, H. (1987). Vascular risk factors and leukoaraiosis. *Arch. Neurol.*, **44,** 42–49.

Ishii, N., Nishihara, Y., and Imamura, T. (1986). Why do frontal lobe symptoms predominate in vascular dementia with lacunes? *Neurology,* **36,** 340–345.

Jagust, W.J., Budinger, T.F., and Reed, B.R. (1987). The diagnosis of dementia with single photon emission computed tomography. *Arch. Neurol.*, **44,** 258–262.

Johnson, K.A., Mueller, S.T., Walshe, T.M., English, R.J., and Holman, B.L. (1987). Cerebral perfusion imaging in Alzheimer's disease: use of single photon emission computed tomography and iofetamine hydrochloride I-123. *Arch. Neurol.*, **44,** 165–168.

Kertesz, A., Black. S.E., Nicholson, L., and Carr, T. (1987). The sensitivity and specificity of MRI in stroke. *Neurology,* **37,** 1580–1585.

Kinkel, W. (1988). Computerized tomography in clinical neurology. In: A.B. Baker and L.H. Baker, eds., *Clinical Neurology,* Vol. 1, Chap. 4, rev. ed. Philadelphia: Harper & Row.

Kirkpatrick, J.B., and Hayman, L.A. (1987). White matter imaging in healthy brains of elderly subjects: a possible pathologic basis. *Radiology,* **162,** 509–511.

Kistler, J.P., Buonanno, F.S., DeWitt, L.D., Davis, K.R., Brady, T.J., and Fisher, C.M. (1984). Vertebro-basilar posterior cerebral territory stroke-delineation by proton nuclear magnetic resonance imaging. *Stroke,* **15,** 417–426.

Kotsoris, H., Barclay, L.L., Hulyalkar, A., and Dougherty, J. (1987). Urinary and gait disturbances as markers for early multi-infarct dementia. *Stroke,* **18,** 138–141.

Ladurner, G., Iliff, L.D., and Lechner, H. (1982a). Clinical factors associated with dementias in ischemic stroke. *J. Neurol. Neurosurg. Psychiatry,* **45,** 97–101.

Ladurner, G., Sager, W.D., and Flooh, E. (1982b). Computer tomography and vascular (multi-infarct) dementia: a qualitative and quantitative investigation. *Exp. Brain Res.* [*Suppl.*] **5,** 264–271.

Leuchter, A.F., and Spar, J.E. (1985). The late-onset psychoses: clinical and diagnostic features. *J. Nerv. Ment. Dis.*, **173,** 488–494.

Lipsey, J.R., Robinson, R.G., Pearlson, G.D., Rao, K., and Price, T.R. (1984). Nortriptyline treatment of post-stroke depression: a double-blind study. *Lancet,* **1,** 297–300.

Liston, E.H., and LaRue, A. (1983). Clinical differentiation of primary degenerative and multi-infarct dementia: a critical review of the evidence. Part I. Clinical studies. *Biol. Psychiatry,* **18,** 1451–1465.

Loeb, C., and Gandolfo, C. (1983). Diagnostic evaluation of degenerative and vascular dementia. *Stroke,* **14,** 399–401.

London, E., de Leon, M.J., George, A., Englund, E., Ferris, S., Gentes, C., and Reisberg, B. (1986). Periventricular lucencies in the CT scans of aged and demented patients. *Biol. Psychiatry,* **21,** 960–962.

Loizou, L.A., Kendall, B.E., and Marshall, J. (1981). Subcortical arteriosclerotic encephalopathy: a clinical and radiological investigation. *J. of Neurol. Neurosurg, Psychiatry,* **44,** 294–304.

Meyer, J.S., Judd, B.W., Tawaklna, T., Rogers, R.L., and Mortel, K.F. (1986). Improved cognition after control of risk factors for multi-infarct dementia. *J.A.M.A.,* **256,** 2203–2207.

Meyer, J.S., Rogers, R.L., Mortel, K.F., and Judd, B.W. (1987). Hyperlipidemia is a risk factor for decreased cerebral perfusion and stroke. *Arch. Neurol.,* **44,** 418–422.

Molsa, P., Paljarvi, L., Rinne, J., and Sako (1985). Validity of clinical diagnosis in dementia: a prospective clinicopathological study. *J. Neurol. Neurosurg. Psychiatry,* **48,** 1085–1090.

O'Brien, M.D.. (1988). Vascular dementia is underdiagnosed. *Arch. Neurol.,* **45,** 797–798.

Olszewski, J. (1962). Subcortical arteriosclerotic encephalopathy. *World Neurol.,* **3,** 359–375.

Perez, F.I., Rivera, V.M., Meyer, J.S., Gay, J.R.A., Taylor, R.L., and Mathew, N.T. (1975). Analysis of intellectual and cognitive performance in patients with multi-infarct dementia, vertebrobasilar insufficiency with dementia, and Alzheimer's disease. *J. Neurol. Neurosurg. Psychiatry,* **38,** 533–540.

Perez, F.I., Stump, D.A., Gay, J.R.A., and Hart, V.R. (1976). Intellectual performance in multi-infarct dementia and Alzheimer's disease: a replication study. *Can. J. Neurol. Sci.,* **3,** 181–187.

Powell, A., Cummings, J.L., Hill, M.A., and Benson, D.F. (1988). Speech and language alterations in multi-infarct dementia. *Neurology,* **38,** 717–719.

Reding, M., Haycox, J., and Blass, J. (1983). Depression in patients referred to a dementia clinic. *Arch. Neruol.,* **42,** 894–896.

Roberts, M.A., McGeorge, A.P., and Caird, F.I. (1978). Electroencephalography and computerized tomography in vascular and non-vascular dementia in old age. *J. Neurol. Neurosurg. Psychiatry,* **41,** 903–906.

Rogers, R.L., Meyer, J.S., Shaw, T.G., Mortel, K.F., Hardenberg, J.P., and Zaid, R.R. (1983). Cigarette smoking decreases cerebral blood flow suggesting increased risk of stroke. *J.A.M.A.* **250,** 2796–2800.

Rogers, R.L., Meyer, J.S., Mortel, K.F., Mahurin, R.K., and Judd, B.W. (1986). Decreased cerebral blood flow precedes multi-infarct dementia, but follows senile dementia of the Alzheimer type. *Neurology,* **36,** 1–6.

Roman, G.C. (1987). Senile dementia of the Binswanger type. *J.A.M.A.,* **258,** 1782–1788.

Rosen, W.G., Terry, R.D., Fuld, P.A., Katzman, R., and Peck, A. (1980). Pathological verification of ischemic score in differentiation of dementias. *Ann. Neurol.,* **7,** 486–488.

Rosenberg, G.A., Kornfeld, M., Stovring, J., and Bicknell, J.M. (1979). Subcortical arteriosclerotic encephalopathy (Binswanger): computerized tomography. *Neurology,* **29,** 1102–1106.

Rothschild, D. (1942). Neuropathologic changes in arteriosclerotic psychosis and their psychiatric significance. *Arch. Neurol. Psychiatry,* **48,** 417–436.

Salgado, E.D., Weinstein, M., Furlan, A.J., Modic, M.T., Beck, G.J., Estes, M., Awad, I., and Little, J.R. (1986). Proton magnetic resonance imaging in ischemic cerebrovascular disease. *Ann. Neurol.,* **20,** 502–507.

Sarpel, G., Chaudry, F., and Hindo, W. (1987). Magnetic resonance imaging of periventricular hyperintensity in a Veterans Administration population. *Arch. Neurol.* **44,** 725–728.

Schiffer, R.B., Cash, J., and Herndon, R.M. (1983). Treatment of emotional lability with low-dosage tricyclic antidepressants. *Psychosomatics,* **24,** 1094–1096.

Schoenberg, B.S., Anderson, D.W., and Haerer, A.F. (1986). Racial differentials in the prevalence of stroke. *Arch. Neurol.*, **43,** 565–568.

Sluss, T.K., Gruenberg, E.M., Rabins, P., and Kramer, M. (1982). Distribution of focal signs in a group of demented men. *Neuropsychobiology,* **8,** 109–112.

St. Clair, D., and Whalley L.J. (1983). Hypertension, multiinfarct dementia and Alzheimer's disease. *Br. J. Psychiatry,* **143,** 274–276.

Steingart, A., Hachinski, V.C., Lau, C., Fox, A.J., Diaz, F., Cape, R., Lee, D., Inzitari, D., and Merskey, H. (1987a). Cognitive and neurological findings in subjects with diffuse white matter lucencies on computed tomographic scan (leuko-araiosis). *Arch. Neurol.*, **44,** 32–35.

Steingart, A., Hachinski, V.C., Lau, C., Fox, A.J., Fox, H., Lee, D., Inzitari, D., and Merskey, H. (1987b). Cognitive and neurological findings in demented patients with diffuse white matter lucencies on computed tomographic scans (leuko-araiosis). *Arch. Neurol.*, **3,** 727–734.

Striano, S., Vacca, G., Bilo, L., and Meo, R. (1981). The electro-encephalogram in dementia. *Acta Neurologica.*, (Napoli), **36,** 727–734.

Sulkava, R., Wikstrom, J., Aromaa, A., Raitasalo, R., Lehtinen, V., Lehtela, K., and Palo, J. (1985). Prevalence of severe dementia in Finland. *Neurology,* **35,** 1025–1029.

Tierney, M.C., Fisher, R.H., Lewis, A.J., Zorzitto, M.L., Snow, W.G., Reid, D.W., and Nieuwstraten, P. (1988). The NINCDS/ADRDA Work Group criteria for the clinical diagnosis of probable Alzheimer's disease: a clinicopathologic study of 57 cases. *Neurology,* **38,** 359–364.

Todorov, A.B., Go, R.C.P., Constantinidis, J., and Elston, R.C. (1975). Specificity of the clinical diagnosis of dementia. *J. Neurol. Sci.*, **26,** 81–98.

Tomlinson, B.E., Blessed, G., and Roth, M. (1968). Observations on the brains of non-demented old people. *J. Neurol. Sci.*, **7,** 331–356.

Tomlinson, B.E., Blessed, G., and Roth, M. (1970). Observations on the brains of demented old people. *J. Neurol. Sci.*, **11,** 205–242.

Torvik, A., Endresen, G.K.M., Abrahamsen, A.F., and Godal, H. Ch. (1971). Progressive dementia caused by an unusual type of generalized small vessel thrombosis. *Acta. Neurol. Scand.* **47,** 137–150.

Tresch, D.D., Folstein, M.F., Rabins, P.V., and Hazzard, W.R. (1985). Prevalence and significance of cardiovascular disease and hypertension in elderly patients with dementia and depression. *J. Am. Geriatr. Soc.*, **33,** 530–537.

Udaka, F., Yamao, S., Nagata, H., Nakamura, S., and Kameyama, M. (1984). Pathologic laughing and crying treated with levodopa. *Arch. Neurol.*, **41,** 1095–1096.

Volpe, B.T., and Petito, C.K. (1985). Dementia with bilateral medial temporal lobe ischemia. *Neurology,* **35,** 1793–1797.

Wolf, J.K., Santana, H.B., and Thropy, M. (1979). Treatment of "emotional incontinence" with levodopa. *Neurology,* **35,** 1793–1797.

Wolf, P.A., Kannel, W.B., and Verter, J. (1984). Cardiovascular diseases in the elderly: epidemiology. In: M.L. Albert, ed., *Clinical Neurology of Aging,* pp. 458–477. New York: Oxford University Press.

Yudofsky, S.C., Stevens, L., Silver, J., Barsa, J., and Williams, D. (1984). Propranolol in the treatment of rage and violent behavior associated with Korsakoff's psychosis. *Am. J. Psychiatry,* **141,** 114–115.

Zimmerman, R.D., Fleming, C.A., Lee, B.C.P., Saint-Louis, L.A., and Deck, M.D.F. (1985). Periventricular hyperintensity as seen by magnetic resonance: prevalence and significance. *Am. J. Neuroradiol,* **7,** 13–20.

8

Dementia Syndrome of Depression in Patients with Stroke

SERGIO E. STARKSTEIN, KAREN I. BOLLA
AND ROBERT G. ROBINSON

Since Broca's (1861) observation that language disturbance was produced by unilateral left hemisphere brain damage, clinical investigators have been searching for specific clinicopathologic correlations between focal brain injury and particular behavioral or neuropsychological deficits. Since the early 1970s a large number of studies have examined the type and severity of language disorders associated with specific sites of brain injury. A great deal of attention has also been devoted to other neuropsychological problems, such as visuospatial deficits, attentional disorders, apraxias, agnosias, and their relation to specific sites of brain damage (Damasio and Geschwind, 1985). Based on these clinicopathologic correlations, it is often possible to determine the location of brain lesions based on the associated neuropsychological findings. It is also well known, however, that exceptions occur. For instance, patients with lesions in similar locations may show different severities or types of neuropsychological impairment (Starkstein et al., 1988), and the same neuropsychological deficits may appear after lesions in atypical locations (Basso et al., 1985). One of the great tasks faced by clinical investigators is to explain the mechanisms by which these atypical clinicopathological correlations may occur. For instance, they might be due to lesions involving postsynaptic connections or to indirect effects (i.e., "diaschisis") of lesions on the primary site of localization. They might also stem from other factors, such as metabolic changes due to another illness, sexual dimorphisms, age, or depression.

We have been examining the manifestations, course, and mechanisms of depression following stroke and have found significant interactions between depression and neuropsychological impairments that could influence the usual clinical pathologic correlations. In this chapter we examine how the presence of post-stroke depression is associated with neuropsychological changes beyond those produced by the lesion itself.

POST-STROKE DEPRESSION

Depression is a common sequela of stroke, and several independent studies have shown a frequency of depression ranging from 25% to 49% (Robinson and Price, 1982; Robinson et al., 1983; Ebrahim et al., 1987; Wade et al., 1987). We have shown that one-half of the patients with post-stroke depression (PSD) show the clinical symptoms of major depression as defined by *DSM-III* criteria (American Psychiatric Association, 1980), and the other one-half have clinical symptoms of minor (dysthymic) depression (Robinson et al., 1983). Major and minor PSD differ in their longitudinal evolution: The former lasts for approximately 1 year without treatment, whereas minor depression lasts more than 2 years without treatment (Robinson et al., 1987). There are also significant differences between major and minor depression in their neuropathologic correlates. There is a strong association between major, but not minor, PSD and lesion location (Robinson and Szetela, 1981; Lipsey et al., 1983; Robinson et al., 1984; Sinyor et al., 1986B, Starkstein et al., 1987). Major PSD is significantly more frequent among patients with left anterior lesions than any other lesion location. (An anterior lesion is defined as having its anterior border proximal to 40% of the anteroposterior distance on CT scan. Anatomically, this definition corresponds to frontal cortex or basal ganglia involvement.) We have demonstrated this association for both cortical and subcortical left hemisphere stroke lesions (Starkstein et al., 1987). In addition, for both cortical and subcortical left anterior lesions, the severity of depression was significantly correlated with the proximity of the lesion to the frontal pole (i.e., the closer the lesion was to the frontal pole, the higher the depression score). Finally, we and others have consistently shown no more than a weak association between PSD and severity of neurologic deficits, impairment in activities of daily living, and social functioning (Folstein et al., 1977; Finkelstein et al., 1981; Robinson et al., 1984; Sinyor et al., 1986a; Starkstein et al., 1987).

DEMENTIA SYNDROME OF DEPRESSION

For many years clinicians have recognized that patients with a variety of functional psychiatric disorders, particularly depression, can show a reversible dementia. Madden and colleagues (1952) found that "symptoms ordinarily considered to be indicative of dementia (disorientation, defects in recent memory, retention, calculation and judgment) . . . may disappear on alleviation of the psychotic picture by means of short-term intensive therapy." Wells (1979) suggested that the main clinical features of dementia of depression consist in intellectual deterioration that begins rather abruptly and rapidly progresses after onset. He considered concentration and memory problems as the main complaints, with less dysfunction, than in other neuropsychological functions.

Caine (1981) suggested that the diagnosis of dementia of depression be based on four criteria: (1) intellectual impairment with a primary psychiatric disorder; (2) features of neuropsychological abnormality resembling neuropathologically induced intellectual deficit; (3) reversibility of intellectual disorder; and (4) no apparent primary neuropathologic process.

Although PSD is secondary to a neuropathological process, there is no a priori reason why depression arising from a brain lesion might not produce dementia of depression. In fact, major PSD is similar to functional (i.e., no known brain lesion) depression in terms of longitudinal evolution (Robinson et al., 1987), clinical profile (Lipsey et al., 1986), and response to treatment (Lipsey et al., 1984).

CONFOUNDING VARIABLES

Before addressing the relation between PSD and cognitive impairment, several methodologic problems must be pointed out. The major methodologic problem when studying the effect of depression on cognitive function in brain-injured patients is that there are two independent variables affecting the same dependent variable. In other words, PSD patients are not only depressed, they also have a brain lesion that, depending on its location, can produce neuropsychological deficits by itself. This one dependent variable must be held constant before the effect of the other dependent variables can be examined. Patients with the same size and location of lesion, with and without depression, may be studied for the effect of depression on cognitive performance, or patients with similar depression can be studied for the effect of lesion location on cognitive functions. This factor makes the study that much more difficult.

Another problem when studying cognitive impairments and depression in brain-injured patients is the existence of aphasia. Aphasic disturbances make the assessment of cognitive functions problematic, as one may have difficulty knowing whether the failure on a cognitive task is due to aphasia or to a specific cognitive impairment. When we have evaluated cognitive functions in brain-injured patients, we excluded patients with aphasia. This exclusion, however, creates a skewed study population, with few patients having left hemisphere inferior parietal or superior temporal or posterior inferior frontal lesions.

Another difficulty is the natural evolution of neuropsychological deficits produced by brain lesions. Several studies have examined the duration of behavioral deficits following left and right hemisphere lesions (Hier et al., 1983; Wade et al., 1987). Because the longitudinal evolution of diverse neuropsychological problems may be different for each deficit and may or may not relate to the longitudinal evolution of PSD, an interaction between time since stroke and neuropsychological deficits may preclude finding intellectual deficits that are related to PSD. It is clear, then, that several important variables such as lesion size, lesion location, aphasia, and time since stroke should be controlled when studying the relation between cognitive impairment and depression. We now summarize several of our studies of dementia and depression in stroke patients, and the way we tried to deal with these methodologic limitations.

DEMENTIA SYNDROME OF POST-STROKE DEPRESSION

In our first study (Robinson et al., 1986), we examined a consecutive series of patients admitted for acute care following stroke. Exclusion criteria were the presence of: (1) decreased level of consciousness; (2) severe comprehension deficits; (3) history of stroke or other brain injury; and (4) computed tomographic (CT) evidence of prior brain injury. Only patients with left hemisphere lesions were included. All patients were administered the Mini-Mental State Examination (Folstein et al., 1975), an 11-item examination found to be reliable and valid for assessing a limited range of cognitive functions in a variety of states including dementia and brain injury. A psychiatric examination was carried out using the Present State Exam (PSE) (Wing et al., 1974), a semistructured psychiatric interview. The severity of depression was quantitated by means of the Hamilton Depression Scale (Hamilton, 1960). Using the symptoms elicited by the PSE, a *DSM-III* diagnosis of a major or minor (dysthymic) depression was made.

No significant background differences were observed among patients with major, minor, or no depression; and a neurologic examination carried out blind to the psychiatric evaluation showed no significant between-group differences in terms of motor and sensory impairments, visual field deficits, frequency and type of aphasia, and frequency of ischemic or hemorrhagic lesions. Finally, no significant between-group differences were observed on the Johns Hopkins Functioning Inventory (Robinson and Szetela, 1981), a scale of activities of daily living.

The first interesting finding that emerged from this study was that patients with major depression had a significantly lower Mini-Mental score than minor and nondepressed patients (mean ± SD: 13.0 ± 5.8 for the major depressed group, 25.0 ± 4.5 for the minor depressed group, and 22.0 ± 6.0 for the nondepressed group; $p < 0.05$). Moreover, whereas *all* the 11 patients with major depression had Mini-Mental scores below 23 (the usual cutoff point for abnormal scores on this scale), only 7 of the 17 nondepressed patients (41%) had abnormal scores, and a hypothesis of unequal frequency of abnormal Mini-Mental scores based on the presence of major depression was statistically substantiated [$\chi^2(1) = 12.6$, $p.<0.001$, Yates correction).

As mentioned above, patients with major, but not minor, PSD showed cognitive impairments (i.e., there were no significant differences in Mini-Mental scores between minor and nondepressed patients). This finding is similar to results in patients with functional depression, in which only patients with *severe* depression were found to have intellectual deficits (Miller, 1975; Stromgren, 1977; McAllister, 1981), and the severity of neuropsychological deficits (e.g., failure in learning) were found to correlate with the severity of depression (Gibson, 1981).

Although these results demonstrate that patients with major depression are significantly more cognitively impaired than nondepressed patients, they do not account for important variables, such as lesion size and location. To account for the lesion, we calculated lesion volumes (expressed as a percentage of total brain volume) from the ratio of the largest cross-sectional area of the lesion on any CT slice, divided by the largest cross-sectional area of total brain on a CT slice passing through the lateral ventricles. Using this procedure, we found a significant negative correlation between lesion size and Mini-Mental scores for the overall group of patients (i.e., the

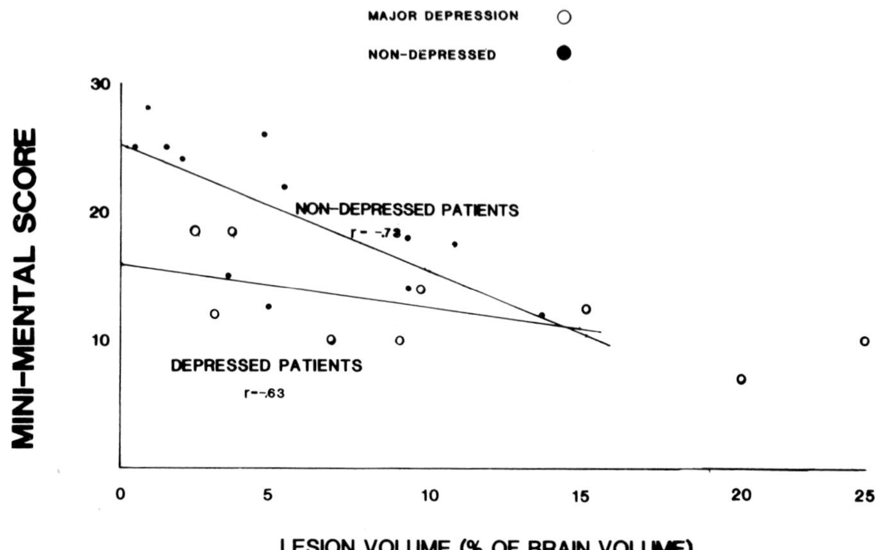

Figure 8–1 Mini-Mental score and brain lesion volume, as measured from CT scans, were found to have a linear relation and to be significantly correlated ($p<0.01$) for nondepressed patients. Larger lesion volumes produced greater degrees of cognitive impairment. (Modified with permission from Robinson et al., 1986.)

larger the lesion size, the greater the intellectual impairment) (Figure 8–1). When patients were divided into major, minor, and nondepressed groups, there were significant correlations between lesion size and Mini-Mental scores for both nondepressed ($r - 0.73$, $p < 0.01$) and major depressed ($r - 0.63$, $p < 0.05$) patients (Fig. 8–1). A multiple linear regression analysis, however, showed that both depression and lesion size were related to Mini-Mental scores. The multiple correlation coefficient was $R = 0.70$, $p < 0.005$, and the partial regression coefficients for the Hamilton depression score and Mini-Mental scores and for lesion size and Mini-Mental scores were -0.55, $p < 0.01$ and -0.42, $p < 0.01$, respectively. There was, however, no significant correlation between the Hamilton depression score and lesion size (r 0.01, NS). These findings suggested that both depression and lesion size independently contributed to intellectual impairment.

This conclusion was further supported when we compared major depressed and nondepressed patients for lesion size after controlling for level of intellectual impairment. When patients with and without depression ($n = 10$ per group) were matched for Mini-Mental score, depressed patients showed significantly smaller lesion volumes (3.3 ± 2.7) than nondepressed patients (6.2 ± 4.0) [$t(19) = 1.9$, $p < 0.05$, one-tailed] (Figure 8–2).

In summary, these results suggest that for a given lesion size depressed patients had greater cognitive impairment than nondepressed patients. Moreover, when cognitive impairment was held constant, depressed patients had significantly smaller lesion sizes than nondepressed patients.

Another important confounding variable in the study of dementia of PSD is lesion location. In an effort to examine the influence of this variable on Mini-Mental scores, we correlated the location of the lesion in the anteroposterior (AP) axis with

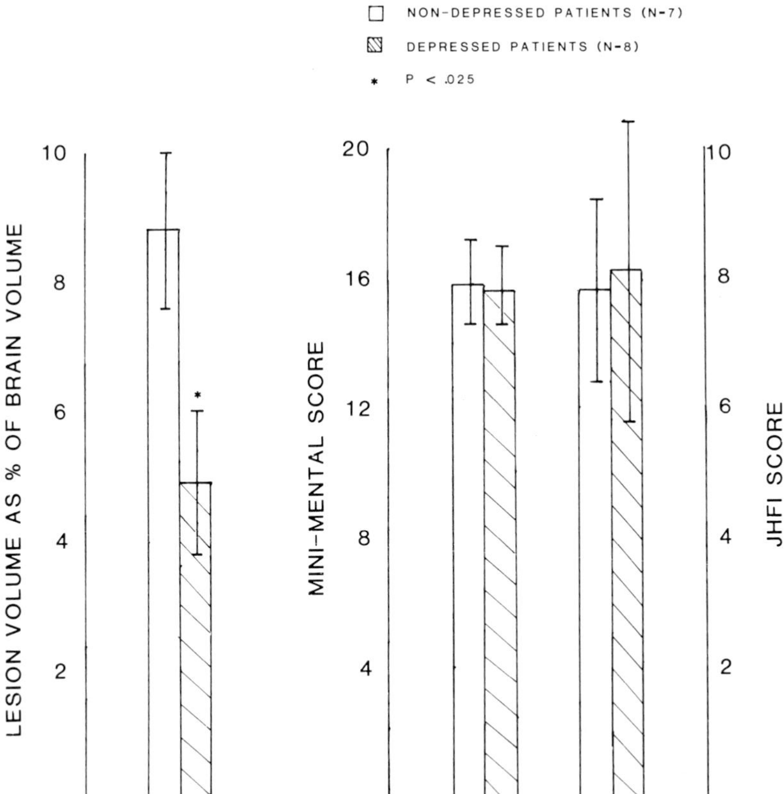

Figure 8–2 Patients with Mini-Mental State scores below 23 were divided into depressed and nondepressed groups. Despite having comparable Mini-Mental State scores and Johns Hopkins Functioning Inventory (JHFI) scores, which measure activities of daily living, depressed patients had a significantly smaller mean lesion volume than nondepressed patients (variability bars represent the SD). (Reproduced with permission from R.E. Hales & S.C. Yudofsky (eds.) *Textbook of Neuropsychiatry,* American Psychiatric Press Inc., Washington, D.C., 1986, page 203).

the Mini-Mental score. The anterior location of each lesion (expressed as a percentage of total AP distance) was defined as the mean distance of the anterior border of the lesion from the frontal pole for all slices in which the lesion was visible. The posterior location of the lesion was defined as the mean distance of the posterior border from the frontal pole. Although no significant correlations were found between the *anterior* border of the lesion and Mini-Mental scores for any of the three groups, significant correlations were observed between the *posterior* border of the lesion and Mini-Mental scores (i.e., the more posterior the lesion, the greater the intellectual impairment), for both nondepressed (r 0.59, $p < 0.05$) and major depressed patients ($r -$ 0.78), $p < 0.05$). The posterior border of the lesion however, did not correlate significantly with severity of depression. This finding demonstrates a relation between lesion location and cognitive function but not between lesion location (i.e., posterior extent of lesion) and depression. The correlation between the posterior border of the lesion and Mini-Mental scores can be interpreted as secondary to the verbal bias of the Mini-Mental examination (Dick et al., 1984), as posterior lesions involve temporoparietal areas related to language comprehension. This finding emphasizes one of the main limitations of this study: Although we were able to control for lesion volume, the effect of lesion location could not be precisely controlled.

In the next study, however, we controlled for both lesion size and location (Starkstein et al., 1988). The study population consisted of 13 pairs of patients who were matched for lesion size and location and time since injury, but one patient had major depression and the other patient was not depressed. Although no significant differences were found in demographic variables, such as age, sex, years of education, and socioeconomic status, depressed patients had significantly lower Mini-Mental scores than nondepressed patients [16.6 $\pm$ 7.8 versus 22.4 $\pm$ 6.6; $t(25) = 3.21$; $p < 0.05$]. Moreover, whereas 9 of 13 patients with depression had Mini-Mental scores below the cutoff point of 23, only 3 patients without depression had Mini-Mental scores below that value. A hypothesis of unequal frequency of "abnormal" (i.e., 23 or below) Mini-Mental score based on the presence or absence of depression was statistically substantiated [$\chi^2(1) = 5.57$, $p < 0.02$]. Moreover, whereas 10 depressed patients had lower scores than their respective matched controls, 2 had the same score and only 1 had a score higher than his respective control [χ^2 (1) = 14.7, $p < 0.001$].

SUBCORTICAL LESIONS AND DEMENTIA SYNDROME OF POST-STROKE DEPRESSION

In our studies on post-stroke depression, we consistently found a significant correlation between the distance of the anterior border of the lesion from the frontal pole and depression scores, so that more anterior lesions were associated with significantly greater frequency and severity of depression. This finding was substantiated in patients with unilateral strokes (Robinson et al., 1984), in those with *bilateral* lesions (in whom the distance from the anterior border of the *left,* but not right, lesion correlated with depression scores) (Lipsey et al., 1983), and in patients with traumatic closed head injury (Robinson and Szetela, 1981). In another study, we examined if this correlation was significant for both cortical and restricted subcortical lesions (Starkstein et al., 1987). We found that patients with cortical lesions (i.e., cortical lesions extending into the subjacent white matter but not involving the deep gray nuclei) showed a frequency of depression similar to that of patients with restricted subcortical lesions (mainly involving the basal ganglia and the anterior limb of the internal capsule). Moreover, patients with anterior subcortical lesions showed the same lateralized phenomena as seen in patients with frontal cortical lesions (i.e., patients with cortical or subcortical lesions of the left hemisphere had a significantly higher frequency of depression than patients with comparable right hemisphere lesions). Finally, we also found a significant AP effect. Patients with left hemisphere cortical (frontal) or subcortical (basal ganglia) lesions were more frequently and severely depressed than patients with lesions in postrolandic (temporo-parieto-occipital) regions of the left hemisphere. A significant correlation between the proximity of the anterior border of the lesion to the frontal pole and depression scores (i.e.,

Table 8–1 Relation of Intellectual Impairment to Depression Scores

Parameter	Abnormal Mini-Mental	Normal Mini-Mental
No. of patients	5	5
Present State Exam[a]	19.8 (8.1)	4.0 (3.2)
Hamilton Depression Scale[a]	10.4 (2.3)	4.1 (2.7)
Zung Depression Scale[a]	57.2 (5.7)	37.2 (5.7)

Standard deviations are shown in parentheses.
[a]$p < 0.01$.

more anterior lesions were associated with more severe depressions) was found for both cortical ($r - 0.52$, $p < 0.05$) and subcortical lesions (r 0.68, p < 0.05).

These findings suggest that because patients with left cortical or subcortical lesions show a similar frequency and severity of PSD, the underlying pathophysiological mechanisms that lead to depression in these two locations of brain injury may be the same.

Because our previous findings of intellectual impairment associated with PSD primarily involved patients with cortical lesions, we examined whether patients with restricted subcortical lesions also showed cognitive impairments associated with depression. In one of the studies described above (Robinson et al., 1986) we examined ten patients with pure subcortical lesions as shown by CT scans. These patients were then divided into those with abnormal Mini-Mental scores (i.e., 23 or less; $n = 5$) or normal (i.e., more than 23; $n = 5$). Patients with abnormal Mini-Mental scores showed significantly higher depression scores than patients with normal Mini-Mental scores (Table 8–1). This finding provides tentative support for the idea that patients with restricted subcortical lesions may also show dementia of PSD.

QUANTITATIVE AND QUALITATIVE DIFFERENCES IN COGNITIVE PERFORMANCE OF PATIENTS WITH AND WITHOUT PSD

Thus far we have presented data from two studies indicating that depression in stroke patients may lead to greater intellectual impairment than could be solely attributed to the lesion. We suggested that major depressive disorders following brain injury may produce an intellectual impairment by itself. Because of the relatively limited number of functions examined by the Mini-Mental examination, however, it was unclear if post-stroke intellectual impairments associated with depression are restricted to specific cognitive processes or represent a more global cognitive decline. We have carried out a study in which we examined the pattern of cognitive deficits in patients with major PSD using a detailed neuropsychological evaluation (Bolla-Wilson et al., 1989). This battery consists of 34 subtests extracted from standardized neuropsychological tests (Wechsler, 1955; Lezak, 1976) and was designed to examine a wide range of functional domains.

Orientation: Orientation (E. Kaplan, personal communication) and General Information (Lezak, 1976, p. 256)

Language: Boston Naming Test (Kaplan et al., 1976); and Verbal Fluency,

Months Forward, Repetition, Reading, Comprehension, and Spontaneous speech tasks from the Boston Diagnostic Aphasia Examination (Goodglass and Kaplan, 1976) and the Multilingual Aphasia Examination (Benton and Hamsher, 1978)

Remote memory: General Information and Famous Faces (Lezak, 1976, pp. 256, 470)

Verbal memory: Logical Memory (Wechsler, 1945), Rey Auditory Verbal-Learning Test (RAVLT), Recurrent Words, and Digit Span (Lezak, 1976, p. 266)

Visual memory: Visual Reproduction (Lezak 1976)

Recognition memory: Recurrent Words (Lezak 1976, p. 436), Logical Memory (E. Kaplan, personal communication), RAVLT (Lezak, 1976, p. 422), and Visual Reproduction (E. Kaplan, personal communication)

Visuoperception-visuoconstruction: Block Design (Wechsler, 1955), Clock Drawing (Lezak, 1976, p. 406), and Hooper Visual Organization test (Hooper, 1958)

Executive/motor: Alternating Fingers, Luria Motor Sequences (Luria, 1966), Praxis (Goodglass and Kaplan, 1976), and Finger Tapping (Reitan and Davison, 1974)

Frontal lobe functions: Verbal Fluency, Alternating Fingers, and Luria Motor Sequences

For this study, we examined a consecutive series of stroke patients with evidence of either a thromboembolic infarct or intracerebral hemorrhage of the left or right hemisphere, with no CT scan evidence or clinical history of prior brain injury. A psychiatric evaluation revealed the existence of either a major depression or no depression; patients with a language deficit, a history of alcoholism, or a metabolic disorder were excluded from the study. Thus we were left with four groups of patients with either left or right hemisphere lesions and either major depression or no depression.

Although no significant differences were found in demographic variables, type and severity of neurologic deficits, and lesion size and location, neuropsychological testing revealed several significant differences. In the left hemisphere lesion group, the presence of depression was associated with significantly lower scores in the following domains: orientation ($U = 109.5, p < 0.01$), language ($U = 80.0, p < 0.05$), executive/motor ($U = 122.0, p < 0.05$), and frontal lobe functions ($U = 109.5, p < 0.02$). In the right hemisphere group, however, no significant differences were observed between depressed and nondepressed patients on any of the nine composite scores.

When we examined the pattern of deficits exhibited by major depressed and nondepressed patients with left hemisphere lesions on each of the subtests, we found similarities between the pattern found in patients with PSD and the pattern of neuropsychological deficits described in patients with functional depression.

In the language domain, deficits were mainly observed in naming ($U = 118.5, p < 0.05$) and repetition ($U = 124, p < 0.01$) tasks. Although language impairment has not been consistently reported in patients with dementia or depression (Nott, 1975; Caine, 1981), more detailed studies have shown naming problems in these patients (Speedie et al., 1988). Moreover, Huff and Corkin (1984) suggested that anomia may be the result of word-retrieval difficulties.

Memory deficits constitute the main neuropsychological problem in patients with functional depression (Caine, 1981). We also found a significantly poorer performance on the Logical Memory Test (in both immediate and delayed recall) for the left major PSD group compared with the left nondepressed group. Because this finding could potentially reflect failures in memory acquisition, retention, and retrieval, we examined differences in the amount of "forgetting" (i.e., immediate recall minus delayed recall) between depressed and nondepressed groups with left hemisphere lesions and found that this difference was not significant. It suggested that both groups forgot at the same rate, and therefore PSD did not appear to be associated with retention difficulties.

Coupled with the finding of no significant between-group differences on cued-recall (recognition) tasks, these results indicate that depressed patients may retain but not be able to retrieve the information. A similar pattern of forgetting was also found for the RAVLT and Visual Reproduction subtests, suggesting that these memory deficits are present for both left hemisphere (verbal) as well as right hemisphere (visuospatial) memory functions even in the presence of a unilateral (left hemisphere) lesion. This finding that patients with major PSD after left hemisphere lesions have cognitive deficits in functions that pertain to both left and right hemispheres is similar to findings in patients with functional depression who show deficits of memory in verbal and visuospatial tasks (Miller and Lewis, 1977; Caine, 1981; Weingartner et al., 1981; Robertson and Taylor, 1985; Calev et al., 1986; Speedie et al., 1988).

We also examined learning curves for depressed and nondepressed stroke patients on the RAVLT. We found that the left hemisphere depressed group showed the least amount of learning over trials, and by trial 5 (a measure of overall learning) they had learned significantly fewer words than the left hemisphere nondepressed group [$t(30) = 2.03$, $p < 0.05$]. This finding suggests that depressed patients have attentional deficits as well as poor sequential learning. Similar findings have also been reported in patients with functional depression. These impairments have been attributed to deficits in using encoding strategies and organizing inputs for subsequent facilitation of recall (Miller and Lewis, 1977; Caine, 1981; Weingartner et al., 1981).

In summary, this detailed neuropsychological study has produced several interesting findings. First, although the patterns of performance of the depressed and nondepressed patients with left hemisphere lesions were similar, the degree of impairment was consistently worse in the depressed group and reached statistical significance on those tasks that have also been reported to be impaired in patients with functional depression (Jorm, 1986). Secondly, dementia of post-stroke depression was a lateralized phenomenon. Patients with major depression after right hemisphere lesions showed no significant differences in cognitive performance compared to nondepressed patients with comparable right hemisphere strokes. Folstein and McHugh (1978) suggested that the dementia of depression may resemble a subcortical dementia. Based on this observation they also suggested that the dementia of depression may be a consequence of pathologic changes in subcortical areas and may be mediated by biogenic amines neurotransmitter pathways. Savard and colleagues (1980) also suggested that depression may be secondary to deficiences in biogenic amines, which have an effect on cognitive function. Roy-Byrne and colleagues (1986) showed that functional depressed patients are impaired on cognitive operations that required effort and showed that these operations are preferentially controlled by dopaminergic systems.

The performance of depressed patients on efforts demanding motor and cognitive tasks showed improvement after levodopa (Roy-Byrne et al., 1986) or amphetamine treatment (Reus et al., 1979). In contrast, other investigators have suggested that cognitive deficits associated with depression may be secondary to distracting thoughts or motivational deficits (see Jorm, 1986, for a review and discussion). The finding, however, that patients with dementia of depression may show improvement in cognition after treatment with biogenic amine precursors (e.g., levodopa or L-tryptophan) even in the absence of mood changes, suggests that depression may be dissociated from the cognitive deficit (Henry et al., 1973; Glass et al., 1981).

We have demonstrated in a rat model of stroke that brain lesions, depending on the side of the lesion, produced significant depletion of norepinephrine and dopamine in cortical areas. Right but not left frontal lesions were associated with biogenic amine depletions (Robinson, 1979). Thus if the biochemical response of the brain is different depending on whether the right or left hemisphere is injured, PSD and dementia of PSD could be the result of asymmetric depletions in biogenic amine concentrations. The lower frequency of depression and the lack of a dementia of depression after right hemisphere lesions may be the consequence of significantly lower biogenic amine levels leading to a conpensatory up-regulation of postsynaptic receptors (Mayberg et al., 1988).

Although the role of biogenic amine depletions in patients with dementia of PSD is still speculative, several other possibly related mechanisms can be proposed based on recent findings. Patients with functional and post-stroke depression may show evidence on CT scans of subcortical atrophy (Schlegel and Kretzschmer, 1987; Starkstein et al., 1988). Kellner and colleagues (1986) have shown a significant correlation between ventricular size and cognitive impairment in patients with major functional affective disorder. Similarly, we have also shown (Starkstein et al., 1988) that patients with post-stroke major depression have significantly more subcortical atrophy and significantly lower MMSE scores than patients matched for age, lesion location, and lesion size. Thus subcortical atrophy may be an important predisposing factor for the production of cognitive deficits in depressed patients. This subcortical atrophy may damage biogenic amine pathways, resulting in lower brain amine concentrations (Standish-Barry et al., 1986).

RELATION OF DEPRESSION TO LONGITUDINAL COURSE OF INTELLECTUAL IMPAIRMENT

We have longitudinally studied a group of 103 patients with acute stroke for the presence of depression and associated variables (Robinson et al., 1986, 1987). These patients underwent evaluation while in hospital during the acute post-stroke period and at 3, 6, 12, and 24 months post-stroke. Eight patients without in-hospital depression who remained nondepressed at 6 months post-stroke were compared for the presence of cognitive deficits with nine patients with in-hospital (major or minor) depression who remained depressed at 6 months' follow-up.

Although the depressed patients had slightly (but nonsignificantly) lower Mini-Mental scores at the time of the initial evaluation, at 6 months follow-up the nondepressed group showed improvmenet in Mini-Mental scores (from 23.2 ± 5.2 to 26.1 ± 4.5), whereas the depressed group showed a slight decline (from 21.8 ± 5.4 to 19.7 ± 5.3). By the end of the 6-month period, Mini-Mental scores of the depressed patients were significnatly lower than those of the nondepressed patients [$t(16) = 2.7$, $p < 0.02$]. Moreover, during this follow-up period only one patient with in-hospital depression spontaneously improved by 6 months' follow-up (from a score of 17 points to 20 points on the Mini-Mental State).

What is the clinical importance of these findings? We and others have demonstrated that PSD is amenable to treatment with tricyclic drugs (Finklestein et al., 1981; Ross and Rush, 1981); Lipsey et al., 1984; Reding et al., 1986), and it is possible that treatment of PSD also has an impact on cognitive impairments. In fact, several patients who received nortriptyline in our treatment study (Lipsey et al., 1984) showed some improvement in cognitive function during the 6 weeks of treatment; and one patient not in the treatment study, whose depression spontaneously remitted, also showed some cognitive improvement. Fogel and Sparadeo (1985) reported the case of a patient who underwent neuropsychological testing during a major depressive episode following a right hemisphere stroke. Although visuoconstructive deficits were present when the patient was depressed, they disappeared after tricyclic treatment.

A caveat should be added, however, as the long-term outcome of treatment of dementia of (functional) depression has not been clearly established. Although cognitive deficits can certainly improve after a therapeutic trial with tricyclic antidepressants (Reynolds et al., 1987), it has also been shown that dementia may not improve in parallel with depression (McAllister and Price, 1982; Rabins et al., 1984), and some patients with dementia of depression show evidence of a degenerative dementia during long-term follow-up.

SUMMARY AND FUTURE DIRECTIONS

Depression is a frequent complication of stroke and is associated with impairments in intellectual function. Several studies have shown that depressed patients get significantly less benefit from physical rehabilitation than nondepressed patients (Sinyor et al., 1986a). Future studies may examine if this lack of recovery in activities of daily living is related to cognitive impairment associated with PSD. Similarly, some aphasic patients fail to respond to speech therapy; and although in some cases it is explained by the type and severity of aphasia (i.e., patients with global aphasia show no benefit from speech therapy), it is also possible that aphasic patients with depression are more difficult to treat because of the simultaneous presence of cognitive impairments. Finally, future studies should demonstrate the impact of treating PSD in the longitudinal recovery of neuropsychological deficits.

Acknowledgments

This work was supported in part by the following NIH grants: Research Scientist Development Award MH-00163 (R.G.R.), MH-40355, NS-15178, NS-15080, a grant from the University of

Buenos Aires (S.E.S.), and a National Alliance for the Research in Schizophrenia and Depression (NARSAD) Fellowship Extension Award (S.E.S.).

REFERENCES

American Psychiatric Association (1980). *Diagnostic and Statistical Manual of Mental Disorders,* 3rd ed. Washington, D.C.: APA.

Basso, A., Lecours, A.R., Moraschini, S., and Hamer, M. (1985). Anatomoclinical correlations of the aphasias as defined through the computerized tomography: exceptions. *Brain Lang.,* **26,** 201–229.

Benton, A.L., and Hamsher, K. (1978). *Multilingual Aphasia Examination,* rev. ed. Iowa City: University of Iowa Press.

Bolla-Wilson, K., Robinson, R.G., Starkstein, S.E., Boston, J., and Price, T.R. (1989). Lateralization of dementia of depression in stroke patients. *Am. J. Psychiatry,* **146,** 627–634.

Broca, P. (1861). Sur la faculte du language articule, suivi d'une observation d'aphemie. *Bull. Anat. Soc. (Paris),* **2,** 330–357.

Caine, E.D. (1981). Pseudodementia. *Arch. Gen. Psychiatry,* **38,** 1359–1364.

Calev, A., Korin, Y., Shapira, B., Kugelmass, S., and Lerer, B. (1986). Verbal and non-verbal recall by depressed and euthymic affective patients. *Psychol.Med.,* **16,** 789–794.

Damasio, A.R., and Geschwind, N. (1985). Anatomical localization in clinical neuropsychology. In: J.A.M. Frederiks, ed., *Handbook of Clinical Neurology, Vol. 1* (45): *Clinical Neuropsychology,* pp. 7–22, rev. ed. Amsterdam: Elsevier.

Dick, J.P.R., Guillof, R.J., Stewart, A., Blackstock, J., Bielawska, C., Paul, E.A., and Marsden, C.D. (1984). Mini-mental state examination in neurological patients. *J. Neurol. Neurosurg. Psychiatry,* **47,** 496–499.

Ebrahim, S., Barer, D., and Nouri, F. (1987). Affective illness after stroke. *Br. J. Psychiatry,* **151,** 52–56.

Finklestein, S., Benowitz, L. I., Baldessarini, R.J., Arana, G.W., Levine, D., Woo, E., Bear, D., Moya, K., and Stoll, A.L. (1981). Mood, vegetative disturbance, and dexamethosone suppression test after stroke. *Ann. Neurol.,* **12,**. 463–468.

Fogel, B.S., and Sparadeo, F.R. (1985). Focal cognitive deficits accentuated by depression. *J. Nerv. Ment. Dis.,* **173,** 120–124.

Folstein, M.F., and McHugh, P.R. (1978). Dementia syndrome of depression. In: R. Katzman, R.D. Terry, and K.L. Bick, eds., *Aging, Vol. 7: Alzheimer's Disease: Senile Dementia and Related Disorders.* New York: Raven Press.

Folstein, M.F., Folstein, S.E., and McHugh, P.R. (1975). Mini-Mental State: a practical method for grading the cognitive state of patients for the clinician. *J. Psychiatr. Res.,* **12,** 189–198.

Folstein, M.F., Maiberger, R., and McHugh, P.R. (1977). Mood disorder as a specific complication of stroke. *J. Neurol. Neurosurg. Psychiatry,* **40,** 1018–1020.

Gibson, A.J. (1981). A further analysis of memory loss in dementia and depression in the elderly. *Br. J. Clin. Psychol.,* **20,** 179–185.

Glass, R.M., Uhlenhuth, E.H., and Hartel, F.W. (1981). Cognitive dysfunction and imipramine in outpatient depressives. *Arch. Gen. Psychiatry,* **38,** 1048–1051.

Goodglass, H., and Kaplan, E. (1976). *The Boston Naming test.* Philadelphia: Lea & Febiger.

Hamilton, M.A. (1960). A rating scale for depression. *J. Neurol. Neurosurg. Psychiatry,* **23,** 56–62.

Henry, G. M., Weingartner, H., and Murphy, D.L. (1973). Influence of affective states and psychoactive drugs on verbal learning and memory. *Am. J. Psychiatry,* **130,** 966–971.

Hier, D.B., Mondlock, J., and Caplan, L.R. (1983). Recovery of behavioral abnormalities after right hemisphere stroke. *Neurology,* **33,** 345–350.

Hooper, H.E. (1958). *The Hooper Visual Organization Test Manual.* Los Angeles: Western Psychological Services.

Huff, F.J., and Corkin, S. (1984). Recent advances in the neuropsychology of Alzheimer's disease. *Prog. Neuropsychopharmacol. Biol. Psychiatry,* **8,** 643–648.

Jorm, A.F. (1986). Cognitive deficit in the depressed elderly: a review of some basic unresolved issues. *Aust. N.Z. J. Psychiatry,* **20,** 11–22.

Kaplan, E., Goodglass, H., and Weintraub, S. (1976). *The Assessment of Aphasia and Related Disorders.* Philadelphia: Lea & Febiger.

Kellner, C.H., Rubinow, D.R., and Post, R.M. (1986). Cerebral ventricular size and cognitive impairment in depression. *J. Affective Disord.,* **10,** 215–219.

Lezak, M.D. (1976). *Neuropsychological Assessment.* New York: Oxford University

Lipsey, J.R., Robinson, R.G., Pearlson, G.D., Rao, K., and Price, T.R. (1983). Moo following bilateral hemisphere brain injury. *Brit. J. Psychiatry,* **143,** 266–273.

Lipsey, J.R., Robinson, R.G., Pearlson, G.D., Rao, K., and Price, T.R. (1984). Nortriptyline treatment for post-stroke depression: a double-blind study. *Lancet,* **1,** 297–300.

Lipsey, J., Spencer, W.C., Rabins, P. V., and Robinson, R.G. (1986). Phenomenological comparison of post-stroke depression and functional depression. *Am. J. Psychiatry,* **143,** 527–529.

Luria, A.R. (1966). *Higher Cortical Functions in Man.* New York: Basic Books.

Madden, J.J., Luhan, J.A., Kaplan, L.A., and Manfredi, H.M. (1952). Non-dementing psychoses in older persons. *J.A.M.A.,* **150,** 1567–1570.

Mayberg, H.S., Robinson, R.G., Wong, D.F., Parikh, R., Bolduc, P.L., Starkstein, S.E., Price, T.R., Dannals, R.F., Links, J.M., Wilson, A. A., Ravert, H.H., and Wagner, H.N. (1988). PET imaging of cortical S2-serotonin receptors following stroke: lateralzied changes and relationship to depression. *Am. J. Psychiatry,* **145,** 937–943.

McAllister, T.W. (1981). Cognitive functioning in affective disorders. *Compr. Psychiatry,* **22,** 572–586.

McAllister, T.W., and Price, T.R.P. (1982). Severe depressive pseudodementia with and without dementia. *Am. J. Psychiatry,* **139,** 626–629.

Miller, W.R. (1975). Psychological deficit in depression. *Psychol. Bull.,* **82,** 238–260.

Miller, E., and Lewis, P. (1977). Recognition memory in elderly patients and depression and dementia: a signal detection analysis. *J. Abnorm. Psychol.,* **86,** 84–86.

Nott, P.N., and Fleminger, J.J. (1975). Presenile dementia: the difficulties of early diagnosis. *Acta Psychiatr. Scand.,* **51,** 210–217.

Rabins, P.V., Merchant, A., and Nestadt, G. (1984). Criteria for diagnosing reve caused by depression. *Br. J. Psychiatry,* **144,** 488–492.

Reding, M.J., Orto, L.A., Winter, S.W., Fortuna, I.M., DiPonte, P., and M (1986). Antidepressant therapy after stroke: a double-blind trial. *Arch. Neurol.,* **43,** 763–765.

Reitan, R.M., and Davison, L.A. (1974). *Clinical Neuropsychology: Current Status and Applications.* New York: Hemisphere Press.

Reus, V.I., Silberman, E., Post, R.M., and Weingartner, H. (1979). d-Amphetamine effects on memory in a depressed population. *Biol. Psychiatry,* **14,** 345–356.

Reynolds, C.F., Perel, J.M., Kupfer, D.J., Zimmer, B., Stack, J.A., and Hoch, C.C. (1987). Open-trial response to antidepressant treatment in elderly patients with mixed depression and cognitive impairment. *Psychiatry Res.,* **21,** 111–122.

Robertson, G., and Taylor, P.J. (1985). Some cognitive correlates of affective disorders. *Psychol. Med.,* **15,** 297–309.

Robinson, R.G. (1979). Differential behavioral and biochemical effects of right and left hemispheric cerebral infarction in the rat. *Science,* **205,** 707–710.

Robinson, R.G., and Price, T.R. (1982). Post-stroke depressive disorders: a follow-up study of 103 patients. *Stroke,* **13,** 635–641.

Robinson, R.G., and Szetela, B. (1981). Mood change following left hemisphere brain injury. *Ann. Neurol.,* **3,** 447–453.

Robinson, R.G., Starr, L.B., Kubos, K.L., Rao, K., and Price, T.R. (1983). A two-year longitudinal study of post-stroke mood disorders: findings during the initial evaluation. *Stroke,* **14,** 736–741.

Robinson, R.G., Kubos, K. L., Starr, L.B., Rao, K., and Price, T.R. (1984). Mood disorders in stroke patients: importance of location of lesion. *Brain,* **107,** 81–93.

Robinson, R.G., Bolla-Wilson, K., Kaplan, E., Lipsey, J.R., and Price, T.R. (1986). Depression influences intellectual impairment in stroke patients. *Br. J. Psychiatry,* **148,** 541–547.

Robinson, R.G., Bolduc, P.L., and Price, T.R. (1987). Two-year longitudinal study of post-stroke mood disorders: diagnosis and outcome at one and two years. *Stroke,* **18,** 837–843.

Ross, E.D., and Rush, A.J. (1981). Diagnosis and neuroanatomical correlates of depression in brain damaged patients. *Arch. Gen. Psychiatry,* **38,** 1344–1354.

Roy-Byrne, R.P., Weingartner, H., Bierer, L.M., Thompson, K., and Post, R.M. (1986). Effortful and automatic cognitive processes in depression. *Arch. Gen. Psychiatry,* **43,** 265–267.

Savard, R.J., Rey, A.C., and Post, R.M. (1980). Halstead-Reitan Category Test in bipolar and unipolar affective disorders: relationship to age and phase of illness. *J. Nerv. Ment. Dis.,* **168,** 297–304.

Schlegel, S., and Kretzschmer, K. (1987). Computed tomography in affective disorders. Part I. Ventircular and sulcal measurements. *Biol. Psychiatry,* **22,** 4–14.

Sinyor, D., Amato, P., Kaloupek, D., Becker, R., Goldenberg, M., and Coopersmith, H. (1986a). Post-stroke depression: relationship to functional impairment, coping strategies, and rehabilitation outcome. *Stroke,* **17,** 1102–1107.

Sinyor, D., Jacques, P., Kaloupek, D.G., Becker, R., Goldenberg, M., and Coopersmith, H. (1986b). Post-stroke depression and lesion location: an attempted replication. *Brain,* **109,** 537–546.

131 Speedie, L., Rabins, P.V., Rothi, L., and Pearlson, G.D. (1988). Language functions of elderly depressed patients: a follow-up report. *J. Clin. Exp. Neuropsychol.,* **10,** 73.

Standish-Barry, M.A.S., Bouras, N., Hale, A.S., Bridges, P.K., and Bartlett, J.R. (1986). Ventricular size and CSF transmitter metabolite concentration in severe endogenous depression. *Br. J. Psychiatry,* **148,** 386–392.

Starkstein, S.E., Robinson, R.G., and Price, T.R. (1987). Comparison of cortical and subcortical lesions in the production of post-stroke mood disorders. *Brain,* **110,** 1045–1059.

Starkstein, S.E., Robinson, R.G., and Price, T.R. (1988). Comparison of patients with and without post-stroke major depression matched for size and location of lesion. *Arch. Gen. Psychiatry,* **45,** 247–252.

Stromgren, L.L. (1977). The influence of depression on memory. *Acta Psychiatr. Scan.,* **56,** 109–128.

Wade, D.T., Legh-Smith, J.E., and Hewer, R.A. (1987). Depressed mood after stroke: a community study of its frequency. *Br. J. Psychiatry,* **151,** 200–205.

Wechsler, D. (1945). A standardized memory scale for clinical use. *J. Psychol.,* **19,** 87–95.

Wechsler, D. (1955). *Manual for the Wechsler Adult Intelligence Scale,* New York: Psychological Corporation.

Wells, C.E. (1979). Pseudodementia. *Am. J. Psychiatry,* **136,** 895–900.

Weingartner, H., Cohen, R.M., Murphy, D.L., Martello, J., and Gerdt, C. (1981). Cognitive processes in depression. *Arch. Gen. Psychiatry,* **38,** 42–47.

Wing, J.K., Cooper, E., and Sartorius, N. (1974). *Measurements and Classification of Psychiatric Symptoms.* Cambridge: Cambridge University Press.

9

Contributions of the Halstead-Reitan Battery in the Neuropsychological Investigation of Stroke

JIM HOM

After heart disease and cancer, cerebrovascular disease (CVD) or stroke is the third most common cause of death in the United States, where approximately 85,000 fatalities occur each year from this cause alone. An additional one million individuals survive strokes with varying degrees of disability (Adams and Victor, 1985; Kurtzke, 1985). Although the incidence and mortality rates for stroke have been falling since the early 1960s, many of the medical problems encountered in a neurologic setting are likely to be related to CVD. For this reason neuropsychologists, clinical psychologists, and other mental health professionals should be aware of the range of brain-behavior problems potentially associated with this important and common neurologic entity.

The study of stroke has provided the fields of neurology and neuropsychology with important information concerning the function of the human brain. To a considerable extent, the understanding of aphasia, apraxia, and the neglect syndrome can be attributed to the study of focal ischemic lesions. Furthermore, information on lateralization and localization of higher cognitive abilities and sensory-perceptual, motor, and emotional functions has been derived from the study of stroke patients. For scientists who study brain-behavior relations, stroke provides an excellent model to understand the behavioral manifestations of brain lesions in humans.

Cerebrovascular disease refers to any abnormality of the brain that results from disorders of the blood supply or blood vessels. Stroke is by far the most common form of CVD (Kurtzke, 1985). Stroke is defined as a "sudden, nonconvulsive, focal neurologic deficit" (Adams and Victor, 1985, p. 530), Also known as apoplexy, apoplectic attack, or cerebrovascular accident, stroke involves disruption of the normal cerebral blood circulation. The brain is highly dependent on a continuous and constant flow of blood to sustain its high metabolic rate; even a short disruption (only a few minutes) in the flow results in brain tissue changes leading to eventual infarction and necrosis.

The two principal mechanisms of parenchymal changes resulting from stroke are ischemia and hemorrhage. Cerebral ischemia is the reduction in blood supply to a local region in the brain as a result of obstruction of a vessel. If the brain tissue distal to the occlusion is not sufficiently supplied by collateral vessels, it eventually becomes infarcted. Obstruction of the blood supply is most commonly the result of progressive atherosclerotic deposits causing stenosis or occlusion. With thrombotic stroke, an accumulation of blood material and tissue becomes incorporated into the atherosclerotic lesion in the vessel wall, causing partial or complete obstruction of blood flow. Fragments of thrombotic material, fatty deposit, or other foreign matter may form and cause embolic strokes. With such strokes the foreign matter usually originates outside the intracranial circulation, most commonly the bifurcation of the internal carotid artery, and obstructs the cerebral blood flow. In contrast to ischemic CVD, hemorrhagic strokes are due to the rupture of cerebral vessels, resulting in destruction of the brain tissue surrounding the area of the bleed. Cerebral hemorrhages are often related to the degree and duration of hypertension but may also result from ruptured aneurysms, arteriovenous malformations, or traumatic brain insult. A detailed description of the anatomy of the cerebral circulation, the pathologic processes involved in the various forms of CVD, and the individual neurovascular syndromes is beyond the scope of this chapter; however, Adams and Victor (1985) provided an excellent overview of these topics.

The type and severity of the neurologic deficit resulting from stroke depend on such factors as the location, size, temporal sequence, and mechanism of the stroke. Although hemiplegia represents the classic sign of stroke, the neurologic sequelae resulting from disruption in blood flow can vary widely in regard to the nature, severity, and persistence of symptoms. Symptoms can range from a comatose state and hemiplegia to negligible, transient neurologic symptoms. Mental confusion, sensorimotor deficits, aphasia, apraxia, seizures, and other dysfunctions are other clinical ramifications of stroke. Most often the apoplectic presentation of stroke allows relatively easy diagnosis. However, sometimes the symptoms are so subtle that the patient is unaware of any neurologic deficit. In such patients the diagnosis of stroke may be missed altogether, or it may be misdiagnosed (Adams and Victor, 1985; Dunne et al., 1986).

In consideration of the frequency and importance of this neurologic problem, there are surprisingly few studies concerned with intellectual, cognitive, and neuropsychological deficits associated with stroke. This lack is likely due to the fact that the major emphasis has been on the use of the clinical symptoms of stroke for diagnosis and identification of the cerebrovascular condition. This orientation reflects the traditions of clinical and behavioral neurology as contrasted with clinical neuropsychology. In general, behavioral neurology focuses on pathology of the nervous system and the specific behavioral deficits associated with that pathology. A strong emphasis is placed on diagnosis using the binary classification of normal versus disordered brain structure and function (Davison, 1974; Rourke and Brown, 1986). As a result, the primary focus of neuropsychological investigations in stroke has been on the identification of specific cognitive deficits.

The behavioral neurologic orientation has had a strong influence on neuropsychological study and methodology as evidenced by the statement of Heilman and Valenstein (1985b, p. 7).

> The understanding of brain-behavior relationships is aided most by the study of behaviors that can be clearly defined and that are likely to be related to brain processes that can be directly or indirectly observed. Behaviors that can be selectively affected by focal brain lesions or by specific pharmacological agents are therefore most often chosen for neuropsychological study. Conversely, behaviors that are difficult to define or that appear unlikely to be correlated with observable anatomical, physiological, or chemical processes in the brain are poor candidates for study. As techniques for studying the brain improve, more kinds of behavior should become amenable to study.

In contrast to the behavioral neurology model, the clinical neuropsychology model emphasizes the behavioral ramifications of brain pathology. This orientation focuses on continuously distributed psychological variables in elucidating clinical brain-behavior relations. Advocates of this approach are interested in understanding the extent and type of neuropsychological dysfunction associated with brain pathology and its effects on the adaptive function of the individual. As a result, the clinical neuropsychological study of stroke investigates many important areas of brain-behavior functions that have not been adequately investigated or have been given a role of secondary importance owing to the lack of clear neuroanatomic correlation (Davison, 1974; Rourke and Brown, 1986).

A number of investigators have advocated more extensive investigation of the extent of cognitive and behavioral changes associated with stroke (Heilman, 1974; Reinvang and Sundet, 1985; Reitan and Wolfson, 1985; Dunne et al., 1986; Hom, 1988; Hom and Reitan, 1990). Although relatively few in number, these clinical neuropsychological investigations have provided some important information concerning the nature of brain-behavior dysfunction resulting from stroke.

The primary focus of this chapter is the clinical neuropsychological study of stroke. The Halstead–Reitan Battery (HRB) (Reitan and Wolfson, 1985) is the most widely used neuropsychological test battery, and has been employed in most neuropsychological studies of stroke. In view of the extensive literature on the validity of the HRB and its previous applications in stroke research, this chapter emphasizes the HRB. In particular, current studies are presented that concern a broad range of brain-behavior functions, including intellectual, cognitive, and sensorimotor abilities that have previously been overlooked in the study of stroke and their effect on human behavior. In addition, comparisons are made with effects of other lesion types. Although stroke has important implications for language and praxic function, it is beyond the scope of this chapter to review the extensive research concerning aphasia, apraxia, or emotional components of stroke; these topics are presented in other chapters in this book, and the reader is referred to Filskov and Boll (1981) and Heilman and Valenstein (1985a) for additional material.

GENERAL VERSUS SPECIFIC NEUROPSYCHOLOGICAL FUNCTION

The clinical symptoms of stroke have significantly aided the clinical diagnosis of a cerebrovascular condition. Based on these symptoms, a neurologist may be able to determine the specific areas in the brain and the site in the cerebral circulation where the neurologic insult has occurred, as well as the probable type of the stroke. Various neurovascular syndromes have been formulated that reflect the sequelae of compromise of the major cerebral arterial distributions (Adams and Victor, 1985). As noted earlier, many investigations of cognitive sequelae in stroke have been concerned with specific cognitive deficits. This focus is useful for providing information about neuroanatomic substrates of particular behavioral deficits. However, it does not provide information about the extent and nature of higher cognitive impairment, the identification of more subtle cognitive deficits, or functions that are dependent on the general integrity of the brain. In fact, such a narrow or circumscribed focus may obstruct understanding of the full behavioral repercussions of stroke.

Cerebral functioning reflects the complex interaction of several factors, including anatomic organization, physiologic function, and experiences of the individual. Impairment of any of these factors may disrupt an individual's cognitive abilities. For example, obstruction of the left middle cerebral artery may lead to infarction of portions of the left cerebral hemisphere, causing right-sided hemiplegia along with various aphasic and apraxic deficits. In addition, cognitive and intellectual abilities, such as memory, attention, problem-solving, and abstraction, may be impaired.

Goodglass and Kaplan (1979) and Reitan and Wolfson (1985) have noted the importance of the effect of cerebral lesions on the general, as well as the specific, functions of the brain. According to these investigators, except for rare "pure" cases, some degree of general or nonspecific deficit typically occurs in association with specific deficits. Whereas measures of some specific functions are dependent on specific sites or areas in the brain, general measures are relatively independent of a particular location of impairment and reflect the overall status of brain functioning. Thus a relatively focal lesion can result in both specific and nonspecific behavioral deficits. The specific deficits may relate to the primary functions of the particular brain area, whereas the nonspecific effects may reflect disruption of a number of neurobehavioral systems to which the lesioned area contributes.

According to Goodglass and Kaplan (1979), general or nonspecific (nonlocalizing) deficits following cerebral damage include (1) impairment of conceptual thinking; (2) slowness of ideational processes; (3) reduced attention; (4) stimulus boundness; and (5) impairment of memory. A conceptual model of hierarchical brain function has been advocated by Reitan and Wolfson (1985) that strongly emphasizes the combined role of general cerebral functions with the more specific functions of the brain. The central features of this theory focus on three stages of central processing. Stage 1 represents registration and integration of incoming material with past experiences, stage 2 involves content specific processing of incoming material, and stage 3 pertains to the highest level of processing concerned with concept formation, reasoning, and logical analysis (Figure 9–1). Six categories of brain function are included in the model: (1) sensory input functions; (2) attention, concentration, and memory; (3) verbal abilities; (4) spatial, sequential, and manipulatory abilities; (5) abstraction, reasoning, logical analysis, and concept formation; and (6) output motor functions. In this model, categories 1 and 6 represent the fundamental input and output components of brain function. Categories 3 and 4 reflect the more specialized functions of the brain and are related to specific brain regions. In contrast, categories 2 and 5 represent general cerebral functions and are related to the equipotentiality

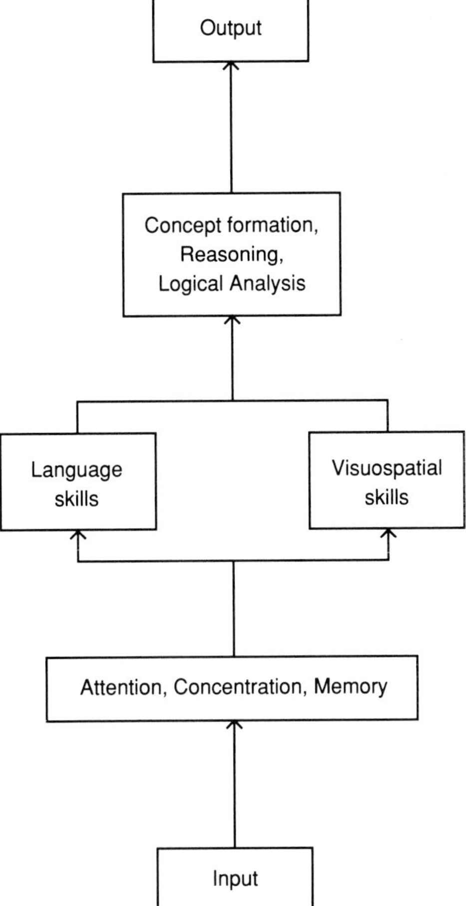

Figure 9–1 Reitan-Wolfson conceptual model of brain-behavior relations. (Reproduced with permission from Reitan and Wolfson, 1985.)

of cerebral cortical tissue. These general functions are considered nonlocalized and are largely independent of a specific brain region. According to Reitan and Wolfson, the understanding of the general functions of the brain is the unique contribution of clinical neuropsychology.

Measurement of general cerebral functions is typically based on the use of a battery of neuropsychological tests, which evaluate both general and specific measures of brain functions (Reitan and Davison, 1974; Goodglass and Kaplan, 1979; Lezak, 1983; Reitan and Wolfson, 1985). The basic assumption of this approach is that systematic measurement of intellectual, cognitive, and sensorimotor functions with an appropriate standardized battery of tests provides a basis from which inferences may be made regarding the organic integrity of the brain. For example, the Halstead-Reitan Neuropsychological Test Battery represents the standardized battery approach and is the most widely used and validated instrument currently available for the assessment of neuropsychological functioning (Reitan and Davison, 1974; Boll,

1981; Reitan and Wolfson, 1985). Neuropsychological batteries of this type allow for more comprehensive specification of various cerebral deficits and the effects of lesions on brain-behavior abilities than can be found in assessments of specific abilities alone. Furthermore, subtle patterns of neuropsychological function and deficits are revealed by the battery approach that are often missed with other less comprehensive methodologies. On the other hand, ability-specific neuropsychological batteries may provide a more in-depth analysis of a particular function, such as memory or language. Nonetheless, the evaluation of general cerebral functions is best accomplished by approaches that utilize a comprehensive and broad behavioral sample of brain function.

NEUROPSYCHOLOGICAL DEFICITS IN STROKE

Neuropsychological studies have revealed the existence of a number of intellectual and cognitive impairments in stroke in addition to sensorimotor and language deficits. The following sections review some of the major findings.

Motor Impairment

The most obvious sign of stroke (particularly involving the middle cerebral artery and its distribution) is hemiplegia. Reitan and Fitzhugh (1971) completed one of the first comprehensive studies on sensorimotor functioning associated with cerebrovascular lesions. Fifteen triads of subjects matched for age, education, and duration of CVD were compared in terms of motor, somatosensory, and psychomotor abilities. Each triad consisted of a subject with a left cerebral hemisphere lesion, one with a right hemisphere lesion, and one with a generalized or diffuse cerebral vascular lesion. Diagnosis was based on a thorough neurologic examination, resulting in groups with the following diagnoses: occlusive cerebrovascular disease—anterior, middle, posterior cerebral artery or internal carotid artery; vascular anomaly—middle cerebral artery; intracranial hematoma; generalized cerebrovascular disease; hypertensive encephalopathy; or bilateral carotid artery insufficiency. Sensorimotor measures from the Halstead-Reitan Neuropsychological Test Battery (HRB) were used, which included the Finger Oscillation Test (tapping), Strength of Grip, Tactual Performance Test (TPT), bilateral simultaneous tactile-, auditory-, and visual-perception, tactile finger recognition, finger-tip number writing recognition, and tactile coin recognition. Patients were also given the Wechsler-Bellevue Intelligence Scale.

Statistical comparisons of motor measures (finger tapping, grip strength, and TPT) were made between groups (left versus right versus diffuse cerebrovascular lesions) and within individuals (right hand versus left hand performance). A relatively consistent and orderly pattern of impairment of motor function was found in relation to the lateralization of the cerebral damage. For both intergroup and intraindividual comparisons, motor function was found to be more impaired contralateral to the side of the cerebral damage. However, intraindividual differences were found to be more reliable in this regard than the intergroup comparisons. In the case of the diffuse or generalized cerebrovascular group, less motor impairment was found relative to the lateralized groups.

Similar findings have been reported by other investigators, indicating greater motor impairment contralateral to the side of cerebral damage for stroke (Reitan, 1970; Finlayson and Reitan, 1980; Haaland and Delaney, 1981; Hom and Reitan, 1982; Hom, 1988), neoplasms (Finlayson and Reitan, 1980; Haaland and Delaney, 1981; Hom and Reitan, 1982, 1984), and traumatic brain lesions (Finlayson and Reitan, 1980; Hom and Reitan, 1982).

Hom (1988) also found that generalized or diffuse cerebrovascular lesions caused less-lateralized motor deficits relative to lateralized cerebrovascular lesions. These findings are not surprising and confirm the relation between the classic anatomic motor pathways and motor function. In addition, in comparison to other neurologic etiologies, motor impairment has been found to be greater in the stroke population than in groups with cerebral neoplasms (Reitan, 1970; Haaland and Delaney, 1981; Hom and Reitan, 1982) or with traumatic brain injury (Reitan, 1970; Hom and Reitan, 1982).

Somatosensory Impairment

In the same study of motor function, Reitan and Fitzhugh (1971) also investigated the somatosensory functions of patients with cerebrovascular lesions. Somatosensory measures from the HRB (see Motor Impairment, above) were compared among the left cerebral hemisphere, right hemisphere, and diffuse cerebral vascular lesion groups. The results indicated that the left cerebral lesion group tended to perform more poorly on the right side of the body than the left. The reverse was true for the right cerebral lesion group; the left side of body tended to be more impaired than the right side. This relation was found to be most significant for bilateral simultaneous tactile perception with less effect for the other somatosensory functions. As was found for motor function, the diffuse group demonstrated a pattern of deficits intermediate to the left and right groups.

Using lesion groups similar to those in the Reitan and Fitzhugh study, Hom and Reitan (1982) compared somatosensory functions in patients with cerebrovascular, neoplastic, and traumatic lateralized cerebral lesions. The same measures from the HRB were used with the exception of the tactile coin recognition measure. Statistical comparisons between those with left versus right cerebrovascular damage indicated greater somatosensory impairment contralateral to the side of the cerebral lesion. A similar relation was found for the neoplastic and traumatic brain lesion groups, although the strength of the relation was least in the traumatic lesion group.

Reitan (1970) investigated the relative neuropsychological performance of patients with cerebrovascular, neoplastic, and traumatic brain lesions and reported findings similar to those of Hom and Reitan (1982). Somatosensory function tended to be more seriously impaired contralateral to the damaged cerebral hemisphere in stroke compared to neoplasms and traumatic brain lesions. Others have shown similar results for tactile perception (Boll, 1974) and tactile sensitivity (Carmon, 1971a) in mixed groups of brain lesions.

Contralateral Versus Ipsilateral Sensorimotor Function

In contrast to the relatively straightforward relation between the classic anatomic pathways and lateralized sensorimotor function, controversy exists in relation to whether one hemisphere or the other has predominant control of sensorimotor functioning. Although existing anatomic evidence points toward basically symmetric sensory and motor representation, numerous studies have suggested differential functional control in the two cerebral hemispheres (Semmes et al., 1960; Vaughan and Costa, 1962; Corkin et al., 1964; Wyke, 1966, 1971; Semmes, 1968; Carmon, 1971a, b; Finlayson and Reitan, 1980; Haaland and Delaney, 1981; Hom and Reitan, 1982). Differential contralateral and ipsilateral sensorimotor functioning for the two cerebral hemispheres has important clinical implications when diagnosing the extent and location of stroke and in regard to residual deficits resulting from stroke. According to Brown and colleagues (1986) in their review of the effects of CVD on higher cortical function, a diagnosis of bilateral cerebral involvement may be falsely made for a unilateral lesion because of differential functional control of sensorimotor abilities between the left and right cerebral hemispheres.

A number of investigators have reported greater sensorimotor control by the left cerebral hemisphere than by the right hemisphere (Semmes et al., 1960; Vaughan and Costa, 1962; Wyke, 1966, 1971; Semmes, 1968). These studies found that left cerebral hemisphere lesions caused both contralateral and ipsilateral sensorimotor deficits, whereas right hemisphere lesions appeared to affect contralateral sensorimotor functions only. Studying patients with penetrating head wounds, Semmes and colleagues (1960) found that right-handed sensorimotor deficits were specifically associated with left hemisphere lesions of the sensorimotor area, whereas no specific area within the right hemisphere was associated with sensorimotor deficits of the left hand. They also presented evidence that left hemisphere lesions resulted in sensorimotor deficits in the ipsilateral as well as the contralateral hand, whereas right hemisphere lesions resulted in a much lower incidence of ipsilateral sensorimotor deficiency. Additional support for these findings was reported by Vaughan and Costa (1962) and Wyke (1966, 1971) in humans and by Glees and Cole (1952) and Semmes and Mishkin (1965) in monkeys. These findings were interpreted by Semmes (1968) to suggest that the cerebral hemispheres are organized differently, with the sensorimotor functions diffusely represented in the right hemisphere and focally represented in the left hemisphere. Furthermore, Semmes postulated that this cerebral organization accounted for the differential higher-level functions of the two cerebral hemispheres, with the more focal representation within the left hemisphere corresponding to the more discrete intrinsic structure of language and the more diffuse organization of the right hemisphere related to nonlanguage abilities.

In contrast to the findings of bilateral sensorimotor control of the left cerebral hemisphere, a number of studies have found no significant asymmetry of ipsilateral function for somatosensory abilities (Corkin et al., 1964; Carmon, 1971a) or motor skills (Carmon, 1971b; Finlayson and Reitan, 1980; Haaland and Delaney, 1981). Furthermore, other studies have shown greater bilateral sensory motor control in the right hemisphere.

Hom and Reitan (1982) compared the contralateral and ipsilateral sensorimotor performances of three groups of 50 adult patients with lateralized cerebrovascular, neoplastic, or traumatic brain lesions. A broad range of motor and somatosensory measures from the HRB were studied, including motor (finger tapping, grip strength, and complex psychomotor function) and somatosensory (bilateral simultaneous tactile, auditory, and visual stimulation, finger recognition, finger-tip number writing perception, and tactile form recognition) measures. These investigators found greater bilateral deficits with right cerebral hemisphere lesions than with left hemisphere lesions. In addition, intergroup comparisons indicated the greatest amount of sensorimotor impairment with cerebrovascular lesions, followed closely by neoplastic lesions; traumatic brain lesions produced significantly less impairment. The pattern of bilateral sensorimotor deficits following a right cerebral hemisphere lesion was determined for each lesion type, with the cerebrovascular group demonstrating the strongest and most consistent pattern, followed by the neoplastic group, with the traumatic groups demonstrating the least strong and most variable pattern. Similar findings have been reported by Boll (1974) for tactile perceptual functioning in a mixed group of patients with cerebrovascular, neoplastic, or traumatic brain lesions.

Hom and Reitan (1982) accounted for the differences in findings, especially from those of Semmes et al. (1960) and Wyke (1966, 1971), as due to differences in patient samples and lesion type and extent. The evidence presented by Semmes et al. was based solely on the performance of patients with long-standing penetrating head injuries inflicted by high-velocity projectiles. A large proportion of patients in the Wyke studies had either meningiomas or temporal lobectomies. Other studies have used patients with a variety of etiologies. It is known that different cerebral lesions are associated with different patterns of neuropsychological deficit (Reitan, 1966). Thus by using patient samples of mixed etiology, the effect of the specific lesion or etiology on sensorimotor function may have been masked. Furthermore, the studies of Semmes et al. and others have attempted to relate patients' deficiencies in sensorimotor function to focal lesions. However, with most naturally occurring lesions of the brain, more extensive areas are damaged rather than only well defined or preselected areas (Courville, 1953). Therefore it is possible that the findings were actually based on impairment that involved large or multiple areas of damage rather than circumscribed lesions of a specific location. In fact, the lesion distribution in the Semmes et al. (1960) patient sample was extensive, frequently involving more than one area of cerebral damage.

In summary, the available studies of sensorimotor functioning after lateralized stroke indicate sensorimotor impairment in accordance with the classic anatomic pathways. Contralateral sensorimotor impairment results from lateralized cerebrovascular lesions. However, in addition, ipsilateral sensorimotor deficits also appear and may be greater with cerebrovascular lesions of the right cerebral hemisphere, as found in the Hom and Reitan (1982) study. This fact may have significant implications for the diagnosis and localization of stroke as described by Brown et al. (1986). Furthermore, this pattern of brain-behavior function may suggest differential strategies for rehabilitation of sensorimotor function after left versus right cerebral hemisphere stroke. For example, right hemisphere lesions may require sensorimotor rehabilitation on both sides of the body, whereas left hemisphere lesions may require only contralateral rehabilitation.

Intellectual Impairment

Surprisingly, few studies of intellectual function after stroke have been conducted. Most investigations of intelligence in relation to cerebrovascular disease pertain to dementia resulting from multiple cerebral infarctions known as multiinfarct dementia (MID). A number of studies have reported significant decrement of intellectual abilities after multiple cerebral infarctions resulting in tissue loss of more than 100 cc (Blessed et al., 1968; Tomlinson et al., 1968, 1970; Cummings and Benson, 1983; Loeb et al., 1988). Those studies are not reviewed in this chapter, but dementia is presented elsewhere in this book.

In general, based on available studies concerning intellectual function and stroke, a relatively consistent pattern of intellectual impairment has been demonstrated for performances on the Wechsler Intelligence Scales (Wechsler, 1944). Reitan and Fitzhugh (1971) found greater impairment of Verbal IQ (VIQ) for the left stroke group than for the right stroke group. No differences were found between the groups on Performance IQ (PIQ). Intragroup comparisons of VIQ minus PIQ discrepancies demonstrated significant differences between the lateralized stroke groups. Left cerebral strokes were found to impair VIQ more than PIQ. The reverse was found for the right stroke group, in which PIQ was more impaired than VIQ. No intragroup differences were found for the diffuse cerebrovascular group; however, their mean difference between VIQ and PIQ occupied an intermediate position of impairment between the lateralized stroke groups.

Brown et al. (1986) noted the lack of a control group in the Reitan and Fitzhugh study. They questioned whether the VIQ performance of the right cerebral stroke group represented normal or impaired function. A similar question can be asked for the PIQ performances of any of the stroke groups. It would be important to determine if intellectual deficits, in comparison with control groups, occur with stroke.

In an earlier study, Reitan (1970) compared three groups of patients with cerebrovascular disease, similar to groups used in the Reitan and Fitzhugh (1971) study, and a control group of patients without evidence of brain damage or disease. The control group was found to perform significantly better than the cerebrovascular groups on all of the individual subtests of the Wechsler-Bellevue Scale, as well as on all measures of sensorimotor function, measures from the Halstead Neuropsychological Test Battery, and the Trail Making Test. These results clearly demonstrated the level and extent of intellectual and neuropsychological impairment in stroke patients in relation to non-brain-damaged controls.

Hom and Reitan (1990) compared the intellectual functioning of three groups of CVD patients with a control group. The three stroke groups were composed of patients with cerebrovascular lesions similar to those in the groups in the Reitan and Fitzhugh (1971) study (left hemisphere, right hemisphere, and diffuse or generalized). The left stroke group consisted of 20 patients with occlusive disease ($n = 16$), arteriovenous malformation ($n = 1$), aneurysm ($n = 2$), and intracranial hemorrhage ($n = 1$). The right lesion group also included 20 cerebrovascular patients primarily with occlusive disease ($n = 18$), and patients with two arteriovenous malformations. Twenty patients with hypertensive encephalopathy, bilateral carotid artery insufficiency, basilar artery occlusion, or generalized atherosclerosis composed the third (diffuse or generalized) stroke group. The control group included seven patients with psychiatric disorders, three patients with noncerebrovascular medical or neurologic problems, and ten normal controls. The subjects in the four groups were matched for age, education, and gender. All subjects were administered the Wechsler Intelligence Scales.

Multivariate analyses of variance yielded highly significant differences among the groups for the summary IQ scores. Univariate analyses indicated that the intellectual

Table 9–1 Group Mean (±SD) Raw Scores and ANOVA Comparisons for Intellectual Abilities of Patients with Cerebrovascular Disease

Measure	Right	Left	Diffuse	Control	F(3,76)	p
VIQ	104.85 ± 16.08	91.05 ± 24.90	96.05 ± 17.14	114.85 ± 6.61	7.20	<0.0005
PIQ	95.55 ± 17.24	100.25 ± 14.03	98.65 ± 14.81	122.25 ± 8.12	15.30	<0.0001
FSIQ	98.80 ± 15.79	93.40 ± 20.68	94.95 ± 17.26	119.15 ± 6.43	11.21	<0.0001
VWS	46.80 ± 14.33	33.90 ± 23.36	37.80 ± 16.53	56.50 ± 5.96	7.66	<0.0005
PWS	29.75 ± 14.34	34.05 ± 14.91	30.30 ± 13.63	52.85 ± 7.31	14.28	<0.0001

functioning of the cerebrovascular groups was significantly poorer than the controls. However, no significant differences were found between the control group and the right stroke group on VIQ. In addition, no significant differences were found among the cerebrovascular groups on any of the measures. Table 9–1 gives the raw score means, standard deviations, and univariate analysis for each intellectual measure. These results clearly indicate that stroke significantly impairs intellectual function in a generalized manner.

Intragroup comparisons of VIQ minus PIQ yielded significant differences between the left and right stroke groups and between the right stroke and control groups. These results are consistent with the VIQ-PIQ pattern found in the Reitan and Fitzhugh study. Verbal intellectual abilities were more impaired relative to perceptual-motor intellectual abilities in the left stroke group, and the reverse was found for the right stroke group. The diffuse stroke group occupied an intermediate position between the left and right stroke groups.

Inspection of the mean IQ performances in the Haaland and Delaney (1981) study indicates a similar tendency toward greater verbal intellectual impairment following left cerebrovascular lesions and greater perceptual-motor intellectual impairment after right lesions. This pattern has also been reported for cerebral neoplasms (Hom and Reitan, 1984). Furthermore, based on the mean IQ performances of the Hom and Reitan (1984) and Haaland and Delaney (1981) samples, the level of intellectual impairment appears to be less with stroke than with neoplasm, although both are impaired in relation to controls. These findings suggest an orderly and fairly consistent pattern of intellectual impairment with lateralized cerebral lesions. However, the strength of this pattern and level of overall impairment depend on the type of neurologic pathology (Andersen, 1950, 1951; Reitan, 1955b; Klove and Reitan, 1958; Doehring et al., 1961; Fitzhugh et al., 1961; Klove and Fitzhugh, 1962; Klove and White, 1963; Satz, 1966; Fields and Whitmyre, 1969).

Overall Brain Impairment

The Halstead Impairment Index (HII) has been thoroughly investigated and was found to be a sensitive indicator of overall brain impairment (Reitan, 1955a; Vega and Parsons, 1967). The HII is a summary value based on the proportion of impaired performances on the Halstead portion of the HRB. The measures contributing to the HII are the Halstead Category Test, Tactual Performance Test (total time, memory, and localization scores), Speech-Sounds Perception Test, Seashore Rhythm Test, and Finger Oscillation Test (dominant hand). The HII is basically a *consistency-of-impairment* value that represents the number of brain-sensitive measures that are in the impaired range (Reitan and Wolfson, 1985). Furthermore, the number of measures in the brain-impaired range likely reflects the amount of difficulty in immediate adaptive abilities. HII values range from 0 to 1.0, with 0 to 0.3 indicating normal brain functioning, 0.4 borderline, and 0.5 to 1.0 indicating brain impairment.

Hom and Reitan (1990) compared the HII values for patients with cerebrovascular lesions and controls. For the left, right, and diffuse cerebrovascular groups, the HII values were 0.82, 0.84, and 0.87, respectively. The control group had an HII of 0.41. All three stroke groups were found to be significantly worse than controls. No significant differences were found among the stroke groups (Table 9–2). These findings clearly indicate a considerable degree of brain dysfunction with stroke. The lateralization of the cerebrovascular lesions did not differentially affect the level of overall brain impairment. These data indicate that in addition to "hemisphere-specific" deficits, CVD also causes impairment of cognitive abilities that are not dependent on the function of a specific hemisphere. Similar findings have been reported for cerebral neoplasms (Hom and Reitan, 1984).

Higher Cognitive Deficits

In addition to studying intellectual abilities, Hom and Reitan (1990) investigated the higher cognitive functions of patients with cerebrovascular lesions. The same three cerebrovascular lesion groups described earlier were compared with a matched control group. Each subject was administered an extensive battery of psychological and neuropsychological tests, including the complete HRB. The neuropsychological test variables were clustered into a priori functional groupings as used by Hom and Reitan (1982, 1984) and Hom and Fulbright (1987). The functional groupings are as follows.

1. *Attention and concentration:* Speech-Sounds Perception Test, Seashore Rhythm Test, Trail Making Test Part A, and Digit Span and Arithmetic from the Wechsler Intelligence Scales
2. *Abstraction:* Halstead Category Test, Tactual Performance Test Total Time, Trail Making Test Part B, and Digit Symbol from the Wechsler Intelligence Scales
3. *Incidental Memory:* Tactual Performance Test Memory and Localization

Multivariate analyses of variance indicated statistically significant group differences beyond the 0.01 level of significance for all three functional groupings. With the exception of one measure (Tactual Performance Test Total Time), univariate analyses indicated differences between the stroke groups and the control group. No significant differences were found among the three stroke groups. Inspection of the mean scores of the control versus the stroke groups in Table 9–2 clearly shows the greater impairment in the stroke groups.

In general, these results demonstrate the extent of higher cognitive impairment exhibited in patients with cerebrovascular lesions. This impairment extends beyond the expected lateralized dysfunctions associated with the damaged cerebral hemisphere. In fact, cerebrovascular lesions, whether lateralized or diffuse, affect complex cognitive processes that depend on the general biologic integrity of the brain. These findings are similar to those found for cerebral neoplasms (Hom and Reitan, 1984) and strongly suggest that impairment of the cerebral hemispheres results in dysfunc-

Table 9–2 Group Mean (±SD) Raw Scores and ANOVA Comparisons for General Neuropsychological and Motor Abilities

Measure	Right	Left	Diffuse	Control	F(3,76)	p
Halstead Impairment Index	0.84 ± 0.20	0.82 ± 0.17	0.87 ± 0.16	0.41 ± 0.20	27.51	<0.0001
Attention & concentration						
Seashore Rhythm	17.55 ± 7.28	17.30 ± 9.89	17.60 ± 7.51	26.8 ± 1.88	8.25	<0.0001
Speech-Sounds Perception	16.20 ± 13.99	20.60 ± 17.11	18.30 ± 12.99	5.50 ± 2.35	5.39	<0.005
Trail Making A	91.95 ± 85.84	88.10 ± 79.07	106.30 ± 87.21	34.45 ± 13.51	3.71	<0.05
Arithmetic	8.75 ± 4.40	5.80 ± 5.38	6.50 ± 4.81	10.85 ± 2.80	5.31	<0.005
Digit Span	7.15 ± 3.71	4.80 ± 4.06	5.95 ± 3.80	9.30 ± 3.36	5.28	<0.005
Abstraction						
Category Test	99.00 ± 27.65	103.90 ± 55.03	96.45 ± 38.43	57.05 ± 22.84	6.44	<0.0005
TPT Total Minute/Block	6.13 ± 6.30	7.60 ± 13.16	5.05 ± 10.49	0.56 ± 0.26	2.28	N.S.
Trail Making B	198.30 ± 85.82	202.45 ± 91.52	216.85 ± 103.73	72.40 ± 22.13	13.39	<0.0001
Digit Symbol	5.54 ± 2.48	5.30 ± 3.79	4.95 ± 3.38	9.15 ± 1.76	8.87	<0.0001
Incidental Memory						
TPT Memory	4.55 ± 2.16	4.45 ± 2.72	4.90 ± 2.83	7.15 ± 1.53	5.78	<0.005
TPT Localization	1.55 ± 1.50	1.00 ± 1.34	1.65 ± 2.03	2.75 ± 1.97	3.56	<0.05
Motor						
Finger Tapping Dominant	45.65 ± 8.92	21.90 ± 19.17	39.50 ± 9.57	47.10 ± 12.19	15.58	<0.0001
Finger Tapping Nondominant	18.60 ± 16.41	38.30 ± 13.05	36.85 ± 10.14	41.70 ± 9.50	13.61	<0.0001

tion of abstraction, memory, problem-solving, attention and concentration, and flexibility of thought not solely attributable to the side of lesion.

CONCLUSIONS

The studies reviewed in this chapter clearly indicate that the effects of stroke on higher cortical function are more extensive than the obvious deficits associated with the side or specific location of the lesion. There is clear evidence that neuropsychological functions that are somewhat independent of the location of cerebral damage, or are dependent on the integrated function of various brain regions, are also impaired. Although there have been relatively few neuropsychological studies concerning the generalized cerebral deficits of stroke patients, those available strongly suggest impairment of a broad range of higher cognitive functions, including intelligence, abstract reasoning, problem-solving, learning, memory, attention and concentration, and flexibility of thought.

In light of the findings presented in this chapter, the understanding of the neuropsychological effects of stroke needs to be broadened to include the effects of stroke on generalized cognitive functions. The deficit-specific model has tended to cultivate the concept of discrete behavioral concomitants following focal brain lesions affecting only a few areas of function with few or no changes to the remainder of the neuropsychological functions. Thus there is an emphasis on identifying the specific deficits and then remediating them. Stroke patients are often referred to rehabilitation for physical therapy and speech therapy for treatment of motor and language deficits. However, the full extent of cognitive dysfunction may be overlooked because of the focus on these discrete dysfunctions.

Many physicians and other health care professionals believe that stroke victims, if they survive the acute neurologic and medical event, recover without significant cognitive or behavioral changes, except possibly residual language or sensorimotor deficits. The effect of post-stroke neuropsychological impairment on immediate adaptive abilities often is poorly understood or incompletely recognized. The erroneous expectation of limited neurobehavioral sequelae after stroke may seriously hinder appropriate treatment and rehabilitation and may thus limit the possible services available to the stroke victim.

Information presented in this chapter provides a basis for drawing conclusions about the comparative effects of stroke in relation to other neurologic conditions. In general, similar brain-behavior relations were found for different types of cerebral lesion. However, the degree of impairment varied with the lesion type. For example, strokes tend to produce a large degree of sensorimotor impairment, followed by neoplasms; traumatic brain lesions result in the least degree of sensorimotor impairment. These findings suggest a "uniqueness" for each lesion type in terms of level of impairment but a similarity in the overall effects.

Additional research, of course, is much needed. In particular, studies of the effects of various types of stroke (e.g., occlusive versus hemorrhagic) on neuropsychological function are essential. Further studies of stroke risk factors, including hypertension, cardiovascular disease, and serum cholesterol, on neuropsychological function would be valuable. We also need to know more about the impact of stroke-related neuropsychological deficits on the adaptive daily function and vocational and psychosocial adjustment of the stroke victim.

REFERENCES

Adams, R.D., and Victor, M. (1985). Cerebrovascular diseases. In: *Principles of Neurology,* (3rd ed.) pp. 530, 569–640. New York: McGraw-Hill.

Andersen, A.L. (1950). The effect of laterality localization of brain damage on Wechsler-Bellevue indices of deterioration. *J. Clin. Psychol.,* **6,** 191–194.

Andersen, A.L. (1951). The effect of laterality localization of focal brain lesions on the Wechsler-Bellevue subtests. *J. Clin. Psychol.,* **7,** 149–153.

Blessed, G., Tomlinson, B.E., and Roth, M. (1968). The association between quantitative measures of dementia and of senile change in the cerebral grey matter of elderly subjects. *Br. J. Psychiatry,* **114,** 797–811.

Boll, T.J. (1974). Right and left cerebral hemisphere damage and tactile perception: performance of the ipsilateral and contralateral sides of the body. *Neuropsychologia,* **12,** 235–238.

Boll, T.J. (1981). The Halstead-Reitan neuropsychological battery. In: S.B. Filskov and T.J. Boll, eds., *Handbook of Clinical Neuropsychology,* pp. 577–607. New York: Wiley.

Brown, G.G., Baird, A.D., and Shatz, M.W. (1986). The effects of cerebral vascular disease and its treatment on higher cortical functioning. In: I. Grant and K.M. Adams, (eds.), *Neuropsychological Assessment of Neuropsychiatric Disorders,* pp. 384–414. New York: Oxford University Press.

Carmon, A. (1971a). Disturbance of tactile sensitivity in patients with unilateral cerebral lesions. *Cortex,* **7,** 83–97.

Carmon, A. (1971b). Sequenced motor performance in patients with unilateral cerebral lesions. *Neuropsychologia,* **9,** 445–449.

Corkin, S., Milner, B., and Rasmussen, T. (1964). Effects of different cortical excisions on sensory thresholds in man. *Trans. Am. Neurol. Assoc.,* **89,** 112–116.

Courville, C.B. (1953). *Commotio Cerebri.* Los Angeles: San Lucas Press.

Cummings, J.L., and Benson, D.F. (1983). *Dementia: A Clinical Approach.* Boston: Buttersworth.

Davison, L.A. (1974). Introduction. In: R.M. Reitan and L.A. Davison, eds., *Clinical Neuropsychology: Current Status and Applications,* pp. 1–18. Washington, D.C.: V.H. Winston & Sons.

Doehring, D.G., Reitan, R.M., and Klove, H. (1961). Changes in patterns of intelligence test performance associated with homonymous visual field defects. *J. Nerv. Ment. Dis.,* **132,** 227–233.

Dunne, J.W., Weedman, P.J., and Edis, R.H. (1986). Inobvious stroke: a cause of delirium and dementia. *Aust. N.Z. J. Med.,* **16,** 771–778.

Fields, F.R.J., and Whitmyre, J.W. (1969). Verbal and performance relationships with respect to laterality of cerebral involvement. *Dis. Nerv. Syst.,* **30,** 177–179.

Filskov, S.B., and Boll, T.J. (1981). *Handbook of Clinical Neuropsychology.* New York: Wiley.

Finlayson, M.A.J., and Reitan, R.M. (1980). Effect of lateralized lesions on ipsilateral and contralateral motor functioning. *J. Clin. Neuropsychol.,* **2,** 237–243.

Fitzhugh, K.B., Fitzhugh, L.C., and Reitan, R.M. (1961). Wechsler-Bellevue comparisons in groups of "chronic" and "current" lateralized and diffuse brain lesions. *J. Consult. Psychol.,* **26,** 306–310.

Glees, P., and Cole, J. (1952). Ipsilateral representation in the cerebral cortex. *Lancet,* **1,** 1191.

Goodglass, H., and Kaplan, E. (1979). Assessment of cognitive deficit in the brain-injured patient. In: M.S. Gazzaniga, ed., *Handbook of Behavioral Neurobiology: Vol. 2 Neuropsychology,* pp. 3–22. New York: Plenum Press.

Haaland, K.Y., and Delaney, H.D. (1981). Motor deficit after left or right hemisphere damage due to stroke or tumor. *Neuropsychologia,* **19,** 17–27.

Heilman, K.M. (1974). Neuropsychologic changes in the stroke patient. *Geriatrics,* **29,** 153–160.

Heilman, K.M., and Valentstein, E. (1985a). *Clinical Neuropsychology.* New York: Oxford University Press.

Heilman, K.M., and Valentstein, E. (1985b). Introduction. In: K.M. Heilman and E. Valenstein, eds., *Clinical Neuropsychology,* pp. 3–16. New York: Oxford University Press.

Hom, J. (1988). Cognitive function in cerebrovascular disease. *Clin. Neuropsychol.,* **2,** 282.

Hom, J., and Fulbright, R.L. (1987). Neuropsychological correlates of early stage Alzheimer's disease. *Clin. Neuropsychol.,* **1,** 279.

Hom, J., and Reitan, R.M. (1982). Effects of lateralized cerebral damage upon contralateral and ipsilateral sensorimotor performances. *J. Clin. Neuropsychol.,* **4,** 249–268.

Hom, J., and Reitan, R.M. (1984). Neuropsychological correlates of rapidly vs. slowly growing intrinsic cerebral neoplasms. *J. Clin. Neuropsychol.,* **6,** 309–324.

Hom, J. and Reitan, R.M. (1990). Generalized cognitive function in stroke. *J. Clin. Exp. Neuropsychol.,* **12,** 644–654.

Klove, H., and Fitzhugh, K.B. (1962). The relationship of differential EEG patterns to the distribution of Wechsler-Bellevue scores in a chronic epileptic population. *J. Clin. Psychol.,* **18,** 334–337.

Klove, H., and Reitan, R.M. (1958). The effects of dysphasia and spatial distortion on Wechsler-Bellevue results. *Arch. Neurol. Psychiatry,* **80,** 708–713.

Klove, H., and White, P.T. (1963). The relationship of degree of electroencephalographic abnormality to the distribution of Wechsler-Bellevue scores. *Neurology,* **13,** 423–430.

Kurtzke, J.F. (1985). Epidemiology of cerebrovascular disease. In: F.H. McDowell and L.R. Caplan, eds., *Cerebrovascular Survey Report for the National Institute of Neurological and Communicative Disorders and Stroke,* pp. 1–34. Washington, DC: NINCDS.

Lezak, M.D. (1983). *Neuropsychological Assessment.* New York: Oxford University Press.

Loeb, C., Gandolfo, C., and Bino, G. (1988). Intellectual impairment and cerebral lesions in multiple cerebral infarcts: a clinical-computed tomography study. *Stroke,* **19,** 560–565.

Reinvang, I., and Sundet, K. (1985). The validity of functional assessment with neuropsychological tests in aphasic stroke patients. *Scand. J. Psychol.,* **26,** 208–218.

Reitan, R.M. (1955a). An investigation of the validity of Halstead's measures of biological intelligence. *Arch. Neurol. Psychiatry,* **73,** 28–35.

Reitan, R.M. (1955b). Certain differential effects of left and right cerebral lesions in human adults. *J. Comp. Physiol. Psychol.,* **48,** 474–477.

Reitan, R.M. (1966). A research program on the psychological effects of brain lesions in human beings. In: N.R. Ellis, ed., *International Review of Research in Mental Retardation,* Vol. 1, pp. 153–218. Orlando: Academic Press.

Reitan, R.M. (1970). Objective behavioral assessment in diagnosis and prediction. In: A.L. Benton, ed., *Behavioral Change in Cerebrovascular Disease,* pp. 155–165. New York: Harper & Row.

Reitan, R.M., and Davison, L.A. (1974). *Clinical Neuropsychology: Current Status and Applications.* Washington, D.C.: V.H. Winston & Sons.

Reitan, R.M., and Fitzhugh, K.B. (1971). Behavioral deficits in groups with cerebral vascular lesions. *J. Consult. Clin. Psychol.,* **37,** 215–223.

Reitan, R.M., and Wolfson, D. (1985). *The Halstead-Reitan Neuropsychological Test Battery: Theory and Clinical Interpretation.* Tucson: Neuropsychology Press.

Rourke, B.P., and Brown, G.G. (1986). Clinical neuropsychology and behavioral neurology: similarities and differences. In: S.B. Filskov and T.J. Boll, eds., *Handbook of Clinical Neuropsychology,* Vol. 2, pp. 3–18. New York: Wiley.

Satz, P. (1966). Specific and non-specific effects of brain lesions in man. *J. Abnorm. Psychol.,* **71,** 65–70.

Semmes, J. (1968). Hemispheric specialization: a possible clue to mechanism. *Neuropsychologia,* **6,** 11–26.

Semmes, J., and Mishkin, M. (1965). Somatosensory loss in monkeys after ipsilateral cortical ablation. *J. Neurophysiol.,* **28,** 473–486.

Semmes, J., Weinstein, S., Ghent, L., and Teuber, H.L. (1960). *Somatosensory Changes After Penetrating Brain Wounds in Man.* Cambridge: Harvard University Press.

Tomlinson, B.E., Blessed, G., and Roth, M. (1968). Observations on the brains of non-demented old people. *J. Neurol. Sci.,* **7,** 331–356.

Tomlinson, B.E., Blessed, G., and Roth, M. (1970). Observations on the brains of demented old people. *J. Neurol. Sci.,* **11,** 205–242.

Vaughan, H.S., and Costa, L.D. (1962). Performance of patients with lateralized cerebral lesions: II. Sensory and motor tests. *J. Nerv. Ment. Dis.,* **134,** 237–243.

Vega, A., and Parsons, O.A. (1967). Cross-validation of the Halstead-Reitan tests for brain damage. *J. Consult. Psychol.,* **31,** 619–625.

Wechsler, D. (1944). *The Measurement of Adult Intelligence.* Baltimore: Williams & Wilkins.

Wyke, M. (1966). Postural arm drift associated with brain lesions in man. *Arch. Neurol.,* **15,** 329–338.

Wyke, M. (1971). The effects of brain lesions on the performance of bilateral arm movements. *Neuropsychologia,* **90,** 33–42.

10

Risk Factors for Stroke and Neuropsychological Performance

ROBERT A. BORNSTEIN AND MARK P. KELLY

Several chapters in this and other volumes (Bornstein, 1986; Brown et al., 1986) have made it clear that there is a strong association between cerebrovascular disease (CVD) and neurobehavioral deficit. When studying the neurobehavioral sequelae of CVD, it is important to assess the influence of other associated conditions that may also affect behavior. Prospective epidemiologic studies such as the Framingham Study, have identified a number of risk factors that are associated with an increased incidence of CVD (Wolf et al., 1978b). The Framingham Study was initially designed to study heart disease and hypertension but has since expanded its scope to consider the epidemiology of CVD. To a large extent, the study of CVD risk factors in the Framingham Study has been influenced by the initial focus of the study. Much of the published epidemiologic data on stroke risk factors has focused on atherothrombotic infarction, as it is the cause of approximately 60% of all strokes and is viewed by some as the cerebrovascular counterpart of myocardial infarction or peripheral vascular disease (Wolf et al., 1978b).

A number of demographic, biomedical, and life style variables have been considered in relation to the incidence of CVD. These variables include age, sex, hypertension, diabetes mellitus, serum hemoglobin, serum lipids (particularly cholesterol), obesity, cardiac disease, and cigarette smoking. Similar to cardiac and peripheral vascular disease, the risk for atherothrombotic stroke, as well as for cerebral embolism and intracerebral hemorrhage, is clearly related to increased age. In contast to cardiac and peripheral vascular disease, there does not appear to be a substantial sex difference in the incidence of stroke. As noted by Brown et al. (1986), many of these risk factors themselves have potential neuropsychological sequelae; and because these disorders occur commonly in stroke populations it becomes important in the study of stroke to understand the relations between risk factors and neuropsychological performance. The purpose of this chapter therefore is to review the literature that has explored these relations. A consideration of the neuropsychology of aging would require entire volumes and thus is well beyond the scope of this chapter. Obesity is a risk factor for stroke as well as for hypertension, diabetes, and hyperlipidemia (Kuller, 1978). When the risks associated with other factors are controlled, the relation between weight and stroke occurrence is no longer significant (Kannel 1984). In any event, there have as yet been no studies of the neuropsychological consequences of obesity. The remainder of the chapter is devoted to a review of studies that have considered the neuropsychological aspects of the previously noted stroke risk factors.

HYPERTENSION

Hypertension has consistently emerged as the strongest medical risk factor for stroke (Shekelle et al., 1974; Kannel et al., 1976; Salonen 1982) and the most extensively studied in regard to neuropsychological sequelae. The risk rises in direct relation to the degree of blood pressure elevation (Dyken et al., 1984) and holds for both sexes and all ages (Wolf et al., 1983). Hypertension increases the risk for both anthero-thrombotic brain infarction and cerebral hemorrhage (Wolfe et al., 1983). Elevations of both systolic and diastolic pressures predict increased stroke incidence (Wolfe et al., 1983). Possible mechanisms by which hypertension may lead to stroke (or neuropsychological deficits) include acceleration of atherogenesis in cerebral blood vessels, mechanical damage to the vessels, reduced perfusion of narrowed cerebral vessels via development of cardiac insufficiency (Lavy, 1979), and metabolic changes at a cellular level (Canessa et al., 1980). Evidence suggests that patients with essential hypertension have altered regional cerebral blood flow (Rodriguez et al., 1987), which is more pronounced in untreated patients with disease of relatively long duration; frontal and temporal areas are maximally involved. Newly diagnosed patients and treated patients with disease of longer duration show less pronounced flow reduction that is confined to the temporal regions.

The importance of hypertension as a risk factor for stroke is amplified by its stature as a major public health problem. Estimates suggest that in the United States 20% of all adults suffer from moderate to severe hypertension (defined as blood pressure of 160/95 mm Hg or higher). Thus roughly 25 million people are likely to be affected in this country alone (U.S. Public Health Service, 1976a, b). It is also well known that the risk of hypertension increases with age. Surveys suggest that by age 64 roughly one-half of the population develops at least mild hypertension (blood pressure of 140/90 mm Hg or higher) (Lew, 1973).

Early Studies

Almost 50 years ago it was reported that a small group of hypertensive patients performed more poorly than controls on a measure of flicker fusion (Enzer et al., 1942). Some 10 years later Apter and colleagues (1951) reported that a group of 14 hypertensive patients showed significant impairment on the Halstead Battery. In the former study no effort was made to exclude patients with complications of hypertension or other medical problems, and the hypertension and control groups were not matched with respect to potentially important background variables (e.g., age, education). In the latter study, no control group was employed; moreover, most of the hypertensive patients had significant psychiatric disease, two were alcoholic, and one had a stroke. The influences of age and education were not explicitly considered when interpreting the neuropsychological results. Neither study considered the possible influence of medication on test performance. Although inconclusive, these early investigations provided an impetus for further study, with greater control for the effects of such factors as concomitant disease, age, background, and medication.

Intellectual Function

Evidence regarding the possibility of intellectual decline related to hypertension comes primarily from studies using the Wechsler Adult Intelligence Scale (WAIS), though other instruments (Wechsler-Bellevue, Ravens Progressive Matrices, Army Alpha Test) have been used. For WAIS studies, despite variations in patient characteristics and design, some degree of impairment has consistently been found. Wilkie and Eisorfer (1971) found that at age 60 to 69 individuals with hypertension (defined as diastolic pressure greater than 105 mm Hg) showed poorer performance than normotensive (diastolic pressure 66–95 mm Hg) or borderline hypertensive (diastolic pressure 95–105 mm Hg) individuals on the WAIS Full Scale and Performance weighted scores. When followed over 10 years (48% return rate), all groups showed stable Verbal scores but the Performance and Full Scale weighted scores decreased for the hypertensive group. A 70- to 79-year-old group was also studied, but no hypertensive patients in this group completed follow-up. Initial diastolic blood pressure values were correlated with initial WAIS scores, and the magnitude of the correlations varied as a function of group composition (age group, whole sample versus returnees only). Boller and colleagues (1977) compared a group of 20 newly diagnosed hypertensive patients to a group of 20 medical clinic controls and found differences on only one of six WAIS subtests (Digit Span).

In the first of a series of studies (Schultz et al., 1979) comparing hypertensive patients to normotensive controls, initial analyses found that the WAIS Verbal composite score was impaired for younger (age 21–39) but not older (age 45–69) hypertensive patients. When the effects of educational level and socioeconomic status were controlled, both younger and older hypertensive patients showed poorer performance than matched normotensive controls on the Performance composite score. Plasma renin levels did not affect WAIS performance. These individuals were followed over a 5- to 6-year period with a 35% return rate (Schultz et al., 1986). No significant change was found in hypertensive patients over time, and they continued to perform more poorly on the Performance composite score at follow-up. Mazzuchi and colleagues (1986) compared three groups of hypertensive patients (diagnosed for 1 year, 3–5 years, and 6–10 years) with a group of individually matched normotensive controls on eight WAIS subtests. As a group, hypertensive patients performed more poorly on the Digit Span, Block Design, and Digit Symbol subtests. However, when individual subgroups of hypertensive patients were considered, only the Digit Span subtest differentiated hypertensive patients in the 3- to 5-year duration disease group from controls. In an uncontrolled study of 15 hypertensive patients (Vanderploeg et al., 1987) negative correlations were found between systolic pressure and the Verbal IQ and all verbal subtests, as well as between diastolic pressures and Digit Symbol and Block Design subtests.

Studies utilizing measures of intelligence other than the WAIS have also suggested a pattern of deficit in hypertension. Francheschi and colleagues (1982) reported that both chronic and recently diagnosed hypertensives performed more poorly than controls on the Ravens Progressive Matrices and WAIS Block Design subtest. Costa and Shock (1980) evaluated hypertensives of three ages (20–39, 40–49, and 50–65 years) and severity [low, average, and high blood pressure (>140/90 mm Hg)] in relation to controls. It was found that hypertension did not influence performance on the Army Alpha Test for any age group. When individuals with serious illnesses or individuals taking medication were eliminated and age groups were collapsed, however, a pattern of deficient performance for the hypertensive group emerged. The performance of the hypertensive group did not deteriorate over an 8-year follow-up.

In summary, controlled studies utilizing the WAIS have consistently found some degree of impairment in hypertensive groups relative to controls, with Performance subtests appearing to be somewhat more vulnerable. This selective vulnerability did not appear in studies by Boller et al., (1977) and Vanderploeg et al. (1987); however, the latter study had no control group, and the former used medically ill (rather than healthy) controls. Some studies failed to explicitly control for the effects of education (Wilkie and Eisdorfer, 1971). The issue of the natural history of impairment is less clear. Data from the two longitudinal studies (Wilkie and Eisdorfer, 1976; Schultz et al., 1986) are conflicting. Because of the high attrition rate in both studies, firm conclusions are unwarranted. Consistent with studies using the WAIS, hypertensives have also been found to be impaired relative to controls on other measures of ability.

Neuropsychological Measures

A number of investigators have utilized portions of the Halstead-Reitan Battery (HRB) for studying neuropsychological concomitants of hypertension. A series of studies (Goldman et al., 1974, 1975; Kleinman et al., 1977) utilized the Category Test to assess neuropsychological change following biofeedback treatment of essential hypertension. In all three studies the average number of errors for hypertensive patients (pretreatment) exceeded the traditional HRB cutoff score for brain dysfunction. However, owing to the lack of a control group and the potential confounding effects of age and educational level, the evidence for impairment related to hypertension is unclear. Pentz and colleagues (1979) found that unmedicated hypertensive patients were impaired relative to normotensive controls on the Category Test, Tactual Performance Test (Memory score), and Finger Tapping Test. For the latter two measures the impairment was significantly more pronounced in the younger (mean age 29 years) than the older (mean age 50 years) hypertensive patients. There were no differences related to previous history of medication. Conclusions regarding the impact of hypertension on neuropsychological performance are clouded, however, as the hypertensive group was significantly less educated than the control group. In contrast to these results, Mazzuchi et al. (1986) found no deficit on Finger Tapping in hypertensive patients relative to well matched controls.

In a study by Elias and colleagues (1986), hypertensive patients and well matched controls were administered the HRB and then followed over a 5- to 6-year period (with the average age at the start of the study in the midfifties). All hypertensive patients were unmedicated initially but were medicated at follow-up. The hypertensive patients exhibited poorer performance than controls on the Category Test, Tactual Performance Test (Memory score), Trail Making Test Part B, and Average Impairment Rating. On follow-up (22% return rate) neither the hypertensive patients nor the controls showed significant change of performance. In a subsequent study (Elias et al., 1987) with larger groups, subjects were further subdivided on the basis of education. For the high education group (mean 16.9 years), hypertensive patients were similar to controls in neuropsychological performance. For the low education group (mean 13 years), hypertensive patients performed more poorly than controls on the Category Test and Tactual Performance Test (Memory and Location scores). When traditional cutoff scores for the Average Impairment Rating were used, there was no significant difference between hypertensive patients and normotensives in the proportion scoring in the abnormal range. The performance of medicated and nonmedicated hypertensives was similar. Vanderploeg et al. (1987) administered the entire HRB to a group of 15 hypertensive veterans. Consensual clinical ratings by two neuropsychologists rated 13 of 15 patients in the study as impaired on baseline testing. Four of the HRB summary measures correlated with systolic blood pressure, but there was no relation with diastolic pressure. The strongest correlation was with the Category Test.

To summarize, all conclusions regarding the effects of hypertension on the HRB must be regarded as preliminary. The two studies that employed appropriate (i.e., age- and education-matched) normotensive control groups (Elias et al., 1986, 1987) suggest impairment in hypertensive patients relative to controls on several measures with the most consistent impairment on the Category Test and the Tactual Performance Test. These results may not be widely generalizable, however, as patients in these two studies were well educated. The issue of longitudinal changes in HRB performance is unresolved. The only longitudinal study (Elias et al., 1986) contained a final sample of only 11 hypertensive patients, and there was a high dropout rate.

Reaction Time/Psychomotor Performance

Timed motor and cognitive tasks are sensitive to cerebral dysfunction and have thus been employed by many investigators in neuropsychological studies of hypertension. Speed of performance was the major parameter studied by Speith (1964). On a composite measure, hypertensive patients (who were undergoing job certification) performed more poorly than a group of healthy controls. In a second group of hypertensive patients who were not undergoing certification (but who were also receiving antihypertensive medication) performance on this composite measure was unimpaired. The groups were not strictly matched for age and education, though all participants in the study fell in the 35- to 59-year age bracket and were "nearly all" in the highest quartile of the population in terms of occupational status and education.

Light (1975, 1978) studied a large group of hypertensive patients and normotensive controls across a wide range of ages, utilizing a set of serial choice reaction time tasks. All hypertensive patients were studied under the influence of a single dose of diuretic medication, though some had a history of treatment prior to the study. Results indicated that the reaction time was significantly reduced for previously medicated hypertensives of all ages but not for previously unmedicated hypertensives. Renin levels were related to reaction time performance only in previously untreated patients. Interpretation of these findings is complicated because both age and duration of illness was greater in the previously medicated group. The study also failed to control for the effects of education and socioeconomic status.

Boller et al. (1977) studied auditory reaction time and several psychomotor measures (Dynamometer, Purdue Pegboard) in newly diagnosed hypertensives. Hypertensive patients were poorer than matched medical controls on the reaction time tasks. In a study by Shapiro and colleagues (1982) there were no differences in reaction time, but hypertensive patients performed more poorly than controls on three measures of motor performance (traverse time and transfer, coordination time, and tapping speed). During a 15-month follow-up to this study, Miller and coworkers (1984) retested roughly 70% of these individuals. Hypertensive patients treated with antihypertensive medication in the interim improved more than controls on one of the six psychomotor tests, whereas untreated hypertensive patients had no improvement and declined significantly on one test (grip strength). The improvement in performance by the treated group accompanied significant blood pressure reduction.

To summarize, studies of reaction time have yielded inconsistent results. Most studies (Light, 1975, 1978; Boller et al., 1977) found abnormalities, but some (Shapiro et al., 1982) did not. Several studies were flawed by the failure to equate hypertension and control groups on the basis of such critical features as age and education. Studies of choice reaction time have reported positive results (Light, 1975, 1978). The studies that found no differences on reaction time measures (Shapiro et al., 1982; Miller et al., 1984) used patients with milder hypertension than those with positive findings (Boller et al., 1977). With respect to performance on measures of psychomotor speed, one study (Boller et al., 1977) provided no evidence for impairment in hypertension, whereas another suggested a decline (Shapiro et al., 1982). In the latter study, patients with hypertension showed impairment on several experimental measures of psychomotor speed. Data from the Miller et al. (1984) studies suggested a slight tendency for untreated hypertensives to decline on psychomotor tasks over time and for treated patients to improve.

Memory

Wilkie and colleagues (1976) found no initial differences between normotensive, borderline hypertensive, and hypertensive patients (age 60–69) on several Wechsler Memory Scale (WMS) subtests including Logical Memory, Visual Reproduction, and Paired Associate Learning. On follow-up averaging 6.5 years (with 34% of participants returning for reevaluation), the hypertension group performed more poorly than the normal or borderline hypertension group on the Visual Reproduction and Logical Memory Subtests. Boller et al. (1977) found no differences on measures of recent memory (Rey Figure and WMS—Logical Memory). Studies by Shapiro et al. (1982) and Miller et al. (1984) found no deficits on the Benton Visual Retention Test. In contrast, Francheschi et al. (1982) reported that recently diagnosed hypertensives performed more poorly than controls on the WMS Memory Quotient and the Logical Memory Subtest. In addition, patients with chronic hypertension (all of whom took medication) performed more poorly than controls on these measures as well as on the Benton Visual Retention Test Form B. Mazzuchi et al. (1986) administered numerous experimental memory measures to hypertensive patients (with subgroups of disease of varying duration) and controls. Patients with shorter duration of illness were impaired on a greater proportion of the measures. The groups were not consistently impaired on any particular measure. When the entire group of hypertensive patients was compared to the entire group of controls, deficiencies were noted on four of the six tests. Vanderploeg et al. (1987) reported significant correlations between systolic pressures and the WMScale Memory Quotient and Visual Reproduction subtest.

Mazzuchi et al. (1986) also included measures of iconic memory for neologisms and nonsense figures. When groups of hypertensive patients were categorized by duration of disease, no impairment was found on either task. When the patient groups were collapsed and compared with controls, however, hypertensive patients tended to perform more poorly on iconic memory for neologisms.

There is no clear consensus regarding the effect of hypertension on recent memory. Three of six controlled studies reported no impairment. Of the three studies that reported impairment, two suggested more substantial impairment later in the course of hypertension, and one suggested more substantial impairment earlier in the course of the illness. Furthermore, some studies suggested deficits in verbal memory, whereas others indicated deficits in nonverbal memory. There has been no consideration of other dimensions of memory function such as recall versus recognition memory or procedural versus declarative memory. No single commonly used memory test showed consistent impairment across studies.

Summary

Although hypertension has been investigated by neuropsychologists more than any other medical risk factor for stroke, the database remains limited. Available evidence suggests that hypertension can be associated with neuropsychological impairment that tends to be subtle. Impaired performance is reported with some consistency on WAIS Performance IQ, Category Test, Tactual Performance Test, and Trail Making Test from the HRB, as well as measures of response speed. It is not surprising that these measures would be impaired, as they are among the most sensitive to cerebral dysfunction generally (Blackburn and Benton, 1955; Benton and Joynt, 1959; Matthews et al., 1966). As such, impairment on these measures provides few clues regarding either the elementary information-processing deficits in hypertension or the location of the underlying neuropathology. In addition, the range of neuropsychological parameters examined is limited.

The onset and natural history of neuropsychological impairment in hypertension are of considerable interest. Several controlled studies (e.g., Boller et al., 1977; Franceschi et al., 1982; Shapiro et al., 1982) have documented neuropsychological impairment in recently diagnosed hypertensives (unmedicated when evaluated); such studies indicate that neuropsychological impairment may occur relatively early in the course of the illness. The issue of progression of neuropsychological impairment is less clear: Three longitudinal studies have found no changes in neuropsychological impairment over time, two have found decline, and one has found improvement in medically treated patients and decline in untreated patients. Conclusions are difficult owing to the inconsistency between studies, small samples, high dropout rate, and variability in medication status of patients in these studies. The finding by Miller et al. (1984) that unmedicated patients decline and medicated patients improve over time is intriguing. Replication of this study would be desirable, as would extension of findings to patients using other forms of antihypertensive medication. Study of the effect of treatment for hypertension on neuropsychological test performance remains in a germinal stage.

Although there are several possible mechanisms that might readily explain the neuropsychological impairment in hypertension, clinical/pathological correlations also remain to be elucidated. The impact of hypertension on the nature and recovery of neuropsychological impairment following acute cerebrovascular events also has undergone little study. When conducting future neuropsychological studies, investigators must attempt to adhere to guidelines for conducting neuropsychological research (Parsons and Prigatano, 1978), including proper controls for the effects of age, education, occupation, and socioeconomic status. Careful attention to the definition of hypertensive groups, including the type of hypertension and specific medication status, is also mandatory if knowledge is to be advanced in this area. Evaluating hypertensive patients with state-of-the-art techniques [magnetic resonance imaging (MRI) or positron emission tomography (PET)] in concert with neuropsychological measures may provide a rich source of data regarding mechanisms of neuropsychological impairment and individual variations in neuropsychological performance.

DIABETES MELLITUS

Diabetes presents an increased risk for stroke in both males and females at most age levels (Wolf et al., 1978b) and has been associated with increased atherosclerotic disease in the circle of Willis (Baker et al., 1961). In addition, fluctuating glucose levels leading to episodes of hypoglycemia (due to excessive control of blood glucose) or ketoacidosis (from inadequate control) have been suggested as possible causes for "diabetic encephalopathy" (Gilhaus et al., 1973; Eeg-Olofssen, 1977; Kaplinsky and Frankl, 1980; Ruderman and Goodman, 1980). Furthermore, hypertension, cerebral atherosclerosis, and peripheral neuropathy are common complications of diabetes (Clarke et al., 1980; Ganda, 1980; Colwell et al., 1981; Moore et al., 1981; Riddle and Hart, 1981). Thus there is a clear rationale for the study of the neurobehavioral correlates of this disease. However, prior to 1980 there were only two studies (Rennick et al., 1968; Bale, 1973) that addressed cognitive function in adults. (Some early studies on intelligence and academic performance in childhood-onset diabetes are not considered here). Since 1980 there have been at least ten studies that have examined neuropsychological performance in adult diabetics.

Rennick et al. (1968) compared groups of diabetics matched for age and education, with and without retinopathy. The groups did not differ in terms of functional vision, but the group with retinopathy had a higher percentage of impairment on neuropsychological tests. The impairments were noted on more complex problem-solving tasks. Bale (1973) compared 100 adult-onset diabetics with matched controls on the WAIS and a word learning test. A higher percentage of diabetics were impaired on the word learning task, and there was an association between impairment on that test and a history of hypoglycemic episodes. A history of stroke, the patient's age, or the duration of illness were not related to deficits on the learning task.

Lawson et al. (1984) examined 48 diabetic patients and matched controls on subtests of the WAIS and several memory tasks, including the WMS, Recurring Figures Test (Kimura, 1963), and a verbal analogue of the Recurring Figures Test. There were relatively few significant differences between the groups, although diabetics obtained significantly lower scores on the WMS Memory Quotient. Diabetics obtained a mean Verbal IQ (VIQ) 8 points lower than controls, and the discrepancy between VIQ and Performance IQ (PIQ) from the WAIS just failed to reach significance. Further analyses indicated that age at onset of illness was negatively correlated with performance on the Recurring Figures Test. These findings were consistent with the suggestion by Meuter and colleagues (1980) that cognitive deficit on tests of reaction time, memory, and concentration may be more commonly associated with adult-onset diabetes. It is unclear how many adult-onset patients were in the Lawson et al. (1984) sample, and there was no attempt to group the patients on the basis of adult versus juvenile onset as was done in the Meuter et al. (1980) study.

Franceschi et al. (1984) examined a group of 37 neurologically asymptomatic patients between the ages of 18 and 35. On virtually all neuropsychological measures the diabetic patients performed more poorly than controls, although the differences reached significance on only the WMS Memory Quotient and the WAIS Block Design and Similarities subtests. The deficits were not related to peripheral neuropathy, duration of illness, or adequacy of metabolic control. Pramming and colleagues (1986) examined performance on a neuropsychological battery in relation to levels of glucose control in 16 diabetic patients. There was a clear relation between decreasing blood glucose levels and declining performance on virtually all tests. In addition, 12 of 16 patients demonstrated decreased neuropsychological performance at glucose levels just below normal (not typically considered hypoglycemic). Performance returned to baseline with restoration of normal serum glucose levels. Although the neuropsychological deficits appeared reversible in this study, the authors raised the possibility of persistent deficit associated with chronic hypoglycemic episodes.

Skenazy and Bigler (1984) compared 39 juvenile-onset diabetics and control groups on an extensive neuropsychological test battery, including the HRB. The diabetic patients were further grouped on the basis of visual impairment. Diabetics without visual impairment fared worse than both control groups on the PIQ and Trail Making Tests (parts A and B). Both diabetic subgroups (with and without visual impairment) made more somatosensory errors than controls. An index of disease severity was employed that reflected duration of illness, number of complications, diabetic comas or severe hypoglycemic episodes, and associated complications. Patients with five or more of these criteria formed a severe disease group and were more impaired on several HRB subtests including Finger Tapping, Trail Making A and B, and the number of visual and somatosensory errors. The less severe group performed more poorly on Tactual Performance Test (Memory and Location scores) and the number of dysphasic errors. Both parts of the Trail Making Test and Finger

Tapping (both hands) were consistently correlated with each of the variables contributing to the severity index. It was concluded that the sensory and motor deficits were related to peripheral neuropathy, but that there was evidence for visual processing and visuopraxic deficits, the mechanism for which was unclear.

Baade (1988) studied 35 patients between the ages of 20 and 49, with age at onset of diabetes between 2 months and 47 years. An extensive neuropsychological battery was employed; and in comparison with matched controls, diabetics were found to have slight but statistically significant differences on a broad range of tests. There were no consistent relations between neuropsychological performance and disease-related variables, including age at onset, duration of illness, and adequacy of metabolic control. It was observed that performance of the diabetic group was more variable, and it was suggested that a subgroup of these patients may have contributed disproportionately to the group differences. This sample contained both juvenile-onset (prior to age 30) and adult-onset patients. In view of previous studies (Meuter et al., 1980; Lawson et al., 1984) the analysis of differences between juvenile- and maturity-onset patients would be of considerable interest.

Holmes and her colleagues have reported several investigations of neuropsychological correlates of juvenile-onset diabetes (Holmes et al., 1983, 1984, 1986; Holmes, 1986, 1990). Consistent with the report by Pramming et al. (1986), hypoglycemic blood levels were associated with impaired performance on tests of verbal fluency (Holmes et al., 1984), speed of recall (Holmes et al., 1983), and rate of decision-making (Holmes et al., 1986). Holmes (1986) reported that patients with poor metabolic control were impaired on several VIQ subtests and simple reaction time measures compared with patients who were well controlled. This finding contrasted with those of previous studies (Franceschi et al., 1984; Lawson et al., 1984; Baade, 1988), which failed to report an association between neuropsychological deficit and adequacy of metabolic control.

These studies provided some evidence of neuropsychological deficits in adults with juvenile-onset diabetes. Only one study (Meuter et al., 1980) explicitly examined maturity-onset patients and found evidence of greater deficit in those patients compared to juvenile-onset patients. Several studies reported a relation between serum glucose levels and neuropsychological performance (Holmes et al., 1983, 1984, 1986; Pramming et al., 1986). Most of these studies have selected younger patients to avoid the potential confounding effects of age on neuropsychological performance. In addition, the principal focus appears to have been in regard to the possible detrimental effects of hypoglycemic episodes. Although these studies provided evidence of neurobehavioral deficit in association with lowered blood glucose, there are other aspects of diabetes that may contribute to the pathophysiologic basis of neuropsychological impairment in patients with diabetes.

Diabetes is associated with accelerated atherogenesis (Lavy, 1979; Kannel et al., 1984) as well as microvessel disease (Redisch et al., 1973). In the Framingham Study (Kannel et al., 1984) the incidence of stroke was significantly associated with antecedent blood glucose and glucose intolerance as well as clinical diabetes. In men this factor was independent of other associated risk factors. If elevated blood glucose is related to increased atherosclerotic changes, it may also be related to the degree of neuropsychological impairment. This point has not been the subject of extensive scientific investigation. In fact, the only studies that have examined the effect of diabetes or serum glucose in CVD patients have been in the context of examining candidates for surgical intervention. Kelly et al. (1980) found that the four patients with evidence of diabetes were not improved on neuropsychological measures following carotid endarterectomy. Bornstein and coworkers (1981) grouped patients on the basis of serum glucose levels below or above 130 mg/dl (mean for the sample was 125.4 mg/dl, range 79–435 mg/dl). The two groups did not differ in regard to age, education, any other risk factor, or the persistence of presenting neurologic deficit [transient ischemic attack (TIA) versus stroke]. On the preoperative neuropsychological examination, the groups did not differ on any test, but it was found that patients with normal levels improved on a broader range of measures than patients with elevated blood glucose. The differences between the two studies may be related to the criteria used for grouping subjects. These studies cannot be used to generalize to the stroke population as a whole because the samples were based on selected criteria (i.e., surgical intervention).

In summary, there is evidence of neurobehavioral deficit associated with hypoglycemia but limited direct evidence of deficits associated with elevated blood glucose. Most of the studies have used young samples, and the results therefore may not generalize to stroke samples in which the patients tend to be considerably older. In the context of studying the potential neurobehavioral effects of elevated blood glucose in stroke populations, it is clear that control for the effects of age is required. Rather than excluding patients older than 45, as is done in many studies, it would be desirable to use an age-matched control group (possibly from some other chronic disease population). This method would permit examination of the effects of elevated serum glucose in the context of advanced age. Furthermore, it seems important to consider the effects of serum glucose at all levels, rather than merely dichotomizing patients on the basis of the presence or absence of clinical diabetes. Elevated serum glucose is a prominent risk factor for stroke, and further investigation of the potential neurobehavioral correlates is clearly indicated.

CHOLESTEROL AND TRIGLYCERIDES

Blood lipids play an important role in the development of cardiac and peripheral vascular disease (Gordon and Kannel, 1972). In contrast, cholesterol and its various lipoprotein fractions and other lipids are relatively weak predictors of stroke (Gordon et al., 1981). The 24-year follow-up data from the Framingham Study found an association between cholesterol and stroke only in men in the 50- to 59-year age group (Wolf et al., 1978b). Although blood lipids appear to have a modest relation with stroke incidence per se, the recognized atherogenic potential and the association with other forms of vascular disease suggest that study of the neuropsychological concomitants of hyperlipidemia may be worthwhile.

There have been few studies of the neurobehaviorial correlates of blood lipids. Reitan and Shipley (1963) examined changes in psychological test performance related to a decrease in serum cholesterol. The study was based on 156 clinically healthy men, and subjects were divided by age (less than or more than 40 years). It was found that older subjects who had at least a 10% decrease in serum cholesterol levels demonstrated significantly greater improvement than older subjects who failed to lower their cholesterol levels. There was no difference in degree of neuropsychological change between the younger groups. Unfortunately, there was no attempt to examine the correlation between test performance and cholesterol levels.

The only study to consider the effects of cholesterol in patients with symptomatic cerebrovascular disease was reported by Bornstein et al. (1981). That study examined neuropsychological test performance in 43 carotid surgery patients grouped on the basis of serum cholesterol levels. There were 26 patients with cholesterol levels below 240 mg/dl and 17 patients with levels above this criterion. The range of levels in the sample was 153 to 324 mg/dl (mean 227 mg/dl). The groups did not differ in regard to demographic or other risk factor variables, or persistence of presenting neurologic deficit (TIA versus stroke). There were no differences between the groups on preoperative performance, but the patients with cholesterol levels in the normal range improved on a broader range of measures following surgery. As in the study of Reitan and Shipley (1963), there was no examination of the correlation between cholesterol levels and preoperative performance.

These studies suggest some relation between cholesterol levels and neuropsychological function. Both studies appear to suggest that lower cholesterol levels may be associated with improved neuropsychological performance. The lack of differences between the groups in the study by Bornstein et al. (1981) suggested that there is no direct relation, as patients grouped on the basis of cholesterol level did not differ on an extensive test battery. On the other hand, the simple dichotomization of subjects around an arbitrary criterion may have obscured a relation. Avoiding such arbitrary criteria and examining the correlation between the full range of cholesterol levels and behavioral variables appear to be important considerations for future studies. As noted by Brown, et al. (1986), the mechanism by which serum cholesterol or other lipids may affect neuropsychological performance is unclear. Assessment of the degree of arterial stenosis in conjunction with serum lipid levels as suggested by Brown et al. (1986) would be useful for determining the mechanism involved.

TOBACCO, HEMOGLOBIN, AND HEMATOCRIT

Similar to the findings on lipids, the relation between cigarette smoking and stroke is much less than the risk for cardiac or peripheral vascular disease (Wolf et al., 1978a,b; Kannel et al., 1984). The risk for stroke associated with smoking could be mediated by a number of mechanisms, including decreased cerebral oxygenation by production of carbon monoxide, stimulation of cardiac arrhythmias, transient nicotine-induced elevation of blood pressure (Kuller, 1978), increased cholesterol associated with smoking (Brackenride and Bloch, 1972), or through the relation between cigarette smoking and hemoglobin (Kannel et al., 1972). The limited literature on the neurobehavioral correlates of smoking in younger subjects is contradictory and reviewed elsewhere (Brown et al., 1986). In contrast to cigarette smoking, elevated levels of hemoglobin and hematocrit are clearly associated with increased risk of stroke in all age groups and in both sexes (Wolf et al., 1978a,b; Kannel et al., 1984). It was particularly true of cases with frank polycythemia (Kannel et al., 1972) but was also true with concentrations within the normal range. There has been relatively little examination of the effects of hemoglobin or hematocrit in patients with symptomatic cerebrovascular disease. The only study that explicitly examined the effect of hematocrit and hemoglobin on neuropsychological performance was conducted with patients who were carotid surgery candidates (Bornstein et al., 1981). That study grouped patients according to levels of increased risk for stroke as suggested by the Framingham Study. Those data suggested increased risk for stroke associated with hematocrit levels above 45% and hemoglobin levels above 15 g/dl of blood (14 g/dl of blood for women). The data from the Bornstein et al. (1981) study related to hematocrit are reviewed here because hemoglobin and hematocrit are closely related, and the Framingham Study data (Kannel et al., 1984) are expressed in relation to hematocrit values.

Hematocrit levels from routine hospital admission investigations were obtained on 44 patients who subsequently undersent carotid endarterectomy. There were 32 subjects with hematocrit levels below 45% and 12 with levels above 45%. As expected, the groups also differed on hemoglobin level, and the high hematocrit–hemoglobin group also reported greater cigarette smoking. The two groups were otherwise similar regarding age, education, other risk factor variables, and the persistence of presenting neurological deficits (TIA versus stroke). There were no differences between the groups on an extensive neuropsychological test battery administered prior to surgery. At follow-up the patients with hematocrits below 45% demonstrated improvement on a broader range of tests than those with hematocrits above 45%. As already noted, these data may not generalize to the stroke population as a whole because it was based on patients selected for surgical consideration. Furthermore, the use of an arbitrary criterion for patient grouping may have been problematic.

The relation between cerebral oxygenation and neuropsychological test performance has been investigated to a much greater extent in the context of patients with chronic obstructive pulmonary disease (COPD). These studies are of interest in relation to stroke risk factors because of the association of COPD with increased hematocrit, cigarette smoking, and risk for polycythemia (Adams et al., 1980; Nocturnal Oxygen Therapy Trial Group, 1980). Because COPD tends to be identified most frequently in patients in their sixties (Hodgkin, 1979), this population may be of value in understanding the relation of stroke risk factors with neurobehavioral status.

Grant and colleagues (1982) examined 203 COPD patients who had a mean hematocrit of 47.5%. The patients performed worse than controls on a broad battery of neuropsychological measures, with higher order or complex cognitive abilities being more severely affected. When compared with an age-matched control group, 42% of patients and 14% of controls obtained scores that were suggestive of impaired cerebral function. Hemoglobin levels were inversely related to impairment on neuropsychological tests, as reflected in clinician ratings and objective summary scores. Prigatano and coworkers (1983) examined 100 mildly hypoxemic COPD patients. The severity of COPD was much less than in the patients reported by Grant et al. (1982) (mean PaO_2 was 66 mm Hg versus 51 mm Hg). Hemoglobin or hematocrit levels were not reported. The qualitative nature of the deficits were similar to those reported by Grant et al. (1982), but the degree of deficit was less severe. In both studies the greater hypoxemia was related to increased neuropsychological impairment.

The data from these two studies were combined in an attempt to examine the neuropsychological performance across the range of hypoxemic COPD patients (Grant et al., 1987). Patients (n = 302) were grouped according to the severity of hypoxemia ($PaO_2 \geq 60$ mm Hg, 50–59 mm Hg, and < 50 mm Hg, respectively). As expected, the severely hypoxemic group also had significantly higher hemoglobin and hematocrit. There was an association between degree of hypoxemia and neuropsychological deficit, with the rate of neuropsychological impairment ranging from 27% in the mildly hypoxemic group to 61% in the severe disease group. Hemoglobin was included with age, education, and other disease variables (including PaO_2) in a multiple regression analysis of neuropsychological performance. In this analysis PaO_2 and respiratory rate, but not hemoglobin, were related to neuropsychological impairment.

Fix and colleagues (1982) examined neuropsychological deficit in a sample of COPD patients with PaO_2 (67.4 mm Hg) levels similar to those of the mildly hypoxemic group reported by Grant et al. (1987). A different neuropsychological test battery was used, and test performance was much more clearly related to PaO_2 levels than to either hemoglobin or hematocrit. Both hemoglobin and hematocrit were negatively correlated with PaO_2, but partial correlations between hemoglobin, hematocrit, and neuropsychological performance (controlling for PaO_2) were not reported.

These studies of COPD patients fail to support any clear relation between hemoglobin, hematocrit, and neuropsychological test performance in hypoxemic patients. In most of these studies, hemoglobin and hematocrit were at levels above those associated with increased risk of stroke in the Framingham Study. Although hemoglobin and hematocrit may increase in response to lowered PaO_2, there were only ten patients with values of hemoglobin and hematocrit that exceeded normal levels. The study of COPD patients may not be ideal for studying the relation between hemoglobin, hematocrit, and neuropsychological performance. The pathophysiologic mechanism for elevations in stroke patients may be different from the compensatory response to lowered PaO_2 that occurs in COPD patients. The only study of the effect of hematocrit on neuropsychological performance (Bornstein et al., 1981) was based on surgical patients. It would be of considerable interest to collect data on hemoglobin and hematocrit levels from an unselected sample of patients with identified cerebrovascular disease. In that context, correlations with neuropsychological performance, as well as matching groups of patients (who differ only on hemoglobin/hematocrit levels) would provide a more direct examination of these relations in cerebrovascular disease.

CARDIAC DISEASE

There is a clear association between various cardiac diseases and increased risk of stroke (Wolf et al., 1977, 1978a; Lavy, 1979; Kannel et al., 1984). Atherosclerotic coronary artery disease, congestive heart failure, atrial fibrillation, and rheumatic heart disease are related to increased stroke risk. In addition, a variety of electrocardiographic (ECG) abnormalities are related to stroke risk, including nonspecific ST and T wave abnormalities, left ventricular hypertrophy (LVH), and intraventricular block. In the Framingham Study, the most powerful ECG predictor of stroke was LVH, even when the risks associated with hypertension were controlled. Several mechanisms have been suggested to explain the increased risk for stroke, and many of these mechanisms could also result in impaired cognitive function. Valvular disease, coronary artery disease, endocarditis, or myocardial infarction can lead to diminished cardiac output, which could result in reduced oxygen availability and cerebral hypoxia related to lowered cerebral arterial perfusion. Abnormal conduction or extreme bradycardia could also result in generalized cerebral ischemia. Intravascular sludging associated with congestive heart failure could also represent a possible mechanism for behavioral impairments.

There is an extensive literature on neuropsychological assessment of patients with various cardiac diseases (see reviews in Becker et al., 1982; Kelleher and Townes, 1982) that has focused primarily on patients undergoing cardiac surgery. Most of these studies have focused on postoperative changes, but a few have reported preoperative comparisons. Bethune (1980) reported delayed memory deficit in patients with aortic valve disease. Zaks (1959) found impaired performance on several tasks in patients with rheumatic heart disease (undergoing mitral commissurotomy) compared to patients undergoing other types of cardiac surgery. Sy and Novelly (1980) found impaired neuropsychological performance in coronary artery bypass patients compared with medically managed cardiac disease control patients. Parker et al. (1984) examined the interactive effects of cardiac and carotid artery disease on neuropsychological performance. Carotid disease patients were impaired compared to patients with cardiac disease only. When the carotid disease group was further subdivided into those with focal (carotid only) and those with generalized cerebrovascular disease, an interaction effect was identified. Patients with generalized cerebrovascular disease and heart disease were more impaired than patients with generalized cerebrovascular disease without evidence of cardiac disease. There was no difference among the subgroups of patients with focal carotid lesions.

All of these studies, in addition to those surgical outcome studies that are not reviewed here, are based for the most part on surgical samples. As such, these samples may not be representative of the general population of cardiovascular disease patients. The patients considered for such procedures may be drawn from the severe end of the disease spectrum. It would therefore be worthwhile for future studies to include patients across a broader range of disease severity. The study by Parker et al. (1984) represents a useful approach for examining the independent and interactive effects of cardiovascular and cerebrovascular disease. Similar studies in patients (not restricted to surgical samples), which also address the influence of different cardiac factors (e.g., type of disease, ECG findings), will be of considerable value in clarifying the role of cardiac disease in neurobehavioral impairment.

SUMMARY

We have reviewed the evidence regarding the relation between stroke risk factors and neurobehavioral deficit. It is presumed that the pathophysiologic mechanisms by which these factors increase the risk of stroke or impaired cerebral function may also be responsible for cognitive, perceptual, or other neuropsychological impairment.

With few exceptions, the behavioral effects of these variables have not been studied to any great extent. The single possible exception is hypertension, in which there is a rather long history of interest in the potential neuropsychological concomitants. To the extent that the other stroke risk factors have been examined, it has been in the context of other primary disease populations (e.g., diabetes mellitus or COPD). It may not be appropriate to generalize to the patients with cerebrovascular disease because of the possibility that there may be different underlying pathophysiology. The other major restriction to generalizing these data to stroke populations is that most of the studies that were performed on patients with identified vascular disease were based on patients selected as candidates for surgical intervention. Whether this selection represents sample bias in terms of disease severity is unclear.

There is at least suggestive evidence that these stroke risk factors may have either a direct or an indirect effect on neuropsychological performance. As pointed out by Brown et al. (1986), these conditions are commonly present in patients with cerebrovascular disease (TIA or stroke) and would be amenable to a number of potentially informative retrospective or prospective investigations. For example, it might be possible to identify patients at risk for stroke and prospectively follow them to determine the relation between duration and severity of disease and the extent of behavioral deficit. Similar to the study by Reitan and Shipley (1963), studies of the effects of treatment of these factors would be of interest. Finally, there is some evidence (Kelly et al., 1980; Bornstein et al., 1981) that these risk factors may moderate the extent of recovery from CVD. Further studies of this possibility in nonsurgical samples would be of considerable value. Because many of these risk factors are interrelated, it will be necessary to accumulate large samples to accommodate groups to study risk factors in isolation, as well as risk factor profiles. The availability of standardized neuropsychological assessment procedures and the ability to pool data across centers have already demonstrated their potential value (Grant et al., 1987); if applied in the investigation of stroke and stroke risk factors, they will represent an important stride forward.

ACKNOWLEDGMENT

The preparation of this manuscript was supported in part by USPHS grant MH42209. (R.A.B.)

REFERENCES

Adams, K.M., Sawyer, J.D., and Kvale, P.D. (1980). Cerebral oxygenation and neuropsychological adaptation. *J. Clin. Neuropsychol.,* **2,** 189–208.

Apter, N.S., Halstead, W.C., and Heimburger, R.F. (1951). Impaired cerebral functions in essential hypertension. *Am. J. Psychiatry,* **107,** 808–813.

Baade, L.E. (1988). Neuropsychological test differences between insulin dependent diabetic adults and controls. Paper presented at the meeting of the International Neuropsychological Society, New Orleans.

Baker, A.B., Kinnard, J., and Iannone, A. (1961). Cerebrovascular disease. VIII. Role of nutritional factors. *Neurology,* **11,** 380–389.

Bale, R. (1973). Brain damage in diabetes mellitus. *Br. J. Psychiatry,* **122,** 337–341.

Becker, R., Katz, J., Polonius, M.J., and Speidel, H., eds. (1982). *Psychopathological and Neurological Dysfunction Following Open-Heart Surgery.* Berlin: Springer Verlag.

Benton, A.L. & Joynt, R.J. (1959). Reaction time in unilateral cerebral disease. *Confin. Neurol.* **19,** 247–256.

Bethune, D.W. (1980). The assessment of organic brain damage following open heart surgery. In: H. Speidel and G. Rodewald, eds., *Psychic and Neurological Dysfunction After Open Heart Surgery.* New York: Grune & Stratton.

Blackburn, H.C., and Benton, A.L. (1955). Simple and choice reaction time in cerebral disease. *Confin. Neurol.,* **15,** 327–338.

Boller, F., Vrtunski, B., Mack, J.L., and Kim, Y. (1977). Neuropsychological correlates of hypertension. *Arch. Neurol.,* **34,** 701–705.

Bornstein, R.A. (1986). Neuropsychological aspects of cerebrovascular disease and its treatment. In: G. Goldstein and R.E. Tarter, eds., *Advances in Clinical Neuropsychology,* Vol. 3, pp. 55–94. New York: Plenum Press.

Bornstein, R.A., Trites, R.L., and Benoit, B.G. (1981). Effects of medical risk factors on extent of improvement following carotid endarterectomy. Paper presented at the meeting of the International Neuropsychological Society, Atlanta.

Brackenridge, C.J., and Bloch, S. (1972). Smoking in medical students. *J. Psychosom. Res.,* **16,** 35–40.

Brown G.G., Baird, A.D., and Shatz, M.W. (1986). The effects of cerebral vascular disease and its treatment on higher cortical functioning. In: I. Grant and K.M. Adams, eds., *Neuropsychological Assessment of Neuropsychiatric Disorders,* pp. 384–414. New York: Oxford University Press.

Canessa, M., Andragna, N., Solomon, H.S., Connolly, T.M., and Tosteson, D.C. (1980). Increased sodium-lithium countertransport in red cells of patients with essential hypertension. *N. Engl. J. Med.,* **302,** 772–776.

Clarke, B., Ewing, D., and Campbell, I. (1980). Clinical features of diabetic autonomic neuropathy. *Horm. Metab. Res.,* [*Suppl.*], **9,** 50–60.

Colwell, J., Lopes-Virella, M., and Halushka, P. (1981). Pathogenesis of atherosclerosis in diabetes mellitus. *Diabetes Care,* **4,** 121–129.

Costa, P.T., Jr., and Shock, N.W. (1980). New longitudinal data on the question of whether hypertension influences intellectual performance. In: M.F. Elias and D.H.P. Streeten, eds., *Hypertension and Cognitive Processes.* Mt. Desert, Maine: Beech-Hill Publishing Company.

Dyken, M.L., Wolf, P.A., Barnett, H.J.M., Bergan, J.J., Hass, W.K., Kannel, W.B., Kuller, L., Kurtzke, J.F., and Sundt, T.M. (1984). Risk factors in stroke. *Stroke,* **15,** 1105–1111.

Eeg-Olofsson, O. (1977). Hypoglycemia and neurological disturbances in children with diabetes mellitus. *Acta Paediatr. Scand.,* [*Suppl.*], **270,** 91–95.

Elias, M.F., Robbins, M.H., Schultz, N.R., Jr., and Streeten, D.H.P. (1986). A longitudinal study of neuropsychological test performance for hypertensive and normotensive adults: initial findings. *J. Gerontol.,* **41,** 503–505.

Elias, M.F., Robbins, M.A., Schultz, N.R., Streeten, D.H.P., and Elias, P.K. (1987). Clinical significance of cognitive performance in hypertensive patients. *Hypertension,* **9,** 192–197.

Enzer, N., Simonson, E., and Blankstein, S.S. (1942). Fatigue of patients with circulatory insufficiency investigated by means of the fusion frequency of flicker. *Ann. Intern. Med.,* **16,** 701–707.

Fix, A.J., Golden, C.J., Daughton, D., Kass, I., and Bell, C.W. (1982). Neuropsychological deficits among patients with chronic obstructive pulmonary disease. *Int. J. Neurosci.,* **16,** 99–105.

Francheschi, M., Tancredi, O., Smirne, S., Mercinelli, A., and Canal, N. (1982). Cognitive processes in hypertension. *Hypertension,* **4,** 226–229.

Franceschi, M., Cecchetto, R., Minicucci, F., Smirne, S., Baio, G., and Canal, N. (1984). Cognitive processes in insulin-dependent diabetes. *Diabetes Care,* **7,** 228–231.

Ganda, O. (1980). Pathogenesis of macrovascular disease in the human diabetic. *Diabetes,* **29,** 931–939.

Gilhaus, K.M., Daweke, H., Lulsdorf, H.G., Sachsse, R., and Sachsse, B. (1973). EEG-veranderungen bei diabetischen kindern. *Dtsch. Med. Wochenschr.,* **31,** 1449–1454.

Goldman, H., Kleinman, K.M., Snow, M.U., Bidus, D.R., and Korol, B. (1974). Correlation of diastolic blood pressure and signs of cognitive dysfunction in essential hypertension. *Dis. Nerv. Syst.,* **35,** 571–572.

Goldman, H., Kleinman, K.M., Snow, M.Y., Bidus, D.R., and Korol, B. (1975). Relationship between essential hypertension and cognitive functioning effects of biofeedback. *Psychophysiology,* **12,** 569–573.

Gordon, T., and Kannel, W.B. (1972). Predisposition to atherosclerosis in the head, heart and lungs. *J.A.M.A.,* **221,** 661–666.

Gordon, T., Kannel, W.B., Castelli, W.P., and Dawber, T.R. (1981). Lipoproteins, cardiovascular disease, and death: the Framingham Study. (1981). *Arch. Intern. Med.,* **141,** 1128–1131.

Grant, I., Heaton, R.K., McSweeny, A.J., Adams, K.M., and Timms, R.M. (1982). Neuropsychological findings in hypoxemic chronic obstructive pulmonary disease. *Arch. Intern. Med.,* **142,** 1470–1476.

Grant, I., Prigatano, G.P., Heaton, R.K., McSweeny, A.J., Wright, E.C., and Adams, K.M. (1987). Progressive neuropsychologic impairment and hypoxemia. *Arch. Gen. Psychiatry,* **44,** 999–1006.

Hodgkin, J.E. (1979). *Chronic Obstructive Pulmonary Disease.* Park Ridge, Illinois: American College of Chest Physicians.

Holmes, C.S. (1986). Neuropsychological profiles in men with insulin-dependent diabetes. *J. Consult. Clin. Psychol.,* **54,** 386–389.

Holmes, C.S. (1990). *Neuropsychological and behavioral aspects of diabetes.* Springer-Verlag, New York.

Holmes, C.S., Hayford, J.T., Gonzalez, J.L., and Weydert, J.A. (1983). A survey of cognitive functioning at different glucose levels in diabetic persons. *Diabetes Care,* **6,** 180–185.

Holmes, C.S., Koepke, K.M., Thompson, R.G., Gyves, P.W., and Weydert, J.A. (1984). Verbal fluency and naming performance in type I diabetes at different blood glucose concentrations. *Diabetes Care,* **7,** 454–459.

Holmes, C.S., Koepke, K.M., and Thompson, R.G. (1986). Visual reaction time: simple versus complex performance impairments during three blood glucose levels. *Psychoneuroendocrinology,* **11,** 353–357.

Kannel, W.B., Gordon, T., Wolf, P.A., and McNamara, P. (1972). Hemoglobin and the risk of cerebral infarction: The Framingham Study. *Stroke,* **3,** 409–420.

Kannel, W.B., Dawber, T.R., Sorlie, P. and Wolf, P.A. (1976). Components of blood pressure and risk of atherothrombotic brain infarction: The Framingham Study. *Stroke,* **7,** 327–331.

Kannel, W.B., Wolf, P.A., and Verter, J. (1984). Risk factors for stroke. In: R.R. Smith, ed., *Stroke and the Extracranial Vessels,* pp. 47–58. New York: Raven Press.

Kaplinsky, N., and Frankl, O. (1980). The significance of cerebrospinal fluid examination in the management of chlorpropamide-induced hypoglycemia. *Diabetes Care,* **3,** 248–249.

Kelleher, W.J., and Townes, B.D. (1982). Neuropsychological and emotional status of cardiac surgery patients: a review of psychometric investigations. *Psychol.Doc.,* No. 2544, pp. 1–77.

Kelly, M.P., Garron, D.C., and Javid, H. (1980). Carotid artery disease, carotid endarterectomy, and behavior. *Arch. Neurol.,* **37,** 743–748.

Kimura, D. (1963). Right temporal lobe damage. *Arch. Neurol.,* **8,** 264–271.

Kleinman, K.M., Goldman, H., Snow, M.Y., and Korol, B. (1977). Relationships between essential hypertension and cognitive functioning. II. Effects of biofeedback training generalized to nonlaboratory environment. *Psychophysiology,* **14,** 192–197.

Kuller, L.H. (1978). Epidemiology of stroke. *Adv. Neurol.,* **19,** 281–310.

Lavy, S. (1979). Medical risk factors for stroke. *Adv. Neurol.,* **25,** 127–133.

Lawson, J.S., Erdahl, D.L.W., Monga, T.N., Bird, C.E., Donald, M.W., Surridge, D.H.C., and Letemendia, F.J.J. (1984). Neuropsychological function in diabetic patients with neuropathy. *Br. J. Psychiatry,* **145,** 263–268.

Lew, E.A. (1973). High blood pressure, other risk factors, and longevity: the insurance viewpoint. *Am. J. Med.,* **55,** 281–294.

Light, K.C. (1975). Slowing of response time in young and middle aged hypertensive patients. *Exp. Aging Res.,* **1,** 209–227.

Light, K.C. (1978). Effects of mild cardiovascular and cerebrovascular disorders on serial reaction time performance. *Exp. Aging Res.,* **4,** 3–22.

Matthews, C.G., Shaw, D.J., and Klove, H. (1966). Psychological test performacne in neurologic and "pseudoneurologic" subjects. *Cortex,* **2,** 244–253.

Mazzuchi, A., Mutte, A., Poletti, A., Pavanetti, C., Novanrini, A., and Parma, M. (1986). Neuropsychological deficits in arterial hypertension. *Acta Neurol. Scand.,* **73,** 619–627.

Meuter, F., Thomas, W., Gruneklee, D., Gries, F., and Lohmann, R. (1980). Psychometric evaluation of performance in diabetes mellitus. *Horm. Metab. Res.,* [*Suppl.*] **9,** 9–17.

Miller, R.E., Shapiro, A.P., King, H.E., Ginchereau, E.H., and Hosutt, J.A. (1984). Effect of antihypertensive treatment on the behavioral consequences of elevated blood pressure. *Hypertension,* **6,** 202–208.

Moore, D., Pope, A., Todd, F., and Lipson, L. (1981). Incidence of hypertension in male diabetic populations. *Diabetes,* **30,** (*Suppl.* 1), **1,** 31a.

Nocturnal Oxygen Therapy Trial Group (1980). Continuous or nocturnal oxygen therapy in hypoxemic chronic obstructive lung disease. *Ann. Intern. Med.,* **93,** 391–398.

Parker, J.C., Seidenberg, M., Granberg, B.W., Nichols, K., Crum, B.S., and Hewett, J.E. (1984). The interactive effects of carotid stenosis and heart disease on neuropsychological performance. Paper presented at the meeting of the International Neuropsychological Society, Houston.

Parsons, O.A., and Prigatano, G.P. (1978). Methodological considerations in clinical neuropsychological research. *J. Consult. Clin. Psychol.,* **4,** 608–619.

Pentz, C.A., Elias, M.F., Wood, W.G., Schultz, N.A., and Dineen, J. (1979). Relationship of age and hypertension to neuropsychological test performance. *Exp. Aging Res.,* **5,** 351–372.

Pramming, S., Thorsteinsson, B., Theilgaard, A., Pinner, E.M., and Binder, C. (1986). Cognitive function during hypoglycemia in type I diabetes mellitus. *Br. Med. J.,* **292,** 647–650.

Prigatano, G.P., Parsons, O., Wright, E., Levin, D.C., and Hawryluk, G. (1983). Neuropsychological test performance in mildly hypoxemic patients with chronic obstructive pulmonary disease. *J. Consult. Clin. Psychol.,* **51,** 108–116.

Redisch, W., Rouen, L.R., Terry, E.N., Opperman, W., Kuthan, F., and Clauss, R.H. (1973). Microvascular changes in early diabetes mellitus. In: R.A. Camerini-Davolos and H. Cole, eds., *Early Diabetes: Advances in Metabolic Disorders,* pp. 383–390. New York: Academic Press.

Reitan, R.M., and Shipley, R.E. (1963). The relationship of serum cholesterol changes to psychological abilities. *J. Gerontol.* **18,** 350–357.

Rennick, P.H., Wilder, R.M., Sargent, J., and Ashley, B.J. (1968). Retinopathy as an indicator of cognitive-perceptual-motor impairment in diabetic adults. In: *Proceedings of the 76th Annual Convention of the American Psychological Association,* pp. 473–474. Washington, D.C.: American Psychological Association.

Riddle, M., and Hart, J. (1981). Unrecognized hyperglycemia precedes stroke and transient ischemic attacks. *Diabetes,* **30,** Suppl. 1, 88a.

Rodriguez, G., Arvigo, F., Marenco, S., Nobili, F., Romano, P., Sardini, G., and Rosadini, G. (1987). Regional cerebral blood flow in essential hypertension: data evaluation by a mapping system. *Stroke,* **18,** 13–20.

Ruderman, N., and Goodman, M. (1980). Brain metabolism in diabetes. *Horm. Metab. Res.* [*Suppl.*] **9,** 1–8.

Salonen, J.T., Pushka, P., Tuomilehto, J., and Homan, K. (1982). Relation of blood pressure, serum lipids, and smoking to the risk of cerebral stroke—a longitudinal study in Eastern Finland. *Stroke,* **13,** 327–333.

Schultz, N.R., Dineen, J.T., Elias, M.F., Pentz, C.A., and Wood, W.G. (1979). WAIS performance for different age groups of hypertensive and control subjects during administration of a diurectic. *J. Gerontol.,* **34,** 246–253.

Schultz, N.R., Elias, M.F., Robbins, M.A., Streeten, D.H.P., and Blakeman, N. (1986). A longitudinal comparison of hypertensives and normotensives on the Wechsler Adult Intelligence Scale: initial findings. *Gerontology,* **41,** 169–175.

Shapiro, A.P., Miller, R.E., Kind, H.E., Ginchereau, E.H., and Fitzgibbon, K. (1982). Behavioral consequences of mild hypertension. *Hypertension,* **4,** 355–360.

Shekelle, R.B., Ostfeld, A.M., and Klawans, H.L., Jr. (1974). Hypertension and risk of stroke in an elderly population. *Stroke,* **5,** 71–75.

Skenazy, J.A., and Bigler, E.D. (1984). Neuropsychological findings in diabetes mellitus. *J. Clin. Psychol.,* **40,** 246–258.

Speith, W. (1964). Cardiovascular health status, age, and psychological performance. *J. Gerontology,* **19,** 277–284.

Sy, M.J., and Novelly, R.A. (1980). Neuropsychological changes following open heart surgery. Presented at the meeting of the International Neuropsychological Society, San Francisco.

United States Public Health Service and Nutrition Examination Survey, 1971–1974, No. 1. Washington, D.C.: Vital and Health Statistics of National Center for Health Statistics, 1976a.

United States Public Health Service and Nutrition Examination Survey, 1971–1974, No. 2. Washington, D.C.: Vital and Health Statistics of the National Center for Health Statistics, 1976b.

Vanderploeg, R.D., Goldman, H., and Kleinman, K.M. (1987). Relationship between systolic and diastolic blood pressure and cognitive functioning in hypertensive subjects; an extension of previous findings. *Arch. Clin. Neuropsychol.,* **2,** 101–109.

Wilkie, F., and Eisdorfer, C. (1971). Intelligence and blood pressure in the aged. *Science,* **172,** 959–962.

Wilkie, F.L., Eisdorfer, C. and Nowlin, J.B. (1976). Memory and blood pressure in the aged. *Exp. Aging Res.,* **2,** 3–16.

Wolf, P.A., Dawber, T.R., Thomas, H.E., Colton, T., and Kannel, W.B. (1977). Epidemiology of stroke. *Adv. Neurol.,* **16,** 5–19.

Wolf, P.A., Dawber, T.R., and Kannel, W.B. (1978a). Heart disease as a precursor of stroke. *Adv. Neurol.,* **19,** 567–576.

Wolf, P.A., Kannel, W.B., and Dawber, T.R. (1978b). Prospective investigations: The Framingham Study and the epidemiology of stroke. *Adv. Neurol.,* **19,** 107–120.

Wolf, P.A., Kannel, W.B., and Verter, J. (1983). Current status of risk factors for stroke. *Neurol. Clin.,* **1,** 317–343.

Zaks, M.S. (1959). Disturbances in psychologic functions and neuropsychiatric complications in heart surgery. In: A.A. Luisaden, ed., *Cardiology: An Encyclopedia of the Cardiovascular System.* New York: McGraw-Hill.

11

Neurobehavioral Correlates of Arteriovenous Malformations and Cerebral Aneurysms

GREGORY G. BROWN, KEVIN B. SPICER, AND GHAUS MALIK

Less is known about the neurobehavioral correlates of cerebrovascular anomalies than of embolic-thrombotic stroke. During the 1980s fewer than a dozen papers published in English contained information about the neuropsychological aspects of arteriovenous malformations (AVMs). A similar number of papers contained information about the neuropsychological effects of cerebral aneurysms. Often these reports are discussions of individual patients or a small series of cases. The sparcity of this literature is in part due to the rarity of AVMs and aneurysms and part to the complications of studying patients with cerebral hemorrhage. Also, cerebral aneurysms and AVMs often do not produce uncomplicated, focal syndromes, making patients with these anomalies less attractive subjects for studies of localization of function than those with ischemic-thrombotic stroke.

Nonetheless, the investigator of neurocognitive questions associated with anatomic anomalies of cerebral vessels confronts a range of interesting issues. These issues include defining the impact of developmental abnormalities on the cerebral organization of behavior, analyzing the neurobehavioral effects of serial damage to the brain, examining the brain systems related to memory and emotion, and monitoring the effects of cerebrovascular surgery. A review of these issues is presented below.

ARTERIOVENOUS MALFORMATIONS

An AVM is a congenital entanglement of blood vessels that forms an abnormal connection between the arterial and venous circulations (Adams and Victor, 1985, p.

622). Some authors have called this entanglement an angioma or an aneurysm; however, the former term inappropriately suggests a tumor, and the latter confuses an abnormality of arteriovenous connection with the balloon-like dilatation of arteries to be discussed in the second half of this chapter.

Arteriovenous malformations are fetal abnormalities arising about 3 weeks after conception, when primitive vessels divide into arteries and veins (Stein and Wolpert, 1980a). An arrest at this early stage in the epigenesis of cerebral vessels produces pipe-like connections or fistulas, which replace the capillary bed. As seen in Figure 11–1A, the core of an AVM, its nidus, is often supplied with blood from several hypertrophied arteries. Arterioles, ranging from 50 to 200 μm, connect the arteries and the AVM (Yamada and Cojocaru, 1987). Blood leaves the core of the AVM through an enlarged draining vein (Figure 11–1C). The smooth muscles and elastic membranes of vessels at the core of an AVM are often severely wasted (McCormick, 1966). The arteries leading to an AVM experience thickening of the smooth muscle and elastic lining; the draining vein is often thin-walled (Yamada and Cojocaru, 1987). The blood contained in the draining vein is frequently much redder than typical venous blood, suggesting reduced extraction of oxygen from the blood passing through the AVM. Presumably the diminished oxygen extraction is in large part due to a loss of functional tissue, as little normal tissue exists within the boundary of an AVM (Mohr et al., 1986b).

Replacement of the capillary bed by fistulas impairs the autoregulation of blood flow through an AVM (Wade and Hachinski, 1987). By virtue of their greater resistance to flow, the smallest cerebral vessels make the largest contribution to the regulation of flow (Wade and Hachinski, 1987). At normal levels of systemic blood pressure, the circulation of blood through vessels less than 300 μm in diameter reduces local blood pressure by 70 mm Hg. The blood's passage through medium and large vessels reduces blood pressure by 20 mm Hg (Wade and Hachinski, 1987). Replacing the capillary bed by looped vessels, typically 0.5 to 2.0 mm in diameter (Yamada, 1982), lowers resistance through the AVM. This lowered resistance can reduce perfusion pressure through the AVM and transmit increased pressure to the venous system. These changes can alter the arteriovenous pressure gradient below the level that can be compensated by vasodilatation.

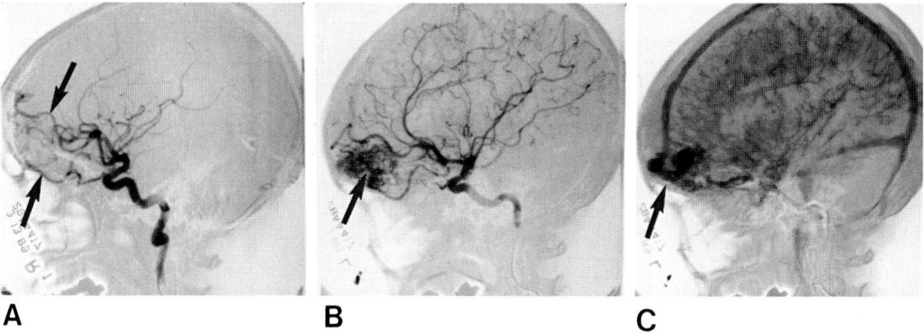

Figure 11–1 Cerebral angiogram of an AVM. (A) Early arterial phase; arrows point to two hypertrophied, feeder arteries. (B) Arterial phase: arrow points to AVM nidus. (C) Venous phase: arrow points to a large draining vein.

Nornes and Grip (1980) have found that pressure in some arteries connected to AVM feeders is below the lower limit of autoregulation. They have also found increased venous outflow pressures. Their results indicated that some patients with AVMs develop critically diminished pressure gradients in regions adjacent to their AVMs. Some authors have speculated that AVMs cause shunting of blood away from neurologically normal tissue (Loeb and Favale, 1962). Homan and colleagues (1986) have argued that this shunting causes some of the neurocognitive abnormalities associated with AVMs.

In addition to AVMs, Stein and Wolpert (1980a) identified three other types of malformation of arteries and veins: (1) capillary telangiectasias; (2) cavernous angiomas; and (3) venous angiomas (varices). Capillary telangiectasias are tiny vascular anomalies, often ranging in size from a pinhead to around 3 mm. They occur deep in the brain and are frequently associated with the Weber-Osler syndrome (Stein and Wolpert, 1980a; Adams and Victor, 1985). They differ from AVMs by involving only capillaries. The cavernous angioma is a type of AVM distinguished only by its dilated sinusoidal shape (Stein and Wolpert, 1980a). Early descriptions of venous angiomas were probably AVMs with a minor arterial contribution (Stein and Wolpert, 1980a). However, pure venous malformations have been described on angiography (Wendling et al., 1976). These three types of vascular anomaly are less common than are AVMs.

Epidemiology

Arteriovenous malformations are relatively rare, with only 2000 new cases identified each year in the United States (Stein and Wolpert, 1980a). Determining the prevalence of AVMs is problematic, however, given the large ratio of asymptomatic to symptomatic cases. McCormick and Schochet (1976) found 196 AVMs among 4530 consecutive autopsies, only 24 (12.2%) of which had been symptomatic. Asymptomatic AVMs are probably much more common than previously believed; nonetheless, the data on history, course, and neurobehavioral effects are dependent on those symptomatic cases eventually presenting to large surgical clinics.

Most of the AVMs that become symptomatic present with hemorrhage, although AVMs are not a frequent cause of hemorrhage. Bleeds from AVMs comprise 2 to 9% of all hemorrhages (Perret and Nishioka, 1966; Perret, 1975; Gross et al., 1984) and about 1% of all strokes (Mohr et al., 1986b). Hemorrhagic AVMs typically do not occur early in life but during the second through fifth decades. The rarity of cases occurring during the first decade might reflect the slow development and evolution of the abnormality (Stein and Wolpert, 1980a).

Presurgical Assessment of Neurobehavioral Functioning

The presurgical impairment of cognitive functioning varies widely in patients with AVMs. The impairment can be manifested as a specific neurobehavioral syndrome or as a general disruption of adaptive functioning (Reitan and Wolfson, 1985). In studies of patients coming to surgery, the reported frequency of cognitive impairment ranges from none (Constans and Assal, 1971) to 50% (Olivecrona and Reeves, 1948). Perhaps the most important limitation of these studies is their methods of measuring neuropsychological functioning. None used well validated measures of cognitive functioning, making it difficult to determine the sensitivity of these methods to cerebral dysfunction.

Waltimo and Putkonen (1974) reported a study that did use well validated behavioral methods. They administered the Wechsler Adult Intelligence Scale (WAIS), Benton Visual Retention Test (BVRT), Token Test, and tests of immediate and delayed memory to 40 patients with AVMs. The average IQ of this group was 106.4; the distribution of IQ did not differ from that of the normal population. When comparing patients with left- or right-sided AVMs, no differences were found on any of the cognitive measures. Additional analyses did not indicate any relation between overall intellectual performance (i.e., Full Scale IQ) and size, laterality, or symptoms of the AVM. However, there was a trend toward an association between neurobehavioral impairment and previous hemorrhage.

In an additional analysis, patients were grouped on the basis of the uniformity of their cognitive performance. Those with obvious cognitive deficits and a large Verbal-Performance IQ difference were placed in one group ("high inequality") and the remainder of patients were placed in a second group. "High inequality" was found to be associated to a greater extent with right-sided malformations. Waltimo and Putkonen concluded that AVMs do not produce the kind of specific cognitive changes typically seen with acute focal lesions involving equivalent areas of the brain.

This conclusion has been supported by the work of others. Dunn and colleagues (1984) evaluated four patients with left hemisphere AVMs. Although findings consistent with AVM location were found (i.e., verbal learning and memory deficits), a visual short-term memory deficit was seen in all patients and was interpreted by the authors as suggesting either poor test specificity or contralateral abnormalities due to the AVM. Neither the Waltimo and Putkonen study nor the one by Dunn and colleagues included a comparison group composed of patients with acute focal lesions. Consequently, they had no independent method to determine the sensitivity of their behavioral measures to focal brain dysfunction. Sass and colleagues (1988a) compared the neuropsychological functioning of AVM patients with the functioning of patients with acute focal lesions. They studied five patients with high flow congenital vascular malformations who had no history of hemorrhage. Patients with high flow abnormalities were identified by digital cerebral angiography (personal communication, 1988). This group was compared with another group of patients who had low flow vascular lesions, e.g., tumor, epilepsy, or tumor with epilepsy. Both groups of patients received a battery of neuropsychological tests consisting of the WAIS—Revised, Wechsler Memory Scale, Selective Reminding Task, Trail Making Test, and other commonly used measures of visuospatial, motor, and adaptive functioniong. The group with high flow congenital malformations were more impaired on general indicators of adaptive functioning than the comparison group.

The study by Sass and colleagues was an advance over previous research because of the inclusion of a focal lesion control group. They also studied a relatively specific subgroup of patients with AVMs—with high flow abnormalities and no hemorrhage. However, no matching was attempted on lesion size, intrahemispheric location of the lesion, irritative versus destructive nature of the lesion, age, or gender.

Despite the general insensitivity of neuropsychological measures to the location of AVMs, case studies and small group studies have suggested that, in some cases, behavioral localization of an AVM is possible (Conley et al., 1980). To pursue this possibility, Brown and colleagues (1989) compared the accuracy of neuropsychological measures for predicting the laterality of AVMs with their accuracy for predicting the laterality of ischemic stroke. The study tested two hypotheses: (1) neuropsychological measures are less accurate for detecting the laterality of an AVM than for detecting the laterality of ischemic stroke; and (2) clear evidence of asymmetric neuropsychological functioniong would be highly accurate for detecting the laterality of either AVMs or ischemic strokes.

Ten patients with left hemispheric AVMs, 14 with right hemispheric AVMs, 11 with left hemispheric ischemic strokes, and 13 with right hemispheric strokes were studied. The AVM patients studied had been referred for neurosurgical treatment; the existence of each AVM was confirmed by cerebral angiogram. The neuropsychological measures used to infer laterality of a lesion were the WAIS or WAIS—Revised, Wechsler Memory Scale, Hand Dynamometer, Finger Oscillation Test, Tactile Finger Recognition Test, Finger Tip Number Writing, and Visual Suppression Test. The Test Index of Lezak (1983) and the Appendix of Reitan and Davison (1974) can be consulted to obtain more detailed information about these measures.

The inference of the laterality of cerebrovascular disease was based upon three methods: discrimination function analysis, actuarial signs, and clinical judgment. The actuarial signs were developed from published literature to minimize false lateralizing signs in samples of subjects without neurologic disease. A rating of the likelihood that a patient had a lateralized lesion was obtained from two judges, who were blind to the patients' diagnoses and to the rating of the other judge. Because the agreement between the two judges was high, the two ratings were averaged.

The discriminant function analysis indicated that neuropsychological measures were significantly related to the laterality of an ischemic stroke but not an AVM. The discriminant analysis correctly classified the laterality of 23 of 24 patients with ischemic stroke. The point biserial correlation between the actuarial measure of functional asymmetry and the laterality of a lesion was significant only for patients with ischemic stroke. Although the point biserial correlation between the clinician's rating of asymmetry and the actual laterality of the lesion was significant for both groups, it was larger for the ischemic stroke group (r .62) than for the AVM group (r .41). All three methods of analysis supported the hypothesis that neuropsychological measures more accurately reflect the laterality of an ischemic stroke than the laterality of an AVM.

When clear evidence of behavioral asymmetry was present, the positive prediction rate of the laterality of cerebrovascular disease was similar for AVM and ischemic stroke. When a preponderance of actuarial signs of behavioral asymmetry was the criterion for predicting laterality, only one AVM case and no ischemic stroke case was misclassified. Furthermore, the laterality of 6 AVMs and 12 strokes was correctly identified. Similarly, when clinical judges decided that the laterality of a cerebrovascular lesion was probable, no AVM patient and only one patient with ischemic stroke were misclassified. The laterality of 4 AMVs and 12 strokes was correctly predicted.

Overall, the results of this study are consistent with the findings of Waltimo and Putkonen (1974) regarding the suggestion that the location of an AVM does not always produce the kind of cognitive effects that might be expected from knowledge of the locus of a lesion. However, the prediction of laterality of an AVM, when neuropsychological signs of asymmetry were clearly present, was highly accurate for both AVMs and ischemic strokes.

Sources of Variability of Neurobehavioral Functioning

A variety of neuropathologic features of AVMs are no doubt responsible for the variability of neuropsychological impairment seen among AVM patients. The contributions made by atypical organization of language functions, hemodynamic factors, and the slowly progressive nature of AVMs toward explaining this variability are discussed below.

Because most AVMs are congenital, they can disrupt the normal development of cerebral organization (Padget, 1956) and complicate behavioral inferences, which usually assume a single, fixed framework of cerebral organization. Some case reports and small-sample studies contain descriptions of the use of the intracarotid sodium amytal technique to evaluate speech organization in patients with AVMs. Wertz and colleagues (1977) described a case of a left-handed patient with a left fronto-parieto-temporal AVM. The sodium amytal test indicated right hemispheric dominance for language, and the patient did not manifest language abnormalities before or after surgery.

The case of Wertz and colleagues might have been a coincidental occurrence of a left hemispheric AVM in a left-handed patient genetically programmed to have right hemispheric language dominance. The following case presents stronger evidence that AVMs can disrupt the typical pattern of speech organization. This patient had an AVM in the left posterior frontal region and showed clear evidence of right hemispheric speech dominance during sodium amytal infusion despite being right-handed, right-eyed, and right-footed (Close et al., 1977). The authors observed no presurgical signs of aphasia on an aphasia screening test, although performance on a series of neuropsychological tests, which included components of the Halstead-Reitan battery, was compatible with mild, chronic, diffuse dysfunction of adaptive abilities. After surgical removal of the AVM, neuropsychological assessment was again negative for language difficulties. At this time, a mild reduction in grip strength, motor slowing, and tactile insensitivity involving the right hand was observed. Unfortunately, none of the data were presented in this report.

Not all studies of right-handed patients with AVMs in the traditional language zones of the left hemisphere have found evidence of right hemispheric dominance for speech. Using the sodium amytal test, Sass and colleagues (1988b) found that right hemispheric dominance for speech was infrequent in a series of patients with left hemispheric vascular malformations. Furthermore, large high flow vascular anomalies in or near language areas were not particularly associated with right hemispheric speech dominance.

When considering patients who do have right hemispheric representation of speech, Sass and colleagues (1988d) speculated that lesion momentum, early childhood hemorrhage, epilepsy, and other "congenital influences" might be more important than lesion size or location in terms of contributing to right hemispheric speech dominance.

Having found evidence that interhemispheric reorganization of language abilities might not be common among patients with AVMs in language areas, Sass and coworkers (1988c) studied intrahemispheric reorganization of language abilities. They mapped the cortical distribution of language areas in the left hemisphere by intraoperative cortical stimulation. Patients with AVMs or neoplasms were studied to contrast the results from AVMs with those from a more rapidly progressive focal lesion. Neoplasms occurring in the posterior temporal region were associated with the displacement of language functions to regions outside the traditional zones, whereas such displacement was not observed among patients wtih AVMs.

Some authors have argued that AVMs often act as fast flow shunts that draw blood from other brain regions, producing ischemia in areas of the brain adjacent to or remote from the AVM (Conley et al., 1980). Variation in the degree of shunting could explain some of the variability in neuropsychological functioning among patients with AVMs. Using single positron emission tomography (SPECT), Homan et al. (1986) found decreased flow in normal brain regions distant from the AVM in 8 of 11 patients. Cases of both ipsilateral and contralateral hypoperfusion were reported. Decreased cerebral blood flow (CBF) measures in areas adjacent to an AVM has been found in studies using SPECT and stable xenon computed tomography (CT). Contralateral electroencephalographic (EEG) and neuropsychological abnormalities have been explained as resulting from contralateral ischemia caused by shunting (Loeb and Favale 1962; Reitan and Wolfson, 1985, p. 208).

The supposition that reduced CBF in areas near an AVM is caused by shunting has been challenged. Indicator dilution methods of measuring flow, i.e., methods for measuring the perfusion rate through brain tissue, assume that the tracer is freely diffusible from blood to tissue (see Chapter 3). Wade and Hachinski (1987) argued that the free movement of tracer across the blood-brain barrier is not always possible within and near AVMs. Changes in radioactive counts with time in these regions might represent the transit times of radioactive isotope through the AVM rather than perfusion rates. Even if perfusion rate is accurately measured, low values might reflect mechanisms other than shunting, such as compression related to hematoma or edema or increased venous pressure (Wade and Hachinski, 1987). Even when an AVM disturbs hemodynamics outside its border, the mechanics of the disturbance are more accurately characterized as changes in resistance gradients than as changes due to the "sucking action" of the AVM, to use Loeb and Favale's (1962) colorful term. To express this difference of emphasis, Wade and Hachinski (1987) have suggested that the term "maldistribution" replace "steal" for describing hemodynamic changes caused by AVMs.

The low values of CBF observed adjacent to or remote from an AVM do not imply ischemic levels of perfusion. The cerebral vasculature can compensate partially for reduced CBF by vasodilation, causing an increase in cerebral blood volume, and by increasing the amount of oxygen extracted from blood (see Chapter 3). Furthermore, resting CBF measures do not convey much information about the autoregulatory status of cerebral vessels. Deutsch (1983) reported on the CBF, measured during rest and activation, of a man with a known posterior left hemisphere AVM. Resting CBF indicated high flow in the region of the AVM, leading to a wide discrepancy in left-right flow in the posterior region. During attention-demanding mental activities, however, blood flow measurements indicated decreased flow in the region of the AVM, and more equivalent left-right posterior flow was observed.

When focal deficits develop as a result of the ischemia associated with AVMs, they often evolve slowly, sometimes over periods of years (Mohr et al., 1986b). Slow-onset lesions, particularly those produced by multiple discrete incidents, each causing only partial damage to a brain region, are often associated with less marked lateralized or focal neuropsychological findings (Fitzhugh et al., 1962; Finger, 1978; Smith, 1981). Variations in the temporal pattern of bleeding could also contribute to the variations in the pattern and level of neuropsychological impairment.

Basic questions about the effects of AVMs on behavior remain unanswered, especially in the areas of organization of language functions and remote effects of AVMs. A simple survey of hand, eye, and foot dominance is needed. More patients need to be studied using the sodium amytal technique and intraoperative stimulation. The possibility should be pursued that ipsilateral subcortical structures and the ipsilateral supplementary speech area make a larger than normal contribution to linguistic functioning in patients with left hemispheric AVMs. Studies using behavioral activation of neuronal activity are needed to detect abnormal organization of function and loss of CBF regulation, as are measurements of blood volume, oxygen utilization, and oxygen extraction to establish the existence of ischemia remote from the site of an AVM. Clearly, a large amount of basic work must be completed to clarify the mechanisms underlying preserved and impaired behavioral functioning in patients with AVMs.

Treatment

Arteriovenous malformations have been treated by radiotherapy, embolization, and surgery. All approaches to treatment attempt to stop flow through the AVM without damaging adjacent brain or vessels (Stein and Wolpert, 1980b). Conventional radiotherapy has not proved effective treatment for AVMs (Stein and Wolpert, 1980b). High dose, focused irradiation utilizing "gamma knife" procedures produces obliteration of small AVMs (< 2.5 cm) in 80 to 85% of patients within a period of 2 years (Steiner, 1985; Lunsford et al., Steiner, 1988). Despite these advances in radiosurgery, most current treatments of AVMs typically combine embolization with surgical removal.

Embolization

Until recently, embolization was accomplished by releasing spherical emboli into the carotid or vertebral circulation following transfemoral catheterization, although balloon techniques were also used (Vinuela and Fox, 1986). The emboli would preferentially flow into an AVM, particularly if it were large, proximal, and supplied by relatively straight vessels (Stein and Wolpert, 1980b). More recent techniques involve placing the catheter proximal to the AVM (Mehta et al., 1986) and releasing the emboli directly into a feeding vessel. In at least one series, emboli that strayed into normal circulation generally caused transient symptoms only (Stein and Wolpert, 1980b). Embolization is used to reduce blood flow to an AVM, particularly from deep arteries, and to prevent the development of collateral channels through the interior of the AVM.

Surgery

Early attempts to surgically remove AVMs generally produced disasters (Stein and Wolpert, 1980b). Dandy (1969, p. 421) asserted that removal of the AVM bed was "too dangerous to life," and hemorrhage of the fistulas in the center of an AVM "may be impossible to control." Surgical treatments that fail to isolate or obliterate the fistulas of an AVM often fail (Parkinson and Bachers, 1980). Ligation of arterial feeders to the AVM is often ineffective when performed as the sole treatment; reduction of blood flow by ligation of an internal carotid artery can be more detrimental to normal brain regions than to the AVM (Stein and Wolpert, 1980b).

Mortality and morbidity associated with complete surgical removal of an AVM has been greatly improved since the publication of Dandy's (1969) paper. For example, in one series of 200 cases, 1% of the patients died and only 6% had deficits that were neurologically severe or limited daily activities to a "modest extent" (Stein, 1986). Malik and colleagues (1988) have shown successful removal of even deep-seated basal ganglia AVMs, with utilization of microsurgical techniques. The improvement in outcome results from a better understanding of the anatomy of AVMs, presurgical embolization, and the use of surgical microscopes (Stein and Wolpert, 1980b). Stein (1986) has discussed in detail surgical methods for removing AVMs. Perhaps the most important detail about the surgery, from a neuropsychological perspective, is that a well defined gliotic plane separating the AVM from healthy tissue can usually be identified by the surgeon (Stein, 1986). By attending to this gliotic plane, even giant malformations can be removed with limited morbidity (Malik, 1982). Dissection through this plane avoids injury to functioning tissue, making possible removal of the AVM with few neuropsychological complications.

Behavioral Effects of Treatment

Conley et al. (1980) studied two patients who had undergone resection of left posterior parietal AVMs. They were evaluated with the Luria-Nebraska battery pre- and postoperatively. Preoperative cognitive findings were believed to be largely consistent with the lesion locus, being primarily speech- and language-related. Improvement in neuropsychological performance following AVM resection was interpreted by the authors as suggesting that AVMs can influence cognitive functions removed from the AVM location, possibly through ischemia produced by a steal phenomenon.

Fogel and Sparadeo (1985) discussed the postsurgical status of a 28-year-old man who had undergone resection of a right parieto-occipital AVM. The patient developed depressed mood 6 months after the surgery; the depression eventually evolved into a major affective disorder. Neuropsychological testing at this point indicated memory and visuoperceptual/visuoconstructive difficulties; language functions were not impaired. Neuropsychological testing was repeated 8 months later following psychotherapy and drug treatment. Memory performance was improved, and qualitative improvement was seen on visuoconstructive tasks. The authors concluded that the cognitive improvement was due to the patient's improved affective status rather than continued postoperative recovery. This case showed that postoperative affective disorders can complicate the assessment of neuropsychological effects of surgery.

Little is known about the range of neuropsychological effects of AVM surgery. Nor is there a significant body of data on rates of recovery from immediate perioperative neuropsychological deficits. More must be learned about which factors predict preservation of neuropsychological functioning with surgery or recovery from immediate postoperative impairment.

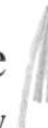

ANEURYSM

An aneurysm is a thin-walled, balloon-shaped dilatation of a vessel. Aneurysms have been classified by their shape (saccular, berry, fusiform, diffuse, or globular) or by their pathologic basis or etiology (congenital, mycotic, traumatic, dissecting, neoplastic, or arteriosclerotic) (Mohr et al., 1986a). Frequently investigators combine the two classifications, and both sets of subtypes seems equally accepted. Patients with aneurysms frequently present with hemorrhage; the rupture of an intracranial aneurysm may cause bleeding into brain parenchyma, the ventricular system, or subarachnoid or subdural spaces. Such patients typically experience a sudden, excruciating headache and progressive loss of consciousness. Many patients die the first day, and 45 to 49% die within the first 3 months of the ruptured aneurysm (Mohr et al., 1986a). Hemorrhages from aneurysms often lead to chronic functional disabilities.

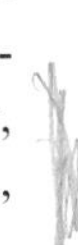

Epidemiology

The prevalence of cerebral aneurysms is estimated from autopsy and imaging studies. Figures from autopsy studies vary, as the criterion defining the minimal size of an aneurysm varies (Mohr et al., 1986a). When arterial defects as small as 2 mm in diameter are considered, 17% of routine autopsies might reveal intracranial aneurysms (Hassler, 1961). When defects only 3 mm in diameter or larger are counted, as few as 4 to 5% of autopsied cases might have aneurysms (Mohr et al., 1986a). Measurements at autopsy of the diameter of an aneurysm are probably underestimates of its in vivo size. In an autopsy study, McCormick and Acosta-Rua (1970) found that reperfusing saccular aneurysms with saline, under conditions modeling normal blood pressure, caused aneurysms to expand by 30 to 60%.

General Issues

Aneurysms can produce disruption of cerebral functioning by rupturing, shedding emboli, and producing mass effects and vasospasm. Hemorrhage associated with aneurysmal rupture generally occurs rapidly, although the occasional slow seepage of blood from an aneurysm can mimic the time course of a cerebral tumor (Sweet, 1941). The hemorrhage disrupts the normal supply of oxygen and glucose to brain tissue and disrupts removal of heat and by-products from metabolic activities. Consequently, areas of infarction develop. The blood itself can disrupt brain metabolism, which may be another source of neuronal dysfunction (Fein, 1975).

The constriction of cerebral arteries following hemorrhage can reduce cerebral blood flow and disrupt energy metabolism. The constriction primarily involves the large cerebral vessels (Powers and Grubb, 1987). Voldby and colleagues (1985) reported that among 38 patients severe diffuse spasm was always associated with global ischemia and subsequent cerebral infarctions identified on CT scans. Patients with less diffuse spasm often displayed focal ischemia or hyperemia. The cerebral metabolic rate of oxygen ($CMRO_2$) decreased in proportion to the diameter of constricted arteries. Furthermore, $CMRO_2$ was more reduced than the rCBF, suggesting that an uncoupling of metabolism and blood flow occurs during spasm. Although uncoupling of flow and metabolism has been found by others, the pattern of uncoupling does not always agree with that seen by Voldby and colleagues (Powers and Grubb, 1987). In the study of Voldby et al. (1985), uncoupling of flow metabolism was associated with increased lactic acid levels measured in cerebro-spinal fluid and with intracranial hypertension. Intracranial hypertension and lactic acidosis were in turn associated with vasoparalysis, detected by measurements of rCBF during hyperventilation. Voldby and colleagues concluded that as vasospasm disrupts the capacity of the arterial system to regulate blood flow in response to changes in neuronal activity, a shift toward anaerobic metabolism occurs.

Little research has focused on the neuropsychological effects of hemorrhage following aneurysmal rupture. Questions regarding the relative ability of neuropsychological tests to localize hemorrhages, particularly in comparison with other focal diseases, and studies of the time course of recovery of functioning from hemorrhage are areas where more research is needed. Given the evidence that abnormalities of pH moderate nerve cell death in ischemic stroke (see Chapter 2), the relation between pH changes and neuropsychological functioning should be examined following cerebral hemorrhage. Brain pH and lactate can be measured noninvasively using ^{1}H and ^{31}P nuclear magnetic spectroscopy (see Chapter 2), making it possible to study neuropsychological correlates of pH changes.

Anterior Communicating Artery Aneurysm

The anterior communicating artery (ACoA) received little attention in Critchley's (1930) discussion of the anterior cerebral artery and its clinical syndromes. However, in 1953 Norlen and Olivecrona described several cases of amnesia in patients with aneurysms of the ACoA. Other case and group studies of patients with AcoA aneurysms have confirmed the presence of memory disorders. Personality changes are also commonly reported, with cognitive signs of frontal lobe involvement and signs of callosal involvement less commonly observed. The clinical features of these abnormalities and their anatomic basis are considered next.

Memory

Patients with hemorrhage of the ACoA often have a history of rapid onset of headache followed by drowsiness, lethargy, and loss of consciousness. As they recover from this stage, they can display disorientation for time, place, and person, nonsensical confabulation, some retrograde amnesia, and more extensive anterograde amnesia (Lindqvist and Norlen, 1966). Disorientation often lessens during the first few weeks after surgery, and the confabulation becomes less fantastic (Parkin et al.,

1988). The chronic long-term disability associated with problems in memory vary greatly. Although some patients require constant supervision and even institutionalization, others live with supervision at home; a third group recovers completely and returns to previous levels of social and vocational functioning. Generally, however, the memory disorder seen during the immediate postoperative period improves during long-term follow-up (Okawa et al., 1980).

The anterograde memory deficit has been studied in the chronic phase more thoroughly than the retrograde abnormality. Verbal memory span is typically normal. (Talland et al., 1967; Vilkki, 1985); however, when the number of items to be recalled exceeds memory span, performance is impaired (Volpe and Hirst, 1983; Alexander and Freedman, 1984). Performacne on memory tasks is also frequently impaired when a second task is interpolated between the presentation of items and their test (Talland et al., 1967; Vilkki, 1985; Parkin et al., 1988).

The anterograde amnesia has been observed on a variety of recall paradigms, e.g., running memory span (Talland et al., 1967), multi-trial free recall tasks (Alexander and Freedman, 1984), incidental learning (Vilkki, 1985), and recall of short stories (Talland et al., 1967). Uncued recall (Volpe and Hirst, 1983) after a delay (Alexander and Freedman, 1984) is particularly impaired. The recall protocols of patients with ACoA are not simply more sparse than normals, they contain an abnormal number of intrusions from previously presented material and other signs of sensitivity to interference effects (Volpe and Hirst, 1983; Parkin et al., 1988). It may be that tests with somewhat less structured verbal materials are more sensitive to the verbal memory impairment in patients with ACoA, provided the amount of information presented exceeds the memory span of the patient. In one case (Alexander and Freedman, 1984, case no. 11) both immediate and delayed recall of the logical memory paragraphs from the Wechsler Memory Scale were within the average range and were compatible with IQ. However, performance on the auditiory verbal learning task, a multi-trial word learning test, was poor. The two patients described by Talland and coinvestigators (1967) were markedly impaired in terms of the recall of consonant trigrams.

Few studies have addressed the question of whether visuospatial information is as poorly recalled as verbal information. The two patients studied by Volpe and Hirst (1983) scored in the borderline range of impairment on the Graham Kendall Memory for Designs. They were also impaired when recalling details of unfamiliar urban scenes. Vilkki's (1985) patients were impaired on the immediate and delayed recall of designs from the Benton Visual Retention Test.

Among the small number of cases reported in the literature, patients with ACoA amnesia scored normally on recognition tests. Volpe and Hirst's (1983) two patients scored as well as normals when recognizing previously studied words or urban scenes. Talland and coworkers (1967) tested their patients for the ability to recognize the glossy covering pages of the *New Yorker* magazine. One patient was impaired during the first 2 months after the hemorrhage but improved into the normal range by the fourth month. The second patient was clearly impaired when tested during the first few months after rupture of the ACoA. However, he developed such an uncritical response bias on subsequent testing that it was difficult to determine how well he could discriminate old from new pictures. The patient examined by Parkin and colleagues (1988) could recognize sentences presented by the examiner, although he could not recall their order of presentation.

Both patients of Talland and colleagues (1967) had retrograde amnesias that extended several years prior to the hemorrhage. However, the first patient experienced gradual recession of his retrograde amnesia and apparently recovered fully after returning home. It is unclear to what degree the second patient recovered from the retrograde amnesia. Butters and coworkers (1984) reported normal performance on the Boston Remote Memory Battery for a patient who was amnesic following rupture of an ACoA. However, this patient's IQs fell into the Very Superior range. The patient presented by Parkin et al. (1988) had a full scale IQ of 115 and performed normally on the British version of the Famous Faces subtest of the Boston Remote Memory Battery. Milberg and colleagues (1988) have reported on two patients with ruptures of ACoA aneurysms who had normal scores on an abbreviated version of the Boston Famous Faces subtest. One patient had an IQ of 103 and the other an IQ of 107. We have studied an amnesic patient, after rupture of an ACoA aneurysm, with low normal IQs: Full Scale IQ 83, Verbal IQ 85, Performance IQ 80. However, he performed normally on an abbreviated version of the Famous Faces Test, scoring 6, 7, 6, 6, 8, and 5 with a maximum score of 8 possible for decades spanning the 1920s, 1930s, 1940s, 1950s, 1960s, and 1970s, respectively. Patients with ACoA aneurysms who hemorrhage and have surgery appear to have intact remote memory. This finding distinguishes them from some other types of patient with brain-related memory dysfunction, e.g., patients with alcoholic Korsakoff syndrome, Huntington's chorea, herpes encephalitis, and Alzheimer's disease (Wilson et al., 1981; Butters and Miliotis, 1985).

The two patients studied by Milberg and colleagues (1988) could learn a complex cognitive rule, despite being severely amnesic. The authors trained their patients to apply a seven-step algorithm to square two-digit numbers. The algorithm simplifies the mental calculation involved by replacing the squaring of the two-digit number with steps involving the multiplication of two numbers that are multiples of ten and the squaring of a single digit number. The algorithm also takes advantage of the result that the middle term of the quadratic equation, implied by the algorithm, drops out of the calculation. Reaction times were measured for trials where the patients were asked to complete only one step of the algorithm and for separate trials where they used the entire algorithm to square a target number. Consequently, the time taken to complete individual components of the algorithm was measured separately from the time required to complete the entire algorithm. Over three sessions, the patients improved their speed of squaring numbers to an equal degree. Similar practice on Hebb's recurring digit task did not show any improvement. One subject's speed improved to the same degree that his speed at performing individual steps of the algorithm improved. However, the second patient's squaring speed improved to a much greater degree than would have been expected from the change in individual steps. The authors concluded that learning a cognitive skill is possible even in severely amnesic individuals. They further concluded that some patients learn such skills by mastering individual steps; others become increasingly proficient at combining the steps into a whole act. Both approaches are found among patients with hemorrhages from ACoA aneurysms, although it is unclear whether either approach is related to a patient's lesion or to premorbid problem-solving styles.

Speculation about the site of damage responsible for the amnesia following ACoA hemorrhage or surgery has focused on damage to the frontal lobe or damage to regions supplied by the perforating branches of the ACoA. Parkin and coinvestigators (1988) argued, in particular, for a primary frontal lobe contribution to their patient's poor memory functioning. Alexander and Freedman (1984) suggested that damage to the anterior hypothalamus or septum, two regions supplied by the perforating branches of the ACoA, might be critical to ACoA amnesia. To support their suggestion, these investigators observed that the paraventricular nucleus of the hypothalamus synthesizes vasopressin, which might contribute to memory functioning, whereas the septal region is a source of cholinergic input into the hippocampus. To settle these issues, correlations of specific patterns of behavioral deficit with the anatomic and metabolic topography of the various lesions seen with ACoA hemorrhage are needed in a series of patients. These topographic studies should be supplemented by manipulations of the neurotransmitters or neuroactive peptides thought to be involved.

Personality Function

In 1966 Lindqvist and Norlen reported that personality changes were seen in some of 33 patients studied after surgical removal of ACoA aneurysms. In one subgroup, mood was mildly elevated with shallow euphoria sometimes present. In another subgroup there were flattening of social ambitions, an indifference about the future, and apathy. These observations are an early reference to the personality changes associated with ACoA aneurysms. However, there was little discussion in the original paper of how the observations were obtained and of the frequency with which various symptoms occurred.

Logue and colleagues (1968) presented a more detailed discussion of personality changes following rupture of anterior cerebral artery (ACA) or ACoA aneurysms in 79 patients. The patients were given a battery of psychological tests and a psychological interview with a spouse or friend present. Seventy items representing demographic, neurologic, psychometric, and personality information were scored or rated for each subject. A principal components analysis performed on items where change in functioning was rated revealed four factors that accounted for 57.7% of the variance. The four factors represented intellectual impairment, mood alterations, changes in affect, and language abnormalities associated with left-sided aneurysms or left-sided surgery. Impairment of intelligence and memory was associated with losses of initiative, interest, and conscientiousness. However, loss of initiative, interest, and conscientiousness did not always occur together with intellectual impairment; in 10 patients these changes were accompanied by only mild intellectual impairment, and in 15 patients no intellectual changes were present. These results indicated that among patients with hemorrhage caused by rupture of ACA or ACoA aneurysms changes in drive can be part of a general dementia or a more specific personality change.

The principal component reflecting mood changes included items assessing irritability and sociability in addition to worry, euphoria, and dysphoria. The changes in mood were bidirectional. Several patients reported increased depression (10 patients), worry (9), or irritability (18), whereas others reported euphoria (15), decreased tendency to worry (25), or decreased irritability (12). Generally, the opinion of the patient's relative agreed with that of the patient. The causes of the depressed-irritable mood changes appeared to be several. Poor adjustment to physical or cognitive disabilities, stressful life events, and direct disruption of brain systems involved in mood appeared to contribute to depressive mood changes.

More often Logue and colleagues found elevations of mood. Occasionally these changes were dramatic. One patient had been depressed for a year prior to her hemorrhage; she would become tearful with little provocation and experienced early morning awakening. The onset of the depression was not associated with any identifiable event, but she had a family history of depression; her brother had committed suicide. After hemorrhage and removal of a left ACA aneurysm, she became happier, more interested in daily activities, and more assertive. Both she and a relative thought these personality changes favorable. The authors speculated that the mechanism of favorable change was similar to frontal leukotomy.

The third component of personality change found by Logue and colleagues involved the expression of affect. Some patients experienced a loss of inhibition with more laughter, crying, sentimentality, irritability, and restlessness present in their behavior. More often patients experienced a reduced capacity to show emotion, with twice as many showing affective flattening than affective release. Generally, both the patient's ratings and the relative's ratings of a particular change loaded on this component. Abnormalities of affect were more closely associated with left-sided than right-sided aneurysms.

The work of Logue and associates indicated that personality changes can follow hemorrhage of aneurysms in either the ACA or ACoA distributions. Although these authors provided information on the role of lesion laterality in producing personality change, they could not contribute evidence about the importance of the location of the lesion along the anterior to posterior axis. Robinson and coworkers (1984) have shown that affective changes following ischemic stroke are more likely the closer the infarction is to the frontal pole. The finding applies to both cortical and subcortical infarction (see Chapter 7). A similar correlation might exist for hemorrhages.

Storey (1967, 1970) provided data on the specific personality changes associated with hemorrhage of the anterior cerebral circulation. He compared personality functionining in 261 patients with subarachnoid hemorrhage associated with aneurysms of the ACoA ($n = 81$), middle cerebral artery (MCA) ($n = 71$), posterior cerebral artery (PCA) ($n = 72$), no known artery, and multiple arteries. Adverse personality changes were associated with the presence of neurologic signs ($\phi = .47$) and the presence of intellectual impairment ($\phi = .57$). An interesting deviation from the above correlations was observed in the ACoA group. All seven ACoA patients with moderate or severe personality alterations had no intellectual changes or only mild change. This finding contrasted significantly with those in MCA and PC patients, in whom moderate or severe personality change was generally associated with intellectual impairment.

Taken at face value, Storey's results suggested that hemorrhage of ACoA aneurysms can selectively change personality functioning. Hemorrhage in other arterial distributions typically alters personality as part of a more general change in cognitive and behavioral functioning. However, in Storey's series, as well as that of Logue and colleagues, it is difficult to know the location and extent of the brain lesions involved. Hemorrhage in the MCA and PCA distributions can involve the frontal lobe. Vasospasm, release of neurotransmitters into the cerebrospinal fluid (CSF), edema, interruption of cerebral blood flow and CSF flow, and disruption of neuronal input into brain regions remote from the hemorrhage complicate determination of the lesion site after hemorrhage.

Okawa et al. (1980) found that patients with ruptured ACoA aneurysms who experienced immediate postoperative personality changes often improved during long-term follow-up. For example, of the 24 patients experiencing a lack of vitality immediately after surgery, only 3 had such symptoms at the end of the follow-up period; and of the 19 patients who were talkative and hyperkinetic immediately after surgery, only one displayed these symptoms at follow-up.

Little recent work has been done on the specific changes in personality that follow hemorrhage from aneurysms. It is an area ready for exploration by the anatomic, metabolic, and neurochemical techniques that have been applied to the study of depression following stroke (Robinson et al., 1984) and to the study of primary affective and anxiety disorders (Carroll and Mendels, 1976; Nesse et al., 1984). Two general models seem worth pursuing. The multivariate model assumes that variability in personality change following hemorrhage from cerebral aneurysms is caused by the additive influences of several neuropathologic, general medical, social, and neurocognitive factors, as well as premorbid personality traits and cognitive abilities. The homeostatic model assumes that the fundamental cause of variability in personality change is the postulated inability of the cortex, particularly the frontal cortex, to regulate levels of drive and mood and to modulate affect. Social factors and adjustment to impairment would play a secondary role in perturbing the neural systems underlying emotion. The primary deficit would be the regulation of these perturbations.

Other Neuropsychological Effects

Typically, patients with rupture of an ACoA aneurysm are not chronically demented (Sengupta, et al., 1975). At 2.5 years after hemorrhage, the patients of Talland et al. (1967) had Verbal IQs of 101 and 102 and Performance IQ scores of 101 and 106, respectively. The 11 cases reported by Alexander and Freedman (1984) had a median Verbal IQ of 94 and a median Performance IQ of 88. One patient, however, had abnormally low scores, with a Verbal IQ of 68 and Performance IQ of 70. This patient also had the lowest Wechsler Memory Quotient and performed much worse than any other patient on the Boston Naming Test. He was lethargic for 6 weeks after surgery and had a large ACA territory infarct. In a series of 20 patients we have studied, the three with the greatest disparity between their predicted and observed IQs had hydrocephalus. Apparently posthemorrhagic depression of the IQ is most likely seen in patients with large infarcts or hydrocephalus.

Although Alexander and Freedman's patients generally had IQs at least in the average range, one-half performed worse than the 10th percentile on an oral verbal fluency task. The task requires subjects to think rapidly of words that begin with the letters F, A, or S. Talland also found that his patients were impaired on verbal fluency. Poor performance on this type of verbal fluency task has been associated with dysfunction of the left frontal lobe involving either inferior or dorsolateral frontal cortex (Milner, 1964). The finding of impaired verbal fluency in the presence of intact verbal intellectual functioning is typical of patients with frontal lobe dysfunction, who are free of a general dementia.

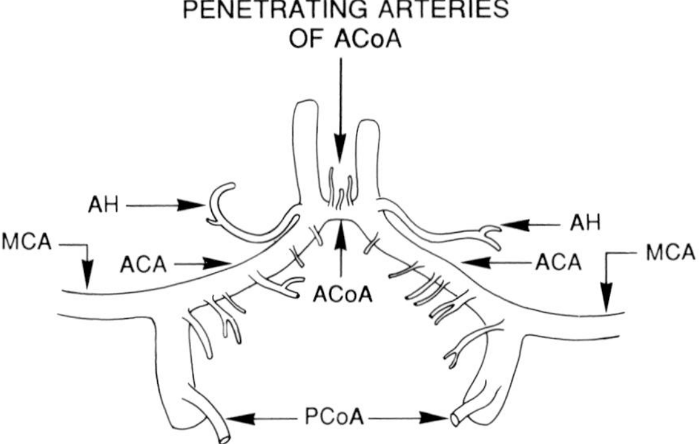

Figure 11–2 Anterior circle of Willis. The small branches of the anterior communicating artery (ACoA) penetrate the brain superiorally. AH = artery of Heubner; ACA = anterior cerebral artery; MCA = middle cerebral artery; PCoA = posterior communicating artery.

Several authors have reported callosal syndromes following hemorrhage from ACoA aneurysms (Sweet, 1941; Beukelman et al., 1980). Left hand apraxia, agraphia, and tactile anomia, as well as left and right hand conflicts have been reported (Sweet, 1941; Beukelman et al., 1980). Generally, these syndromes are associated with infarction of the anterior two-thirds of the corpus callosum.

Surgery

Dunker and Harris (1976) reported that the ACoA has three superiorally penetrating branches (Figure 11–2). Gade (1982) has argued that surgical approaches to ACoA aneurysm that preserve blood flow through these branches reduce the likelihood of amnesia following surgery. In particular, he compared two surgical procedures, ligation and trapping. The first procedure involved stopping blood flow to the aneurysm by tying shut the neck of the aneurysm (Figure 11–3). This approach does not reduce blood flow through the penetrating arteries. The second procedure traps the aneurysm by tying shut both ends of the ACoA (Figure 11–3). This approach stops flow through the aneurysm and the penetrating branches. Gade found that only 6 of 37 patients whose aneurysms were ligated at the neck developed amnesia, whereas 9 of

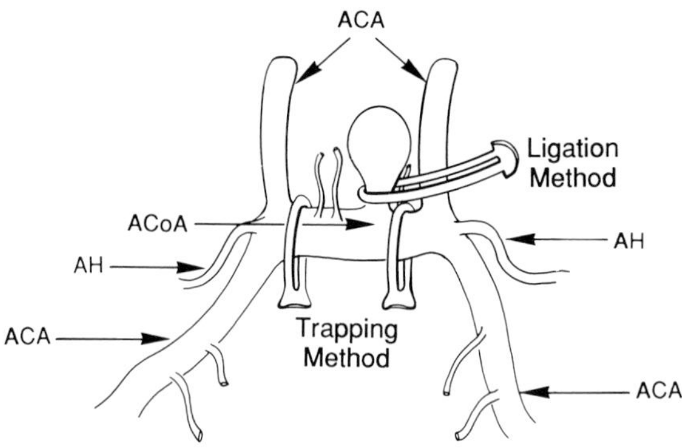

Figure 11–3 Ligation and trapping methods of surgically treating an anterior communicating artery (ACoA) aneurysm. AH = artery of Heubner; ACA = anterior cerebral artery.

11 patients whose aneurysm was trapped developed amnesia. The difference is significant ($\chi^2 = 13.60$, $p < 0.001$). Gade's work not only bears on how surgery on ACoA aneurysms should be performed, it is strong evidence that some regions supplied by the penetrating branches of the ACoA, such as the anterior hypothalamus and septum, make important contributions to memory functioning (Alexander and Freedman, 1984).

Another important advance in improving outcome after ACoA surgery involves use of the surgical microscope. The microscope simplifies detection of the location of the small penetrating arteries, the dissection of small arteries from blood clots, and the identification of the neck of the aneurysm. Okawa et al. (1980) found less mortality and morbidity in a series where the microscope had been used compared with a series where the microscope was not used.

FUTURE DIRECTIONS

Research on memory pathology following rupture of ACoA aneurysms is likely to make substantial contributions to a general neuropsychological theory of memory. Behavioral studies are needed to determine if some or all of this type of memory disorder is primary amnesia or derivative of a more general disruption of personality or executive functioning. Behavioral studies of ACoA amnesia might help answer the question of whether there is one type of amnesia or several. Pharmacologic manipulations of cholinergic metabolites, vasopressin, and other transmitters would add to our understanding of the neurochemistry of memory.

Studies are needed to identify the critical structures associated with personality change and amnesia following rupture of ACoA aneurysms. Anatomic research needs to be supplemented by studies that correlate changes in brain energy metabolism and pH with neurobehavioral symptoms. We need better data on the contribution of vasospasm to long-term functional disability following hemorrhage. The range of clinical neuroscience techniques that have successfully elucidated brain-behavior relations following ischemic stroke need to be more widely applied to the study of brain functioning following rupture of ACoA aneurysms. Unique insights into the biologic basis of memory, personality, and frontal lobe functioning appear to await those who are willing to study the rupture of this tiny artery.

REFERENCES

Adams, R.D. and Victor, M. (1985). *Principles of Neurology,* 3rd ed. New York: McGraw-Hill.

Alexander, M.P., and Freedman, M. (1984). Amnesia after anterior communicating artery aneurysm rupture. *Neurology,* **34,** 752–757.

Beukelman, D.R., Flowers, C.R., and Swanson, P.D. (1980). Cerebral disconnection associated with anterior communicating artery aneurysm: implications for evaluation of symptoms. *Arch. Phys. Med. Rehabil.,* **61,** 18–23.

Brown, G.G., Spicer, K.B., Robertson, W.M., Baird, A.D., and Malik, G. (1989). Neuropsychological signs of lateralized arteriovenous malformations: comparison with ischemic stroke. *Clin. Neuropsychol.,* **3,** 340–352.

Butters, N., and Miliotis, P. (1985). Amnesic disorders. In: K.M. Heilman and E. Valenstein, eds., *Clinical Neuropsychology,* pp. 403–451. New York: Oxford University Press.

Butters, N., Miliotis, P., Albert, M.S., and Sax, D.S. (1984). Memory assessment: evidence of the heterogeneity of amnesic symptoms. In: G. Goldstein, ed., *Advances in Clinical Neuropsychology,* Vol 1, pp. 127–159. New York: Plenum Press.

Carroll, B.J., and Mendels, J. (1976). Neuroendocrine regulation in affective disorders. In: E.J. Sachar, ed., *Hormones, Behavior and Psychopathology,* pp. 193–244. New York: Raven Press.

Close, R.A, O'Keefe, A.M., and Buchheit, W.A. (1977). The determination of speech organization in a patient with an arteriovenous malformation. *Neurosurgery,* **1,** 111–113.

Conley, F.K., Moses, J.A., Jr., and Helle, T.L. (1980). Deficits of higher cortical functioning in two patients with posterior parietal arteriovenous malformations. *Neurosurgery,* **7,** 230–237.

Constans, J.P., and Assal, G. (1971). Evolution de la symptomatologie neuropsychologique d'une sérié d'anévrismes arterio-veineux opérés. *Neurochirurgia,* **14,** 201–216.

Critchley, M. (1930). The anterior cerebral artery, and its syndromes. *Brain,* **53,** 120–165.

Dandy, W.E. (1969). *The Brain.* New York: Harper & Row.

Deutsch, G. (1983). Blood flow changes in arteriovenous malformation during behavioral activation. *Ann. Neurol.,* **13,** 38–43.

Dunker, R.O., and Harris, A.B. (1976). Surgical anatomy of the proximal anterior cerebral artery. *J. Neurosurg.,* **44,** 359–367.

Dunn, W., Rosen, W.G., Malamut, B., and Zappulla, R.A. (1984). Memory deficits in left hemisphere arteriovenous malformations. *INS Bull.* p. 13.

Fein, J.M. (1975). Cerebral energy metabolism after subarachnoid hemorrhage. *Stroke,* **6,** 1–8.

Finger, S. (1978). Lesion momentum and behavior. In: S. Finger, ed., *Recovery from Brain Damage: Research and Theory,* pp. 135–164. New York: Plenum Press.

Fitzhugh, K.B., Fitzhugh, L.C., and Reitan, R. (1962). Wechsler-Bellevue comparisons in groups of "chronic" and "current" lateralized and diffuse brain lesions. *J. Consult. Psychol.,* **26,** 306–310.

Fogel, B.S., and Sparadeo, F.R. (1985). Focal cognitive deficits accentuated by depression. *J. Nerv. Ment. Dis.,* **173,** 120–124.

Gade, A. (1982). Amnesia after operations on aneurysms of the anterior communicating artery. *Surg. Neurol.,* **18,** 46–49.

Gross, C.R., Kase, C.S., Mohr, J.P., Cunningham, S.C., and Baker, W.E. (1984). Stroke in south Alabama: incidence and diagnostic features—a population based study. *Stroke,* **15,** 249–255.

Hassler, O. (1961). Morphological studies on the large cerebral arteries with references to aetiology of subarachnoid hemorrhage. *Acta Psychiatr. Neurol. Scand.* [*Suppl. 154*], **36:** 5–145.

Homan, R.W., Devous, M.D., Stokely, E.M., and Bonte, F.J. (1986). Quantification of intracranial steal in patients with arteriovenous malformation. *Arch. Neurol.,* **43,** 779–785.

Lezak, M.D. (1983). *Neuropsychological Assessment,* 2nd ed., New York: Oxford University Press.

Lindqvist, G., and Norlen, G. (1966). Korsakoff syndrome after operation on ruptured aneurysm of the anterior communicating artery. *Acta Psychiatr. Scand.,* **42,** 24–34.

Loeb, C., and Favale, E. (1962). Contralateral EEG abnormalities in intracranial arteriovenous aneurysms. *Arch Neurol.,* **7,** 121–128.

Lindqvist G., and Norlen, G. (1966). Korsakoff's syndrome after operation on ruptured aneurysm of the anterior communicating artery. *Acta Psychiatr. Scand.,* **42,** 24–34.

Logue, V., Durwald, M., Pratt, R.T.C., Piercy, M., and Nixon, W.L.B. (1968). The quality of survival after rupture of an anterior cerebral aneurysm. *Br. J. Psychiatry,* **114,** 137–160.

Lunsford, L.D., Flickinger, J.C., and Steiner, L. (1988). The gamma knife. *J.A.M.A.*, **259,** 2544.

Malik, G.M. (1982). Surgical treatment of large cerebral arteriovenous malformations. In: R.R. Smith, A. Haeren, and W.E. Russell, eds., *Vascular Malformations,* pp. 77–99. New York: Raven Press.

Malik, G.M., Umansky, F., Patel, S., and Ausman, J.I. (1988). Microsurgical removal of arteriovenous malformations of the basal ganglia. *Neurosurgery,* **23,** 209–217.

McCormick, W.F. (1966). The pathology of vascular ("arteriovenous") malformations. *J. Neurosurg.,* **24,** 807–816.

McCormick, W.F., and Acosta-Rua, G.J. (1970). The size of intracranial saccular aneurysms: an autopsy study. *J. Neurosurg.,* **33,** 422–427.

McCormick, W.F., and Schochet, S.S., Jr. (1976). *Atlas of Cerebrovascular Disease.* Philadelphia: Sanders.

Mehta, B., Jack, C.R., Jr., Boulos, R.S., Patel, S.C., Ausman, J.I., and Malik, G.M. (1986). Interventional neuroradiology: Henry Ford Hospital experience with transcatheter embolization of vascular lesions in the head, neck, and spine. *Henry Ford Hosp. Med. J.,* **34,** 19–30.

Milberg, W., Alexander, M.P., Charness, N., McGlinchey-Berroth, R., and Barrett, A. (1988). Learning of a complex arithmetic skill in amnesia: evidence for a dissociation between compilation and production. *Brain Cogn.,* **8,** 91–104.

Milner, B. (1964). Some effects of frontal lobectomy in man. In: J.M. Warren and K. Akert, eds., *The Frontal Granular Cortex and Behavior,* pp. 313–334. New York: McGraw-Hill.

Mohr, J.P., Kistler, J.P., Zabramski, J.M., Spetzler, R.F., and Barnett, H.J.M. (1986a). Intracranial aneurysms. In: H.J.M. Barnett, J.P. Mohr, B.M. Stein, and F.M. Yatsu, eds., *Stroke Pathophysiology, Diagnosis, and Management,* Vol. 2, pp. 643–677. New York: Churchill Livingstone.

Mohr, J.P., Tatemichi, T.K., Nichols, F.C., III, and Stein, B.M. (1986b). Vascular malformations of the brain: clinical considerations. In: H.J.M. Barnett, J.P. Mohr, B.M. Stein, and F.M. Yatsu, eds., *Stroke: Pathophysiology, Diagnosis, and Management,* Vol 2, pp. 679–719. New York: Churchill Livingstone.

Nesse, R.M., Cameron, O.G., Curtis, G.C., McCann, D.S., and Huber-Smith, M.J. (1984). Adrenergic function in patients with panic anxiety. *Arch. Gen. Psychiatry,* **41,** 771–776.

Norlen, G., and Olivecrona, H. (1953). The treatment of aneurysms of the circle of Willis. *J. Neurosurg.,* **10,** 404–415.

Nornes, H., and Grip, A. (1980). Hemodynamic aspects of cerebral arteriovenous malformations. *J. Neurosurg.,* **53,** 456–464.

Okawa, M., Maeda, H., Nukui, H., and Kawafuchi, J. (1980). Psychiatric symptoms in ruptured anterior communicating aneurysms: social prognosis. *Acta Psychiatr. Scand.,* **61,** 306–312.

Olivecrona, H., and Reeves, J. (1948). Arteriovenous aneurysms of the brain: their diagnosis and treatment. *Arch. Neurol. Psychiatry,* **59,** 567–602.

Padget, D.H. (1956). The cranial venous system in man in reference to development, adult configuration, and relation to the arteries. *Am. J. Anat.,* **98,** 307–355.

Parkin, A.J., Leng, N.R.C., Stanhope, N., and Smith, A.P. (1988). Memory impairment following ruptured aneurysm of the anterior communicating artery. *Brain Cogn.,* **7,** 231–243.

Parkinson, D., and Bachers, G. (1980). Arteriovenous malformations: summary of 100 consecutive supratentorial cases. *J. Neurosurg.,* **53,** 285–299.

Perret, G. (1975). The epidemiology and clinical course of arteriovenous malformations. In:

H.W. Pia, J.R.W. Gleave, E. Grote, and J. Zierski, eds., *Cerebral Angiomas: Advances in Diagnosis and Therapy,* pp. 21–26. New York: Springer-Verlag.

Perret, G., and Nishioka, H. (1966). Report on the cooperative study of intracranial aneurysms and subarachnoid hemorrhage. Section VI. Arteriovenous malformations. *J. Neurosurg.,* **25,** 467–490.

Powers, W.J., and Grubb, R.L., Jr. (1987). Hemodynamic and metabolic relationships in cerebral ischemia and subarachnoid hemorrhage. In: J.H. Wood, ed., *Cerebral Blood Flow: Physiologic and Clinical Aspects,* pp. 387–401. New York: McGraw-Hill.

Reitan, R.M., and Davison, L. (1974). *Clinical Neuropsychology: Current Status and Applications.* Washington, D.C.: V.H. Winston & Sons.

Reitan, R.M., and Wolfson, D. (1985). *The Halstead-Reitan Neuropsychological Test Battery.* Tucson, Az: Neuropsychology Press.

Robinson, R.G., Kubos, K.L., Starr, L.B., Rao, K., and Price, T.R. (1984). Mood disorders in stroke patients: importance of location of lesion. *Brain,* **107,** 81–93.

Sass, K.J., Spencer, D.D., Novelly, R.A., and Chyatte, D. (1988a). Neocortically based, congenital vascular malformations. I. Level of neuropsychological functioning and localization of impairments. *J. Clin. Exp. Neuropsychol.,* **10,** 86.

Sass, K.J., Spencer, D.D., Novelly, R.A., Chyatte, D., and Barr, W. (1988b). Neocortically based, congenital vascular malformations. II. Speech lateralization via the intracarotid amytal procedure. *J. Clin. Exp. Neuropsychol.,* **10,** 86.

Sass, K.J., Spencer, D.D., Novelly, R.A., and Chyatte, D. (1988c). Neocortically based, congenital vascular malformations. III. Intrahemispheric localization of language functions. *J. Clin. Exp. Neuropsychol.* **10,** 86–87.

Sass, K.J., Spencer, D.D, Novelly, R.A., and Chyatte, D. (1988d). Neocortically based, congenital vascular malformations. IV. Right-hemisphere speech dominance in patients with arteriovenous malformations. *J. Clin. Exp. Neuropsychol.,* **10,** 87.

Sengupta, R.P., Chiu, J.S.P., and Brierley, H. (1975). Quality of survival following direct surgery for anterior communicating artery aneurysms. *J. Neurosurg.,* **43,** 58–64.

Smith, A. (1981). Principles underlying human brain functions in neuropsychological sequelae of different neuropathological processes. In: S.B. Filskov and T.J. Boll, eds., *Handbook of Clinical Neuropsychology,* Vol. 1, pp. 175–226. New York: Wiley.

Stein, B.M. (1986). Surgical decisions in vascular malformations of the brain. In: H.J.M. Barnett, J.P. Mohr, B.M. Stein, and F.M. Yatsu, eds., *Stroke: Pathophysiology, Diagnosis, and Management,* Vol. 2, pp. 1129–1172. New York: Churchill Livingstone.

Stein, B.M., and Wolpert, S.M. (1980a). Arteriovenous malformations of the brain. I. Current concepts and treatment. *Arch. Neurol.,* **37,** 1–5.

Stein, B.M., and Wolpert, S.M. (1980b). Arteriovenous malformations of the brain. II. Current concepts and treatment. *Arch. Neurol.,* **37,** 69–75.

Steiner, L. (1985). Radiosurgery in cerebral arteriovenous malformations. In: J.M. Fein and E.S. Flamm, eds., *Cerebral Vascular Surgery,* Vol. 4, pp. 1161–1215. New York: Springer Verlag.

Storey, P.B. (1967). Psychiatric sequelae of subarachnoid hemorrhage. *Br. Med. J.,* **3,** 261–266.

Storey, P.B. (1970). Brain damage and personality change after subarachnoid haemorrhage. *Br. J. Psychiatry,* **117,** 129–142.

Sweet, W.H. (1941). Seeping intracranial aneurysm simulating neoplasm: syndrome of the corpus callosum. *Arch. Neurol. Psychiatry,* **45,** 86–104.

Talland, G.A., Sweet, W.H., and Ballantine, H.T. (1967). Amnesic syndrome with anterior communicating artery aneurysms. *J. Nerv. Ment. Dis.,* **145,** 179–192.

Vilkki, J. (1985). Amnesic syndromes after surgery of anterior communicating artery aneurysms. *Cortex, **21,** 431–444.*

Vinuela, F., and Fox, A.J. (1986). Interventional neuroradiology. In: H.J.M. Barnett, J.P., Mohr, B.M. Stein, and F.M. Yatsu, eds., *Stroke Pathophysiology, diagnosis, and management,* Vol. 2, pp. 1173–1189. New York: Churchill Livingstone.

Voldby, B., Enevoldsen, E., and Jensen, F.T. (1985). Regional CBF, intraventricular pressure, and cerebral metabolism in patients with ruptured intracranial aneurysms. *J. Neurosurg.,* **62,** 48–58.

Volpe, B.T., and Hirst, W. (1983). Amnesia following the rupture and repair of an anterior communicating artery aneurysm. *J. Neurol. Neurosurg. Psychiatry,* **46,** 704–709.

Wade, J.P.H., and Hachinski, V.C. (1987). Cerebral steal: robbery or maldistribution? In: J.H. Wood, ed., *Cerebral Blood Flow: Physiologic and Clinical Aspects,* pp. 467–480. New York: McGraw-Hill.

Waltimo, O., and Putkonen, A.-R. (1974). Intellectual performance of patients with intracranial arteriovenous malformations. *Brain,* **97,** 511–520.

Wendling, L.R., Moore, J.S., Jr., Kieffer, S.A., Goldberg, H.I., and Latchaw, R.E. (1976). Intracerebral venous angioma. *Radiology,* **119,** 141–147.

Wertz, R.T., Messert, B., Collins, M., Rosenbek, J.C., and Kao, C.C. (1977). Right-hemisphere language dominance in a case of left-hemisphere arteriovenous malformation. *J. Speech Hear. Disord.,* **42,** 106–112.

Wilson, R.S., Kaszniak, A.W., and Fox, J.H. (1981). Remote memory in senile dementia. *Cortex,* **17,** 41–48.

Yamada, S. (1982). Arteriovenous malformations in the functional area: surgical treatment and regional cerebral blood flow. *Neurol. Res.,* **4,** 283–322.

Yamada, S., and Cojocaru, T. (1987). Arteriovenous malformations. In: J.H. Wood, ed., *Cerebral Blood Flow: Physiologic and Clinical Aspects,* pp. 580–590. New York: McGraw-Hill.

12

Deficits in Auditory Comprehension and Brain Lesions in Left Hemisphere Ischemic Stroke

DAVID KNOPMAN, OLA SELNES, AND ALAN RUBENS

The study of aphasia due to stroke has provided unique insights into some of the physical principles that govern the representation of linguistic functions in the brain. For example, Wernicke's first case of "sensory aphasia" to come to autopsy had an infarction of the first temporal gyrus of the left hemisphere (Wernicke, 1874/1969). Sixty percent of the aphasics in Weisenburg and McBride's (1964) classic study had vascular disease; about one-half of the patients reported by Goldstein (1948) had strokes. A broad discussion of the contribution of stroke to our knowledge of aphasia would require a general review of focal aphasic syndromes; however, a thorough general review requires a book in itself. Instead, we deal here with one part of the history of aphasia: the nature of auditory comprehension deficits. Many of the linguistic and anatomic issues to be considered when studying auditory comprehension deficits have implications for general aphasic theory. The view of aphasia secondary to stroke appears somewhat different than that emanating from the cortical stimulation literature (Ojemann, 1983) or the positron emission tomography literature (Petersen et al., 1988). Each technique has its strengths and weaknesses, and one should not expect absolute concordance across widely differing methodologies.

AUDITORY COMPREHENSION DEFICITS IN APHASIA

Wernicke (1874/1969) believed that the first temporal gyrus is a memory center for sound images. He further believed its destruction in the left hemisphere would cause a loss of memory for the sound images of the names of objects. He argued that although the sound image of a name would be lost with such a lesion, the concept associated with this image could persist with complete clarity. His argument was based on the belief that concepts are essentially related to visual and tactile images; therefore disruption of the auditory representation of words need not impair symbolic thinking or intelligence. Many theorists (Bastian, 1887; Henschen, 1926; Luria, 1964) joined Wernicke in attributing speech comprehension deficits to a disorder of the analysis of speech sounds. However, more recent studies (Blumstein et al., 1977; Varney and Benton, 1979) have found that the severity of speech comprehension deficits in patients with Wernicke's aphasia correlates only modestly with the severity of the phonemic deficit. To further understand the principles underlying auditory comprehension deficits, we studied a series of consecutive patients with ischemic cerebral infarctions of the left hemisphere. The goal of this chapter is to present an analysis of the relation between comprehension deficits and imaging findings obtained from computed tomography (CT) of the head.

HENNEPIN COUNTY RECOVERY FROM APHASIA STUDY

The Hennepin County study was initiated in 1978 and continued to 1983. Unlike most studies of aphasia, we evaluated patients longitudinally, following them beyond the acute phase of their stroke. A longitudinal study can determine the qualitative features of a patient's aphasia that change over time. Longitudinal studies can also provide prognostic indicators of recovery of function.

The Hennepin County study evaluated the anatomic correlates of aphasia from a psycholinguistic perspective with little emphasis on traditional aphasic nosology. We and many others (Schwartz, 1984; Benson, 1985; Marshall 1986; Knopman et al., 1989) have criticized the syndrome approach to the study of aphasia as a model that has serious methodologic flaws and seems to preclude integration with psycholinguistic models. As clinicians, we are aware of the motivation for the use of syndrome labels in bedside practice. However, the syndrome approach is awkward within a psycholinguistic analysis as well as within an anatomic analysis. There are several negative aspects to the use of the syndrome approach. In particular, most patients are not readily classified, and within some syndromes there is vast heterogeneity. In addition, the syndrome approach makes it much more difficult to utilize, as fully as possible, the information contained in a continuous variable such as comprehension.

While investigating the neuroanatomy of auditory comprehension deficits, we were confronted by several problems using CT scans to localize strokes. Therefore we discuss next our approach when using CT scanning for clinicoanatomic analysis.

CT Scanning

Computed tomography was performed using a Siemens Somatom II instrument at 5 months post-stroke. The slices were 4 mm thick with 2 mm of overlap. Lesion volume was determined using software supplied by Siemens. For the regional analysis, the left hemisphere was subdivided into 40 regions with explicitly defined boundaries. If the area of infarction included a particular subregion, the degree to which the region was minimally to totally destroyed was rated on a 5-point scale. [See Rubens et al. (1984), Knopman et al. (1989), and Knopman et al. (1983) for further discussion of these anatomic methods.] Lesion localization and volume were both determined by a neuroradiologist who had no knowledge of the clinical information on the patients.

Although all of our patients had CT scans performed as part of their clinical evaluation during the immediate post-stroke period, our study was unique in that all patients had scans as well at 5 months post-stroke. Therefore we were able to minimize variability in CT data that occurs when patients are studied at different points in time. Edema and mass effects can confuse the interpretation of a lesion's location and size. These effects are most evident on scans done during the acute post-stroke period, so that later scanning yields more distinct localization of the infarct. We were also able to standardize the scanning protocols across subjects, so that such factors as variations in scan angle did not introduce further variability in the CT data.

The methodology of lesion volume determination and lesion localization by CT scanning has limitations, even under the best of circumstances. Even with motor function, in which the clinicoanatomic relations are clearly defined, we have found less than perfect correlations between CT lesion localization in the corticospinal tract and weakness (Knopman and Rubens, 1986). Occasionally, it was difficult to distinguish viable and functional brain tissue from nonfunctional tissue within a zone that appeared to be hypodense radiographically. As there is known to be substantial interindividual variability of relations between major fissures (Rubens et al., 1976), a reliance on simple, stereotyped measurements can lead to incorrect localization. For instance, if a particular patient's left sylvian fissure turned upward early in its course rather than extending occipitally, as it does in most right-handers, a lesion that was actually in the infrasylvian region of the supramarginal gyrus might be incorrectly localized to the suprasylvian supramarginal gyrus. Moreover, differences between the two hemispheres in the anatomy of the posterior sylvian region (Cunningham, 1892; Geschwind and Levitsky, 1968) make problematic a reliance on landmarks in the uninfarcted hemisphere. Whenever possible, the neuroradiologic raters utilized sagittal or coronal CT scan reconstructions to check localizations in order to minimize such problems.

Our experience with this large series of aphasics showed that the effects of individual variability plus inevitable variations in scan interpretation cannot be ignored. Basso and colleagues (1985) have also noted considerable variability in localization of aphasia-producing lesions. Many of the historical claims for cerebral localization were based on only one or two cases examined at autopsy. As our studies with a consecutive series of patients showed, the interindividual variability was substantial enough to raise questions about claims based on small numbers of patients. A major advantage of a study that utilizes a large sample of patients is that both positive and negative instances of linguistic–anatomic relations are considered in the analysis.

For analysis of localization data, we used predictive accuracy as the metric. Predictive accuracy is a concept borrowed from analysis of 2×2 contingency tables in which one axis represents the outcome variable (e.g., performance on a comprehension task) and the other axis represents the predictor variable (e.g., presence of a lesion in a specific CT subregion). Predictive accuracy is a ratio that refers to the sum of the true positives plus the true negatives, divided by the total number of cases. As we have discussed elsewhere (Knopman et al., 1989), this type of analysis captures both the positive cases as well as the negative cases. Other than as case reports, the latter type of instances have tended to be ignored in most treatises on localization of aphasic deficits.

Patients

The patients studied had single left hemisphere ischemic strokes. They were all right-handed native English speakers with at least an eighth grade education. Ninety-nine individuals who were referred to us met those criteria; 54 of them returned for at least six monthly follow-up visits. We could not identify any disease factors that preselected those who remained with the study. Therefore they represented a consecutive and unbiased series of aphasics. The average age of the 54 patients who formed the study group was 61 years (range 35–71 years). Only two patients were under 50 years of age. There were 15 women and 39 men. For the degree of initial deficit, the entry criteria was the presence of aphasia at 30 days post-stroke, as defined by a score of 93 or less on the Western Aphasia Battery (Kertesz and McCabe, 1977).

Language Assessment

The patients were tested monthly for at least the first 6 months post-stroke. Because of the limitations of the syndrome approach, we have adopted a clinical approach to patients with aphasia that we believe is consistent with a psycholinguistic formulation. Rather than considering "comprehension" as a single entity that was either normal or abnormal, we chose to focus on definable subunits, such as phoneme identification, word comprehension, and sentence comprehension. This function by function approach to aphasia was not so much a radical departure as it was simply a restructuring of our thinking about the patients' clinical deficits. Numerous studies have shown that deficits in auditory comprehension do not distinguish between syndromes (Poeck et al., 1972; Riedel, 1981). In fact, the classic subtypes of aphasia are defined mainly on the basis of the patient's verbal output. It therefore seemed reasonable to focus on auditory comprehension deficits independently of speech production deficits, again a departure from the syndrome approach. The theme of the following discussion centers on the question: "What are the anatomic correlates of linguistically defined components of auditory comprehension?"

RESULTS AND DISCUSSION

Our interpretation of the representation of the function of language comprehension in the left hemisphere was most consistent with a multifocal localization of the lexicon, or access to it, in the perisylvian cerebral cortex. The data also suggested that the complex processing of multiword expressions was localized in a multifocal fashion.

Single Word Comprehension

Selnes and colleagues (1984) have reported on single word comprehension. Deficits in the comprehension of single words were most closely related to the amount of left hemisphere perisylvian brain tissue destroyed and were less dependent on the specific localization of the lesion within the perisylvian zone. We used the Word Discrimination subtest of the Boston Diagnostic Aphasia Examination (BDAE) (Goodglass and Kaplan, 1972) as the measure of word comprehension. There were 36 items from six semantic categories: actions, objects, letters, forms, numbers, and colors. The Word Picture Matching subtest of the BDAE was used for the assessment of reading comprehension of single words. The auditory comprehension of single words and the reading comprehension of single words were highly correlated (*r* .93). Thus deficits in word comprehension were supramodal in nature in our group of aphasics.

The phoneme discrimination test was modeled after that described by Blumstein et al. (1977). Normal performance on this test was defined by an independent group of normal age-matched controls (Rubens et al., unpublished observations). The lower end of the normal range was 95% correct on the phoneme discrimination test. We found that word comprehension deficits were not specifically related to deficits in phoneme discrimination (Table 12–1). Of the 36 patients who had complete testing at 6 months post-stroke, only 13 had deficits in phoneme discrimination. In 6 of these 13, single word comprehension was normal. Among the other seven with both phoneme discrimination deficits and word comprehension deficits, five had impaired word reading as well. In these five patients, the combination of impaired reading and impaired auditory word comprehension suggested that the phoneme discrimination deficits were not the cause of the word comprehension deficits. At most, then, in only 2 of 13 could a case be made that phoneme discrimination deficits might have been the cause of the word comprehension deficits. Furthermore, of the 23 patients with normal phoneme discrimination, three had deficits in single word comprehension. It was not possible to define an anatomic basis for deficits in phoneme discrimination in our patient sample. There is, of course, ample evidence from patients with the syndrome of pure word deafness that critically situated lesions deep in the left temporal lobe may leave hearing relatively intact but impair the ability to comprehend speech (Kanshepolsky et al., 1973; Michel and Peronnet, 1980).

Therefore the two functions, word comprehension and phoneme discrimination, appeared easily dissociable. When deficits in the comprehension of single words were present in the aphasic patients, the deficits probably reflected impaired semantic access or analysis rather than deficits in phonologic analysis. We concluded that

Table 12–1 Relation Between Phoneme Discrimination and Auditory Word Comprehension

	Single Word Comprehension	
Phoneme Discrimination Performance	Impaired	Normal
Impaired	7	6
Normal	3	20

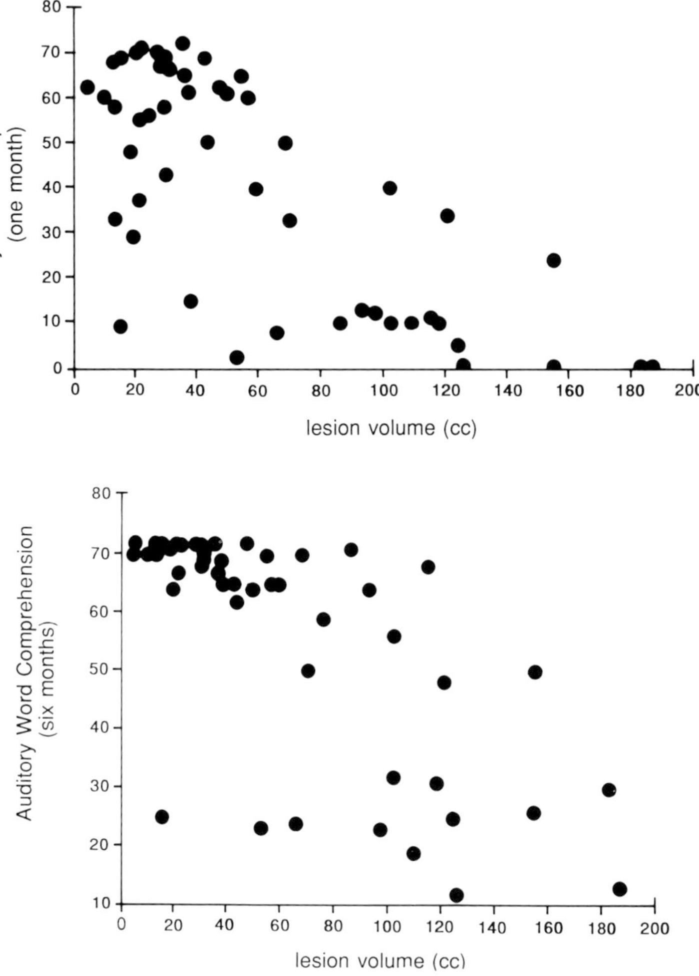

Figure 12–1 Lesion volume versus scores on single word comprehension test at (A) 1 month post-stroke and (B) 6 months post-stroke.

access to the meaning of words, rather than phonemic hearing, was the predominant function of the left perisylvian region. The function of accessing meaning appears to occur throughout this zone. The widespread distribution of semantic analysis, compared to phonemic analysis, appears logical given that the number of lexical items far exceeds the number of phonemes in any language. We disagree with Luria (1964) on the relative importance of phonological processing. Analyses have suggested that his procedures to test phoneme identification actually utilized semantic properties of words (Blumstein et al., 1977), exposing the basis of his mistaken belief.

By 6 months post-stroke there was a strong correlation (r — .75) between lesion volume and severity of deficits in single word comprehension (Figures 12–1B and 12–2). An infarction whose volume was more than 100 cc was almost invariably associated with a profound deficit. The one exception was a patient whose lesion included the distribution of the anterior cerebral artery; the lesion volume estimate

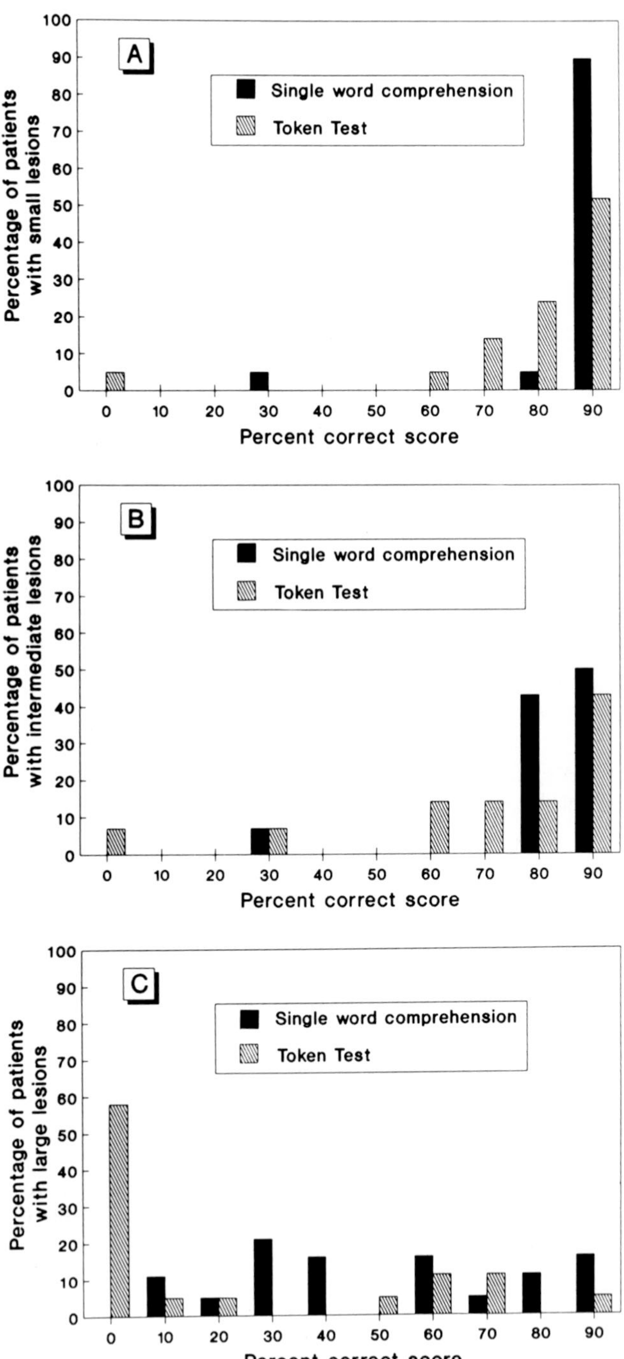

Figure 12–2 Distributions of scores on single word comprehension and Token Test for patients with (A) small lesions, $N = 21$ (volumes ≤ 30 cc); (B) intermediate size lesions, $N = 14$ (volumes 31–60 cc); and (C) large lesions, $N = 19$ (volumes ≥ 60 cc).

included a considerable region outside of the perisylvian zone. For patients with lesions between 60 and 100 cc, there was some variability. With lesions of less than 60 cc, 5 of 35 patients failed to score in the normal range on single word comprehension. Only two of these five were dramatically out of the normal range. The two "exception" patients with profound deficits and small lesions by volume may have been examples of a methodologic deficiency in CT analysis. Lesions in the frontoparietal white matter may render large areas of overlying cortex nonfunctional. Even though the cortical areas remained normal radiographically, their function might have been grossly impaired. An alternative hypothesis that would account for these exceptional patients would be that their lesions were critically placed within some key set of pathways. However, because other patients had lesions in similar locations and were not as impaired, we believed that it was unlikely that some critical region was included in the zone of infarction in these exceptional patients. Instead, the picture that emerged from the pattern seen in the vast majority of the patients was that performance on word comprehension was related to the amount of infarcted perisylvian brain tissue. It must be emphasized that the effect of lesion volume was independent of the patients' fluency or their syndrome classification.

Analysis of regional localization of single word comprehension deficits did not demonstrate any critical region which, if lesioned, was invariably associated with normal performance. Because patients with large lesions could potentially confound the discovery of a regional effect, we also performed an analysis of correlations between deficits in single word comprehension and regional involvement using only patients with lesions of less than 60 cc. Again, lesions in no specific region appeared related to the deficit in word comprehension.

On the basis of these two analyses, regional correlations and lesion volume correlations, we concluded that the lexicon, or access to the lexicon, was represented in a diffuse or multifocal fashion in the perisylvian region. A similar conclusion suggested itself from the analysis of confrontation naming (Knopman et al., 1984) even though naming performance is confounded by potential deficits limited to motor output. Positron emission tomographic findings have demonstrated that lexical access may involve multiple discrete regions (Petersen et al., 1988). Because there are indeed multiple processes involved in the accessing of meaning, the label "multifocal" may be more accurate than "diffuse." From a theoretical point of view, this simple relation seemed consistent with emerging models of distributed memory (McClelland and Rumelhart, 1985). Although there are well described patients with deficits in comprehension limited to certain semantic classes (Goodglass et al., 1966), our experience with a consecutive series of aphasics suggests that the typical pattern was one of diffuse representation of the lexicon. The existence of a word frequency effect in aphasics (Tweedy and Schulman, 1982) was also compatible with the principle of diffuse localization of access to the lexicon. One would expect that common words would be more strongly represented, and therefore impairment in their comprehension would be less vulnerable to lesions of less than 60 to 100 cc.

Sentence Comprehension

Selnes and colleagues (1983b) have studied sentence comprehension. In patients with normal or near-normal comprehension of single words, deficits in comprehension of sentence-length material were even more sensitive to the effects of increasing lesion volume but also showed some regional specificity to the posterosuperior temporal lobe.

The Token Test (DeRenzi and Vignolo, 1962) was the primary instrument used to assess sentence comprehension. This widely used test required the subjects to point to a series of tokens of different colors and shapes. In the first five parts of the Token Test, the spoken commands varied in length and complexity from "Point to a square" to "Point to the red square and the large blue circle." In the final section of the test, the commands also involved some degree of syntactic complexity. Based on our normal controls, a score of 90% or greater correct was considered to be in the normal range.[1]

A ten-item written version of the final section of the Token Test was also given. The correlation between the oral and written versions was only moderately high (*r* .63) in the aphasics. Part of this lack of correlation might have been due to ceiling effects in the reading task. Nonetheless, patients did somewhat better on written sentence comprehension than on oral sentence comprehension. Because there was a modality specificity to sentence comprehension in our patients, the subsequent discussion should be considered relevant to spoken sentence comprehension and not necessarily applicable to written sentence comprehension. With written sentences, the additional time available to study the sentence may be a great advantage to an aphasic.

For patients with lesion volumes in any particular range (small, medium or large), the distribution of patients' scores on the Token Test was shifted downward compared to the distribution for single word comprehension (Figure12–2). Among patients with lesion volumes of less than 60 cc, 95% had scores in the normal or near-normal range on single word comprehension, whereas only 43% also had normal Token Test performance. Among patients with lesions larger than 60 cc, only 1 of 19 scored in the normal range on the Token Test, whereas five had normal or near-normal single word comprehension. Therefore normal or near-normal performance on the test of single word comprehension did not predict success on sentence comprehension. Normal word comprehension was necessary for normal sentence comprehension but was not sufficient.

Only the 33 patients with normal or near-normal single word comprehension and lesion volumes less than 60 cc were considered for analysis of the regional localization of sentence comprehension deficits. Indeed, of patients with impaired single word comprehension, all had severe deficits on sentence comprehension. Furthermore, by eliminating five patients with the largest lesions, among those with normal single word comprehension, we hoped to enhance the specificity of the regional analyses. Four of the five had moderate to severe deficits on the Token Test, and their inclusion could have slanted the conclusions toward more widespread localization of the Token Test deficits.

It has been argued that the posterior temporal lobe plays a critical role in auditory comprehension (Wernicke, 1874/1969; Luria, 1964). Our previous report (Selnes et al., 1983b) of performance on the Token Test on a subsample of the patients described here supported that view. However, when the current, larger sample of patients was considered, the results were less clear-cut. Consider the patients with lesions of less than 60 cc who had normal or almost normal single word comprehension. Three patients with posterior infrasylvian lesions (including the two subregions from our 40-region parcellation of the left hemisphere, the "posterior superior temporal" and the "infrasylvian supramarginal gyrus" subregions) had Token Test scores over 90%. Furthermore, there were seven patients without posterosuperior temporal lesions who had impairment on the Token Test. The predictive accuracy of a lesion in the posterosuperior temporal or infrasylvian supramarginal subregions for a deficit on the Token Test was only 70% when the cutting score was 90% correct. If a deficit was instead defined less stringently as a score of 80% correct or less, the predictive accuracy rose to 79%. Although impairment in sentence comprehension appeared to be less strongly correlated with posterior infrasylvian lesions than we previously thought, no other regions achieved as high a predictive accuracy.

One criticism of our interpretation of the relation between lesion characteristics and sentence comprehension was that the Token Test confounds deficits related to sentence length with deficits specific to syntactic (e.g., word order, relational expressions) demands. Patients who had only an auditory verbal short-term memory deficit but no comprehension deficit might have been penalized on the latter parts of the test. Therefore we also administered a test that specifically focused on processing of syntactically complex material in which sentence length was controlled.

The type of syntactically complex material in the Receptive Syntax Test (Selnes et al., 1983a) was a sentence/picture verification task in which a series of 42 subject-object sentences were presented in active, passive, or negative forms and in which the two nouns were reversible. That is, the meaning of the sentence could be changed by reversing the order of the two noun phrases but without making the sentences semantically anomalous. An equal number of nonreversible sentences that used some of the same nouns but different verbs served as control material (Table 12–2). A series of four pictures (target and three foils) accompanied each sentence. For the

Table 12–2 Receptive Syntax Test: Nonreversible Sentences

Base sentences

Reversible

The man is pushing the boy.
The dog is chasing the cat.
The car is following the truck.

Nonreversible

The boy is hitting the ball.
The nurse is examining the child.
The dog is eating the bone.

Derivative syntactically complex sentences for a base nonreversible sentence (examples of 5 of the 12 sentences)

The young nurse is examining the child.
The young nurse is examining the small child.
The nurse isn't examining the child.
The child is being examined by the nurse.

Derivative syntactically complex sentences for a base reversible sentence (examples)

The cat is chasing the black dog.
The cat isn't chasing the dog.
The cat is being chased by the dog.
The dog is being chased by the cat.
The dog that is chasing the cat is black.

reversible sentences, one foil was always the reverse of the correct choice; the other foils were related to the choice of the correct adjective. The patients were instructed to point to the correct picture.

The 36 normal controls (mean age 53 years) scored a mean of 97% correct (range 81–100%) on the nonreversible sentences and 97% correct (range 86–100%) on the reversible sentences. For the subgroup of normals over age 65 years, the means for both types of sentence were somewhat lower, at 94% correct. The wide range of performance among the normal controls made it somewhat difficult to assign a meaningful cutoff score for normal performance among the aphasics. With that caveat in mind, we defined the normal range by a score of 93% correct or better (38 correct) on the nonreversible sentences, and 83% correct or better (35 correct) on the reversible sentences.[2] Performance by the aphasics on the nonreversible sentences was highly correlated with performance on the Token Test (*r* .94); in only a few cases did large discrepancies arise. These results suggest that poor performance by aphasics on the Token Test was generally due to syntactic, rather than mnestic, demands.

Although few of our normal controls had any difficulty with the reversible sentences, the specificity of the deficits in comprehension of reversible sentences for aphasia must be questioned. Some of these changes may have been age-related (Feier and Gerstman, 1980). Perhaps the nonspecific effects of perseveration, impulsiveness, or slight impairment of attentional focusing were sufficient to account for these deficits. Further work with other brain-damaged patients is necessary before we can be certain that the results we and others have seen with syntactically complex sentence comprehension are specific to aphasia. Other studies involving patients with right hemisphere lesions have suggested that such lesions might also be associated with deficits in some aspects of linguistic processing. Performance on the Token Test itself (Swisher and Sarno, 1969), problem solving (Caramazza et al., 1976), the comprehension of humorous material (Wapner et al., 1981), and the syntactic reassign-

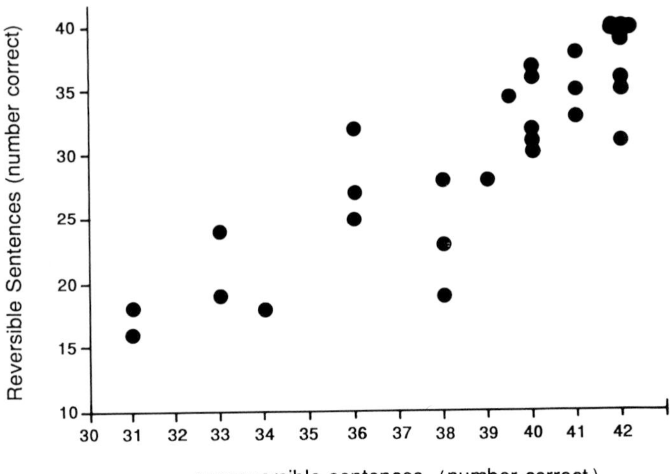

Figure 12–3 Scores on the Receptive Syntax Test for nonreversible and reversible sentences. Only subjects with normal single word comprehension and scores on the nonreversible sentences over 75% correct were included.

ment of words in sentences (Schneiderman and Saddy, 1988) were among the tasks where deficits were identified in patients with right hemisphere damage.

At 6 months post-stroke there were 20 patients who scored in the normal range on nonreversible sentences. All had lesion volumes of less than 60 cc. Of these 20 patients, 11 performed in the normal range[2] on the reversible sentences. The reversible sentences were more difficult than the nonreversible ones for these aphasics, but perhaps only quantitatively rather than qualitatively. As performance dropped in comprehension of the nonreversible sentences, performance on the reversible sentences dropped even more precipitously (Figure 12–3). Among the patients who scored more than 96% correct on the nonreversible sentences, most did well on the

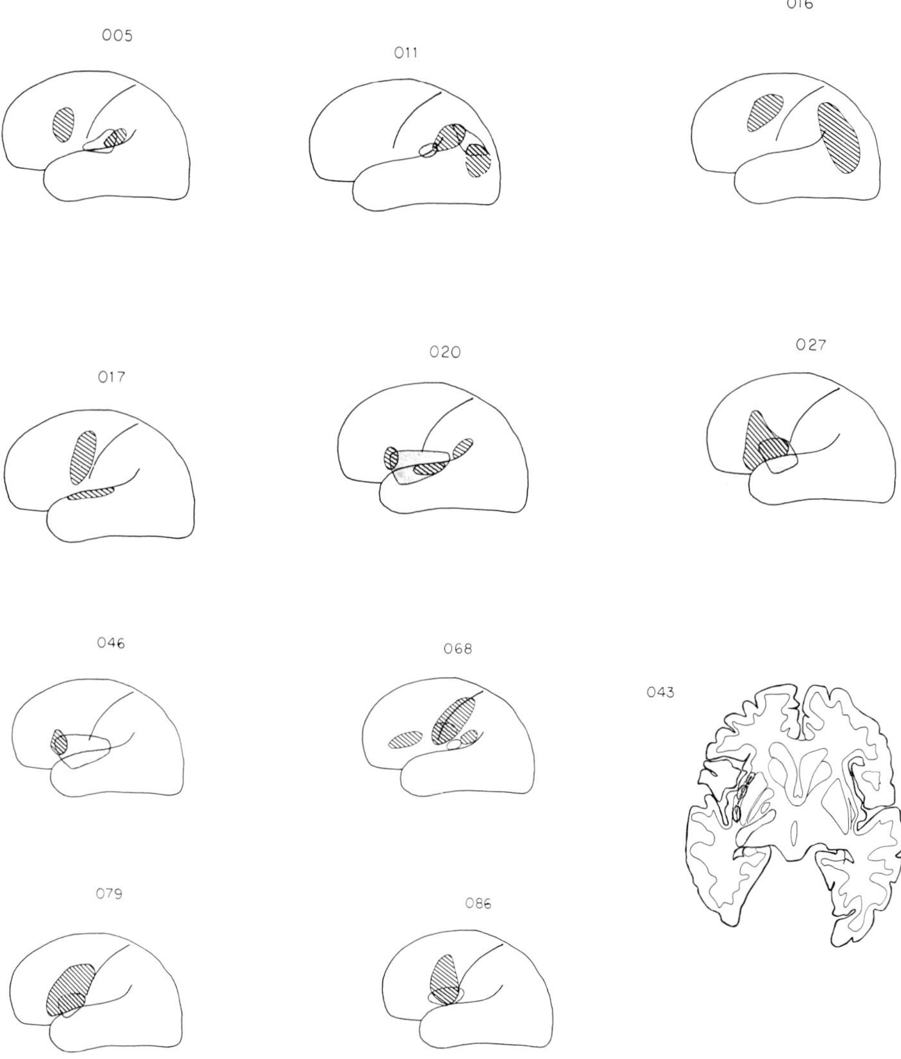

Figure 12–4 Approximate lesion location of patients with normal performance on reversible sentences.

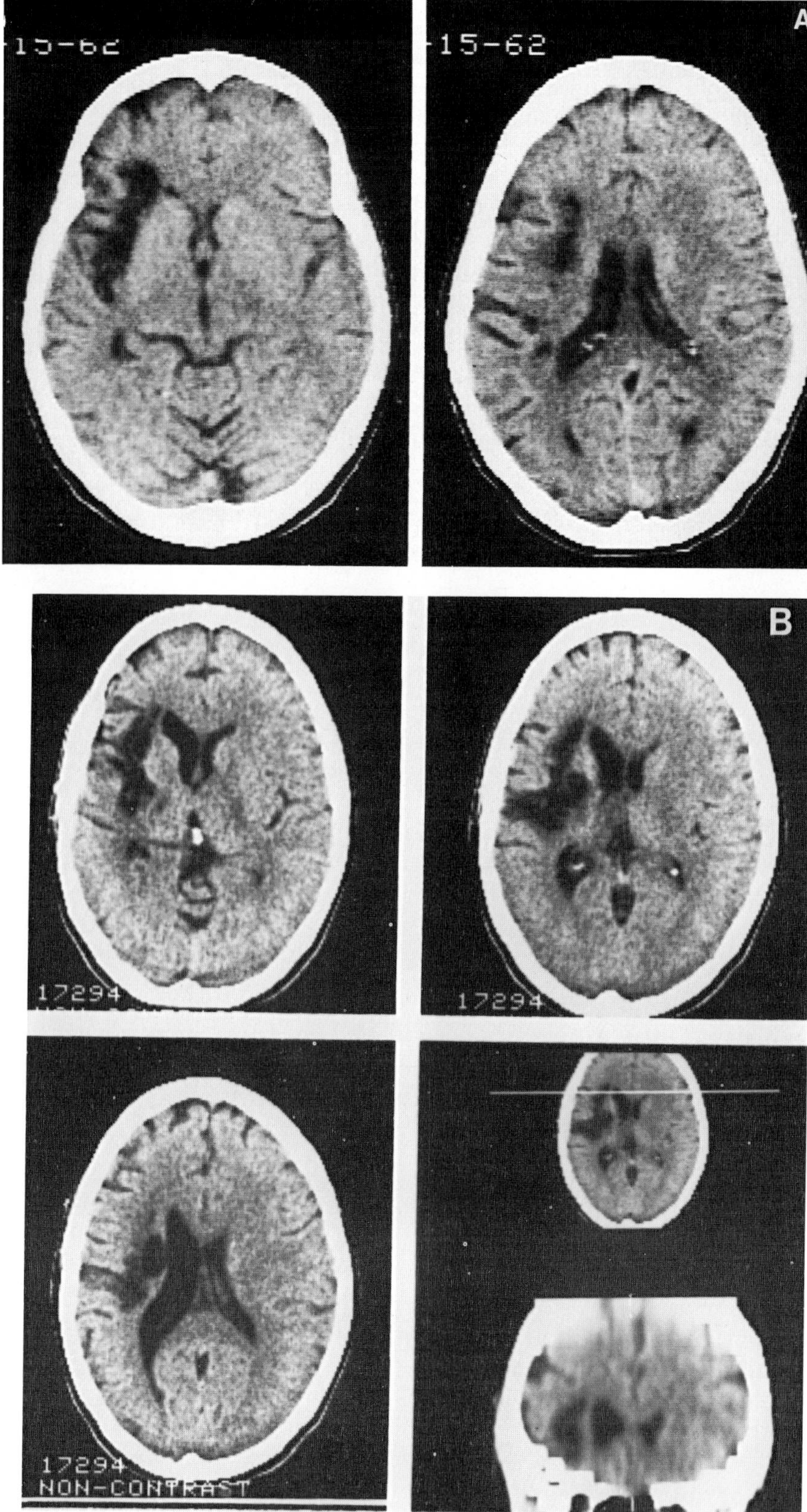
A
15-62
15-62
B
17294
17294
17294
NON-CONTRAST

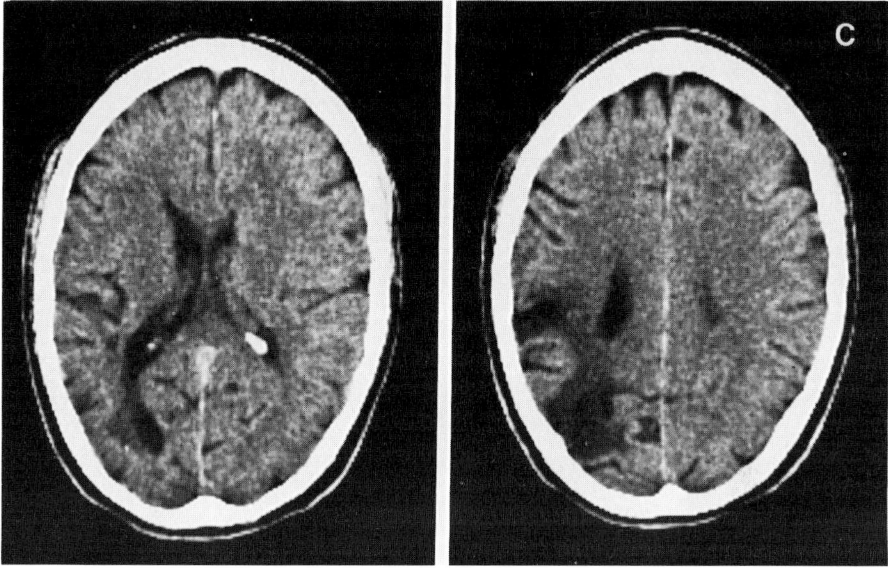

Figure 12–5 CT scans of patients with normal performance on the reversible sentences of the Receptive Syntax Test. (A) Patient 046. (B) Patient 020. (C) Patient 011.

reversible sentence comprehension. However, in the patients who scored less than 96% correct on the nonreversible sentences, only a few achieved a normal score on the reversible sentences. Among almost all of the patients scoring below 92% correct on the nonreversible sentences, performance on the reversible sentences was dramatically lower.

Of the patients with normal range performance on the reversible sentences, all but one had small *supra*sylvian lesions (Figures 12–4 and 12–5). The one exception

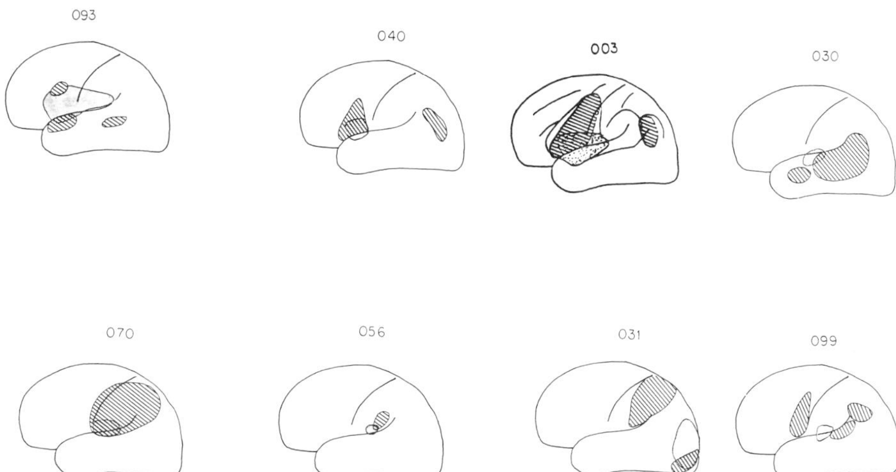

Figure 12–6 Approximate lesion locations in eight of the nine patients with impaired performance on reversible sentences but normal nonreversible sentence comprehension. The ninth patient is shown in Figure 7B.

had a lesion in the posterosuperior temporal region; it was rather small and of questionable significance. It was of note that several patients with circumscribed inferior frontal lesions (patients 027, 046, and 079) had normal range performance. Figure 12–5 shows frontal opercular and supramarginal lesions that did not interfere with successful comprehension of the complex sentences.

Three of the nine patients (Figures 12–6 and 12–7A) with definite impairment on comprehension of the reversible sentences had clear-cut lesions in the posterior temporal region. Four had lesions in the insular cortex and putamen with extension frontally, and two had lesions restricted to the supramarginal gyrus (Figures 12–6 and 12–7B). Thus there was considerable individual variability in the effects of nontemporal lobe lesions on the comprehension of syntactically complex sentences. Patients with inferior frontal lesions and impaired comprehension of reversible sentences tended to have lesions with deeper insular, putamenal, or subcortical white

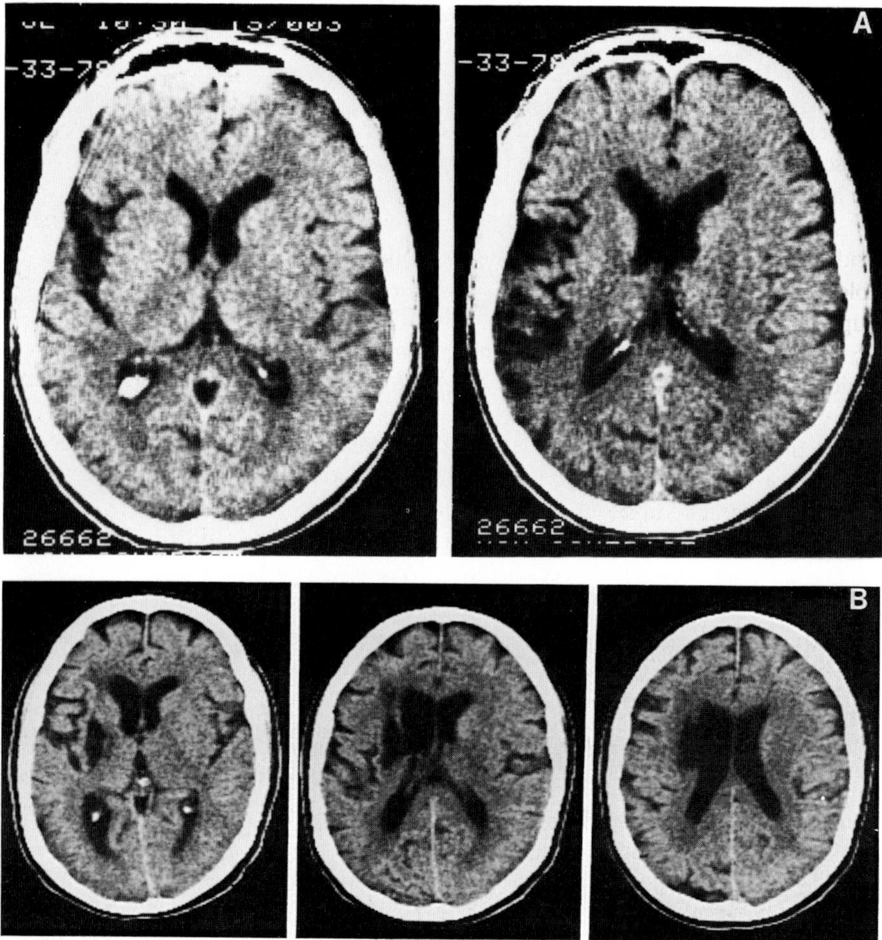

Figure 12–7 CT scans showing three lesion locations associated with impaired performance on reversible sentences but normal performance on nonreversible sentences. (A) Patient 099. (B) Patient 058.

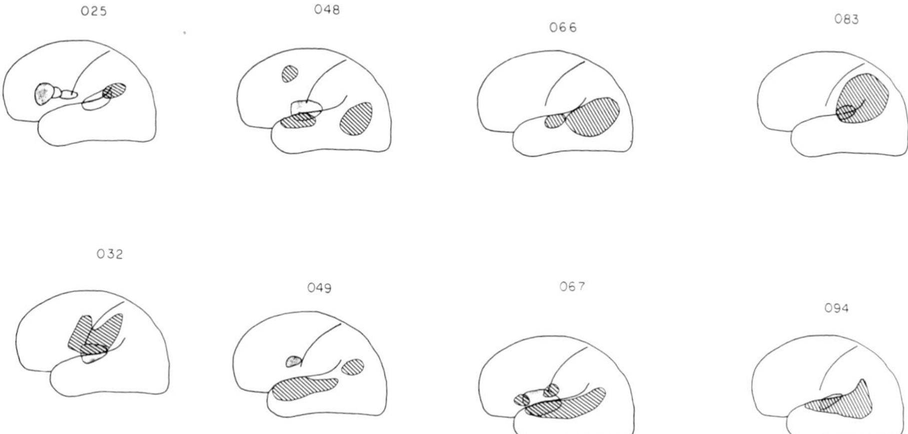

Figure 12–8 Approximate lesion locations in patients with impaired performance on both reversible and nonreversible sentences in the presence of normal single word comprehension.

matter involvement than unimpaired patients with inferior frontal lesions. However, these anatomic differences were often subtle, as can be seen by comparing patients 20 and 46 in Figure 12–5 with patient 58 in Figure 12–7B.

Among patients who were mildly to moderately impaired (scoring between 75 and 92% correct) on the nonreversible sentences (all of whom did poorly on reversible sentences), there were a number with posterior temporal lesions, one with a supramarginal lesion, and one with a centrally placed lesion (Figures 12–8 and 12–9). Three of these patients were nonfluent and had large inferior frontal opercular lesions that extended into underlying subcortical regions. The rest of the patients in this group were fluent.

Deficits in the processing of syntactically complex material therefore occurred with lesions in a variety of locations. The boundaries of the critical region were not entirely clear. The posterosuperior temporal regions, supramarginal gyrus, central operculum, insular regions, and deep structures such as the putamen appeared to be

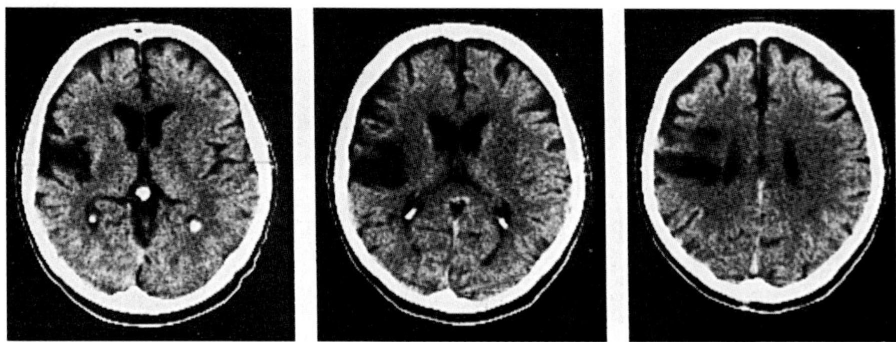

Figure 12–9 CT scan of patient 032, who had markedly impaired performance on reversible sentences and nearly normal performance on nonreversible sentences.

part of the functional system involved in the comprehension of complex sentences. Whether the inferior frontal region should be included was unresolved, but it appeared that discrete lesions in the inferior frontal cortex were more likely *not* to impair sentence comprehension. In suggesting that a large part of the temporal and parietal lobes were involved, our assessment was similar to Luria's (1964) that the localization of "complex simultaneous and spatial synthesis" was in the temporo-parietal association areas.

The relation between lesions of the posterior temporal lobe and deficits in sentence comprehension may be accounted for, in part, by an auditory/verbal short-term memory deficit, a mechanism suggested by the association of lesions in the posterosuperior temporal region with sentence repetition deficits (Selnes et al., 1985). The latter association was so robust that we believe that auditory verbal short-term memory deficits might well explain some deficits in complex sentence processing (Caramazza et al., 1981). If subvocal repetition is an important component of the comprehension of syntactically complex sentences, its disruption could lead to impaired sentence comprehension, which may be one function that can be localized to the posterior temporal lobe. On the other hand, of the nine patients with poor performance (below 80% correct) on reversible sentence comprehension but normal nonreversible sentence comprehension, four had scores in the normal range on sentence repetition. The converse also occurred: One patient with near-normal performance on the reversible sentences had a severe repetition deficit. Therefore there must have been mechanisms other than failure of auditory verbal short-term memory by which sentence comprehension failed.

Complex sentence comprehension must involve the simultaneous semantic processing of multiword expressions. Components of this activity that have been shown to be impaired in aphasia include semantic processing of the meaning of "closed class" words (Bradley et al., 1980), the assignment of thematic roles to nouns (Caplan and Futter, 1986), and appreciation of the spatial relations between words (Luria, 1964). There are other definable components as well. Whether these independent components operate in parallel or in series, the integrity of the individual cognitive activities is critical to achieving the successful end-product, correct sentence comprehension. Because small lesions in a variety of perisylvian regions were capable of producing deficits in the comprehension of syntactically complex material, these various activities must be represented in multiple locations in the perisylvian region. Susceptibility to failure in patients with left hemisphere lesions would be high because competent performance requires that most or all the brain regions supporting the several components of sentence comprehension be intact.

The lack of clear distinctions, on the basis of lesion volume and lesion location, between patients with normal performance and those with impaired performance on complex sentences might have reflected methodologic flaws in measurement or definition of lesion boundaries. Another possibility was that there may have been considerable individual variability in the specific localization of this function (Caplan, personal communication, 1987). The determinants of localization of language functions across individuals could be environmental or genetic. By this hypothesis, mere chance might determine if a lesion of given size and location produces a deficit in a particular individual. Either explanation—multiple components or individual variability—seems plausible, and our data do not allow us to choose one over the other. They are not mutually exclusive, so both could be operative.

Comprehension Deficits During the Early Post-Stroke Period

All of the above conclusions concerning the relations between deficits in comprehension and lesion configuration were based on analyses of language performance 6 months post-stroke. However, the same conclusions may be drawn from analysis of data obtained at 1 month post-stroke. The relation between lesion volume and comprehension was even more striking at the earlier time after onset.

At 1 month, lesion volume correlated (−.72) with scores on the Word Discrimination Subtest (Figure 12–1A). The effect of lesion volume on word comprehension was greater than any effects specific to one region (Selnes et al., 1984; Knopman et al., 1989). Furthermore, the effects of lesion volume on recovery seemed somewhat greater than the effects of the initial severity of the deficits. If one inspects the scattergrams of lesion volume and word comprehension (Figure 12–1), patients with worse deficits at 1 month than at 6 months post-stroke were more common among those with small lesions. Only 37% of patients with lesions less than 60 cc had scores in the normal range for word comprehension at 1 month, compared to more than 90% at 6 months. With lesions larger than 60 cc in volume, all patients had severe deficits at 1 month post-stroke, and only 15% recovered to the normal range by 6 months. Large lesions thus carried a much worse prognosis than lesions less than 60 cc.

A similar effect was seen for sentence comprehension (Selnes et al., 1983b; Knopman et al., 1989). Only three patients (5%) of the entire group scored in the normal range on the Token Test at 1 month post-stroke, compared to 33% at 6 months. Even if the analysis was restricted to patients scoring in the normal range on single word comprehension at these two time points, a smaller portion of patients achieved normal range scores at 1 month than at 6 months post-stroke. The same findings were evident in the Receptive Syntax Test at 1 month post-stroke. For patients with lesions larger than 60 cc, severe impairment on the Token Test was the rule at 1 month post-stroke, and recovery into the normal range was unlikely, occurring in only 1 of 19 patients by 6 months. Only two others managed to achieve scores in the mildly impaired range (75–80% correct); the remainder were left with severe deficits. Therefore, despite the consistently poor performance on sentence comprehension across all patients at 1 month post-stroke, it was only those with lesions less than 60 cc who showed later recovery of sentence comprehension.

One possible mechanism of recovery of auditory comprehension was that reversibly dysfunctional areas gradually regained normal activity. At 1 month post-stroke, large areas of brain were probably impaired owing to mass effect, recovery from ischemia, and possibly transsynaptic depression (Metter et al., 1981). Recovery may have occurred as these effects ameliorated. An alternative mechanism of recovery, which might have occurred simultaneously, was that over the first several months post-stroke nonlesioned areas assumed functions they had not previously supported.

Our data suggest that both mechanisms may be operative. If one considers either single word or sentence length comprehension deficits, there were clear lesion volume thresholds over which there were virtually no examples of individuals who recovered into the normal range. Recovery of normal or near-normal sentence comprehension critically depended on left perisylvian cortex; and if the lesions damaged a sufficient amount of the region, the return of normal function was precluded. Nonetheless, in most of the patients with large perisylvian lesions, even though virtually none recovered into the normal range, some recovery of single word comprehension did occur. The partial recovery offered support for the contention that there exists an accessible lexicon in the right hemisphere, as was suggested by the findings of Zaidel (1976). In addition, among less severely affected patients, the possibility remained that some assumption of function by the right hemisphere facilitated recovery. Serial xenon 133 cerebral blood flow studies (see Chapter 3) in our patients provided support for this contention (Knopman et al., 1984). Other serial studies of patients with multiple lesions, first in the left and then in the right hemisphere, also suggest that the right hemisphere may assume some comprehension functions (Lee et al., 1984).

Involvement of Other Brain Regions in Auditory Comprehension

Because of the nature of our study, certain types of brain lesion were not well represented. In particular, we had no examples of patients with aphasia due to thalamic lesions (Gorelick et al., 1984). Such lesions can lead to specific linguistic deficits, perhaps because thalamic function is integrally related to cortical function. Our emphasis in this chapter on the perisylvian cortex was simply based on the patients who entered our study.

Our findings of the pivotal role of lesion volume in auditory comprehension deficits, be they in the setting of single word or multiword comprehension failure, suggested that the neural substrates of single word comprehension and sentence comprehension were co-localized and relied on multiple neural systems throughout the perisylvian region. The two functions differed in their sensitivity to lesion volume. Single word comprehension was more resistant to lesions of the perisylvian core, whereas sentence comprehension was disrupted even with small lesions. In the only other study of which we are aware that measured lesion volume in aphasics, Naeser et al., (1981) also noted that aphasia severity, within which word and sentence comprehension would clearly be subsumed, was closely related to lesion volume.

Analysis of the changes in deficit–lesion relations over the course of recovery also suggested that the critical region for both word and sentence comprehension was largely but not completely confined to the perisylvian core. Although some recovery of word comprehension occurred in patients with virtually complete perisylvian destruction, suggesting support for the function elsewhere, the performance of these patients was markedly deficient.

The exact manner in which the lexicon and the rules that govern analysis of multiword expression are realized in the neurons of the perisylvian region is not known. We might speculate that specific linguistic functions can be localized to a series of cortical bands located throughout the perisylvian cortex in a fashion comparable to that of the distribution of visual functions in the visual association areas (Livingstone and Hubel, 1988). The neurophysiologic definition of the components of language comprehension is just beginning to occur (Petersen et al., 1988) at the single word level. Much more work needs to be done in patients with brain lesions as well as in normal subjects studied with physiologic techniques.

ACKNOWLEDGMENTS

The authors are deeply indebted to our colleagues in the Hennepin County Recovery from Aphasia project, Drs. Gail Risse, Nancy Niccum, and Loren Jordan. This work was supported by NINCDS N01-2378.

NOTES

1. The definition of "normal" for Token Test scores in this chapter is slightly lower than we have used elsewhere (Knopman et al., 1989) and differs from the definition we used in our original publication on these results (Selnes et al., 1983b). However, the conclusions we have drawn are virtually independent of exactly where the cutpoint for normal is placed.
2. In a prior publication (Knopman et al., 1989) a slightly more stringent definition of normal performance on reversible sentences was used. As with the Token Test scores, this slight difference did not alter the conclusions.

REFERENCES

Basso, A., Lecours, A.R., Moraschinis, S., and Vanier, M. (1985). Anatomoclinic correlations of the aphasias as defined through computerized tomography: exceptions. *Brain Lang.*, **26,** 201–229.

Bastian, H.C. (1887). On different kinds of aphasia with special reference to their classification and ultimate pathology. *Br. Med. J.*, **2,** 931–936.

Benson, D.F. (1985). Aphasia. In: K.M. Heilman and E. Valenstein, eds., *Clinical Neuropsychology*, 2nd ed., pp. 17–47. New York: Oxford University Press.

Blumstein, S.E., Baker, E., and Goodglass, H. (1977). Phonological factors in auditory comprehension in aphasia. *Neuropsychologia*, **15,** 19–30.

Bradley, D.C., Garrett, M.F., and Zuriff, E.B. (1980). Syntactic deficits in Broca's aphasia. In: D. Caplan, ed., *Biological Studies of Mental Processes*, pp. 269–286. Cambridge, MA: MIT Press.

Caplan, D., and Futter, C. (1986). Assignment of thematic roles to nouns in sentence comprehension by an agrammatic patient. *Brain Lang.*, **27,** 117–134.

Caramazza, A., Gordon, J., Zurif, E.B., and DeLuca, D. (1976). Right-hemispheric damage and verbal problem solving behavior. *Brain Lang.*, **3,** 41–46.

Caramazza, A., Berndt, R.S., Basili, A.G., and Koller, J.J. (1981). Syntactic processing deficits in aphasia. *Cortex*, **17,** 333–348.

Cunningham, D.F. (1892). *Contribution to the Surface Anatomy of the Cerebral Hemispheres.* Dublin: Royal Irish Academy.

DeRenzi, E., and Vignolo, L.A. (1962). The Token Test: a sensitive test to detect receptive disturbances in aphasics. *Brain*, **85,** 665–678.

Feier, C.D., and Gerstman, L.J. (1980). Sentence comprehension abilities throughout the adult life span. *J. Gerontol.*, **35,** 722–728.

Geschwind, N., and Levitsky, W. (1968). Left-right asymmetries in temporal speech region. *Science*, **161,** 186–187.

Goldstein, K. (1948). *Language and Language Disturbances.* New York: Grune & Stratton.

Goodglass, H., and Kaplan, E. (1972). *The Assessment of Aphasia and Related Disorders.* Philadelphia: Lea & Febiger.

Goodglass, H., Klein, B., Carey, P., and Jones, K. (1966). Specific semantic word categories in aphasia. *Cortex,* **2,** 74–89.

Gorelick, P.B., Hier, D.B., Benevento, L., Levitt, S., and Tan, W. (1984). Aphasia after left thalamic infarction. *Arch. Neurol.,* **41,** 1296–1298.

Henschen, S.E. (1926). On the function of the right hemisphere of the brain in relation to the left in speech, music and calculation. *Brain,* **49,** 110–123.

Kanshepolsky, J., Kelley, J.J., and Waggener, J.D. (1973). A cortical auditory disorder. *Neurology,* **23,** 699–705.

Kertesz, A., and McCabe, P. (1977). Recovery patterns and prognosis in aphasia. *Brain,* **100,** 1–18.

Knopman, D.S., and Rubens, A.B. (1986). The validity of computed tomographic scan findings for the localization of cerebral functions. *Arch. Neurol.,* **43,** 328–332.

Knopman, D.S., Selnes, O.A., Niccum, N., Rubens, A.B., Yock, D., and Larson, D. (1983). A longitudinal study of speech fluency in aphasia: CT correlates of recovery and persistent nonfluency. *Neurology,* **33,** 1170–1178.

Knopman, D.S., Rubens, A.B., Selnes, O.A., Klassen, A.C., and Meyer, M.W. (1984). Mechanisms of recovery from aphasia: evidence from serial xenon 133 cerebral blood flow studies. *Ann. Neurol.,* **15,** 530–535.

Knopman, D.S., Selnes, O.A., Niccum, N., and Rubens, A.B. (1984). Recovery of naming in aphasia: relationship to fluency, comprehension, and CT findings. *Neurology,* **34,** 1461–1470.

Knopman, D.S., Selnes, O.A., and Rubens, A.B. (1989). CT scanning and new perspectives in aphasia. In: E. Bigler, Y.A. Yeo, and E. Turkheimer, eds., *Brain Imaging and Neuropsychology,* pp. 139–159. New York: Plenum Press.

Lee, H., Nakada, T., Deal, J.L., Lin, S., and Kwee, I.L. (1984). Transfer of language dominance. *Ann. Neurol.,* **15,** 304–307.

Livingston, M., and Hubel, D. (1988). Segregation of form, color, movement and depth: anatomy, physiology and perception. *Science,* **240,** 740–749.

Luria, A.R. (1964). Factors and forms of aphasia. In: A.V.S. DeReuck and A.M. O'Connor, eds., *Ciba Foundation Symposium, Disorders of Language,* pp. 143–161. Boston: Little, Brown.

Marshall, J.C. (1986). The description and interpretation of aphasic language disorder. *Neuropsychologia,* **24,** 5–24.

McClelland, J.L., and Rumelhart, D.E. (1985). Distributed memory and the representation of general and specific information. *J. Exp. Psychol.,* **114,** 159–188.

Metter, E.J., Wasterlain, C.G., Kuhl, D.E., Hanson, W.R., and Phelps, M.E. (1981). FDG positron emission computed tomography in a study of aphasia. *Ann. Neurol.,* **10,** 173–183.

Michel, F., and Peronnet, F. (1980). A case of cortical deafness: clinical and electrophysiological data. *Brain Lang.,* **10,** 367–377.

Naeser, M.A., Hayward, R.W., Laughlin, S.A., and Zatz, L.M. (1981). Quantitative CT scan studies in aphasia. *Brain Lang.,* **12,** 140–164.

Ojemann, G.A. (1983). Brain organization for language from the perspective of electrical stimulation mapping. *Behav. Brain Sci.,* **2,** 189–230.

Petersen, S.E., Fox, P.T., Posner, M.I., Mintun, M., and Raichle, M.E. (1988). Positron emission tomographic studies of the cortical anatomy of single word processing. *Nature,* **331,** 585–589.

Poeck, K., Kerschensteiner, M., and Hartje, W. (1972). A quantitative study language understanding in fluent and nonfluent aphasia. *Cortex,* **8,** 299–304.

Riedel, K. (1981). Auditory comprehension in aphasia. In: T. Sarno, ed., *Acquired Aphasia,* pp. 215–269. New York: Academic Press.

Rubens, A.B., Mahowald, M., and Hutton, T. (1976). Asymmetry of the lateral (sylvian) fissures in man. *Neurology,* **26,** 620–624.

Rubens, A.B., Jordan, L., Niccum, N., Risse, G., Selnes, O., and Knopman, D. (1984). *A Comprehensive Study of the Language Recovery Process in Adults with Aphasia Following a Cerebrovascular Accident* (Report to NINCDS. Contract N01-NS-2378). Minneapolis: Hennepin County Medical Center, Department of Neurology.

Schneiderman, E.I., and Saddy, J.D. (1988). A linguistic deficit resulting from right-hemisphere damage. *Brain Lang.,* **34,** 38–53.

Schwartz, M.F. (1984). What the classical aphasia categories can't do for us and why. *Brain Lang.,* **21,** 3–8.

Selnes, O., Knopman, D., Risse, G., and Rubens, A. (1983a). *Comprehension of Syntactically Complex Sentences in Aphasia: CT-Correlates.* Poster presentation at the meeting of the Academy of Aphasia, Minneapolis.

Selnes, O.A., Knopman, D.S., Niccum, N., Rubens, A.B., and Larson, D. (1983b). Computed tomographic scan correlates of auditory comprehension deficits in aphasia: a prospective recovery study. *Ann. Neurol.,* **13,** 558–566.

Selnes, O.A., Niccum, N., Knopman, D.S., and Rubens, A.B. (1984). Recovery of single word comprehension: CT-scan correlates. *Brain Lang.,* **21,** 72–84.

Selnes, O.A., Knopman, D.S., Niccum, N., and Rubens, A.B. (1985). The critical role of Wernicke's area in sentence repetition. *Ann. Neurol.,* **17,** 549–557.

Swisher, L.P., and Sarno, M.T. (1969). Token Test scores of three matched patient groups: left brain damaged with aphasia; right brain damaged without aphasia; non-brain damaged. *Cortex,* **5,** 264–273.

Tweedy, J.R., and Schulman, P.D. (1982). Toward a functional classification of naming impairments. *Brain Lang.,* **15,** 193–206.

Varney, N.R., and Benton, A.L. (1979). Phonemic discrimination and aural comprehension among aphasic patients. *J. Clin. Neuropsychol.,* **1,** 65–74.

Wapner, W., Hamby, S., and Gardner, H. (1981). The role of the right hemisphere in the apprehension of complex linguistic materials. *Brain Lang.,* **14,** 15–33.

Weisenburg, T., and McBride, K.E. (1964). *Aphasia: A Clinical and Psychological Study.* New York: Hafner.

Wernicke, C. (1969). The symptom complex of aphasia: a psychological study on an anatomical basis. In: R.S. Cohen and M.W. Wartofsky, eds., *Boston Studies in the Philosophy of Science,* Vol. 4, pp. 34–97. Boston: D. Reidel Publishing Company. (original work published in 1874).

Zaidel, E. (1976). Auditory vocabulary of the right hemisphere following brain bisection or hemidecortication. *Cortex,* **12,** 191–211.

13

Localization of Function: A Perspective from Cognitive Neuropsychology

PATRICIA A. REUTER-LORENZ AND MICHAEL S. GAZZANIGA

Research on patients with cerebrovascular damage has contributed immeasurably to the progress in neuropsychology over the past two decades. Stroke provides an opportunity to study cognition in the context of focal brain injury. After the acute phase, the behavioral deficits are relatively stable and can be correlated with the locus of structural damage. Other chapters in this volume discuss the merits and drawbacks of studying cognition in stroke patients. Our concern in this chapter is with the problem of relating cognitive functions to brain structures.

Cognitive neuropsychology is a discipline at the boundary between cognitive psychology, neurology, and neuroscience. In the effort to understand the functional organization of cognitive systems, cognitive neuropsychologists apply theories and research methods from cognitive psychology to the investigation of neurologic populations. Cognitive neuropsychologists generally hold the view that cognitive abilities, such as memory, attention, and imagery, are not indivisible "mental faculties" but, rather, functional systems comprised of interactive subcomponents that are functionally and structurally distinct (Luria, 1966). The cognitive neuropsychological approach differs from the more traditional approach to neuropsychology primarily in the conceptualization of what is localized. The aim is to specify the mental operations needed to perform cognitive tasks and to describe the functioning of a particular brain region in terms of the processing operations they perform. These operations are understood as component parts of a network distributed throughout the brain that makes up a particular cognitive system. Tasks designed to measure specific mental operations can be used to determine the components that are dysfunctional. Cognitive models that specify the components and organization of a functional system provide a framework through which to analyze patterns of behavioral deficit. Research with neurologic populations has also proved to be a valuable means of testing cognitive models (e.g., Martin and Caramazza, 1986; Ellis, 1987).

This chapter has three goals, each of which corresponds to a major subdivision of the chapter. The first goal is to illustrate how well specified cognitive models can guide the analysis of neurologic deficits and assist in localizing the components comprising a complex cognitive system. This section discusses how Kosslyn's model of mental imagery (Kosslyn, 1980) and Posner's model of spatial attention (Posner et al., 1982) have been used in the analysis of neuropsychological deficits. The second goal is to illustrate how the application of cognitive/experimental methods has led to the reevaluation of traditional conceptions of the functions subserved by various cortical regions. This section focuses on research in neurolinguistics to highlight the changing views about the function of Broca's and Wernicke's areas. The final goal is to evaluate, from the perspective of cognitive neuropsychology, two paradigmatic principles—the disconnection theory and the syndrome approach—which have had central roles in the development of traditional accounts of structure-function relations.

COMPONENTIAL APPROACH TO COGNITIVE FUNCTIONS

Localization of Imagery

Until recently, investigations of the neurologic basis for visual imagery have produced a confusing picture. Early reports recognized the importance of occipital areas for imagery (Neilsen, 1946; Brain, 1950; Spalding and Zangwill, 1950; Humphrey and Zangwill, 1951) yet revealed little consistency in the laterality of lesions producing imagery impairment. Bilateral damage was common in imagery loss, but impairment after unilateral right hemisphere and left hemisphere lesions was also reported (for reviews see Ehrlichman and Barret, 1983; Farah, 1984).

The type of imagery loss also varies. Some patients lose the ability to imagine objects or faces while spatial imagery remains intact, whereas others show the opposite pattern (see Levine et al., 1985, for review). Neilsen (1946) reported the selective loss of the ability to imagine inanimate objects. Visual agnosia accompanies imagery loss in some cases (Neilsen, 1955; Taylor and Warrington, 1971; Wapner et al., 1978), whereas in others visual recognition is intact (Neilsen, 1946; Brain, 1950; Spalding and Zangwill, 1950).

As of 1980, there was no coherent account of the neurologic basis for imagery. However, by that time Kosslyn (1980) had developed a cognitive theory of imagery that breaks down the "faculty" of imagery into components, each of which is essential to the mechanics of the imaging process. The theory is supported by research with normal populations and sufficiently well specified to be instantiated in a computer model. Furthermore, the theory has implications for a neuropsychological model of imagery. It predicts that different types of imagery impairment should result from damage to different components of the imagery system, which could reside at different neural loci (Kosslyn, 1980; Farah, 1984).

For present purposes the general outlines of this detailed model suffice. According to Kosslyn (1980, 1981) the "picture-like" representation that we experience while imaging is formed by the process of image *generation.* This process converts information from *long-term visual memory* (LTVM) into the "picture-like" representation that is configured in the *visual buffer.* The model specifies subprocesses that make up the process of image generation. Other processes, such as *inspection* and *transformation,* operate on the contents of the visual buffer and support the various ways that imagery can be used in the service of other cognitive abilities.

Some of the model's components, such as *image generation,* are unique to imagery, whereas others are also part of visual perception. For example, LTVM is necessary for recognition of visually presented objects in addition to providing the information for the generation of an image. The *visual buffer* and the processes that operate on its contents, such as the *inspection* process, are utilized for both perception and imagery.

The neuropsychological viability of this model was evaluated in a retrospective investigation of the neurologic literature on imagery loss (Farah, 1984). According to the model, the imagery and perceptual systems share some components but not others. Therefore comparison of performance on perceptual and imagery tasks permits inferences about which components of the system are damaged. Using the information about task performance provided in published case reports, Farah (1984) identified constellations of behavioral deficits that related to particular components of the imagery model. Three distinct deficits were inferred: an image generation deficit, a long-term visual memory deficit, and an image inspection deficit. Kosslyn's model provided theoretical motivation for distinguishing between patterns of task performance and separating patients into subgroups that were relatively homogeneous with respect to competence on certain perceptual and imagery tasks.

Was there any consistency in the lesion locations among these groups? The greatest consistency in lesion site was found for the group with the inferred deficit in image generation. Most of these cases had left posterior involvement. More recently the lateralization of an image generation process to the left hemisphere has been supported by our work with commissurotomy patients (Farah et al., 1985; Kosslyn et al., 1985) and by reports of imagery loss after left posterior infarction verified with computed tomography (CT) (Grossi et al., 1986).

The group with the inferred deficit in image inspection had bilateral or diffuse injury. For the most part, these patients had severe perceptual impairments in addition to their imagery loss. The third subgroup whose deficit was attributed to impairment in the LTVM system tended to have bilateral lesions, content-specific imagery impairment, and visual agnosia. A content-specific deficit implies that the image-generation and inspection components of the system are intact, as some types of images can still be formed. As Farah noted, content-specific deficits also suggest that LTVM may itself be divisible into subcomponents that can be selectively impaired. If these subcomponents are represented in distinct neural loci, selective deficits in LTVM could result from damage to different regions of the brain, thus leading to the anatomic heterogeneity of this group. Although a great deal remains unknown about how images are formed by the brain, this work represents a valuable step toward the development of a comprehensive neuropsychological model of mental imagery. Kosslyn's model offered guidelines for distinguishing the patients with imagery loss due to a circumscribed deficit in the image-generation process from those with both perceptual and imagery impairments due to damage to components shared by both systems. By specifying relatively homogeneous functional deficits, evidence was found for the neuroanatomic localization of at least one component of the imagery system, the image-generation process. Future research can use these taxonomic guidelines to select subtypes of imagery impairment in order to carry out more in-depth psychological and neuroanatomic investigations.

Localization of Attention

Attention can refer to a variety of psychological states. Therefore it is not surprising that numerous pathologies involving diverse structures can impair attentional functioning. Clearly, in order to relate the attentional processes to particular neural loci we must begin by distinguishing between types of attention. Psychologists have distinguished empirically between the components of attention associated with alertness, concentration, and stimulus selection (e.g., Posner and Boies, 1971). The present discussion focuses on the selective processing of visual information based on its spatial location.

The notion that attention can function as a focal, mobile mechanism that is directed and distributed selectively in space is perhaps best expressed by the "spotlight" metaphor (Hernandez-Peon, 1964). Early on, Head and Holmes (1911) suggested that parietal damage can affect attention in the following manner: "When (local attention) is disturbed some impulses evoke sensation, but others from lack of attention, do not affect consciousness. Attention no longer moves freely over the sensory field to be focused successively on fresh groups of sensory impressions" (p. 189).

Within the last 10 years, Posner and his colleagues have developed a model of this aspect of attention and found evidence that its components can be localized to different areas of the brain (e.g., Posner, 1980; Posner et al., 1982, 1984; Posner and Presti, 1987). This model was developed through use of an experimental paradigm that measures the effects of covert attention.

In this task, subjects keep their eyes focused steadily on a fixation point while a cue appears on the screen. The cue informs them which of two locations will most likely contain the next target. A target then appears in one of the two locations, and subjects respond to it by rapidly pressing a key. When the cue provides valid information about the target's location, response times are fast relative to trials in which the wrong location is cued. Because subjects refrain from moving their eyes during this task, any advantage (benefits) or disadvantage (costs) in response time relative to trials in which no location information is given in advance can be attributed to covert shifts of attention to the location of the cue. The rate at which attention is allocated to the cued location can be assessed by varying the time between the onset of the cue and the onset of the target (stimulus onset asynchrony, SOA). Posner specified three component operations that make up the attention-shifting process: *engage, disengage, move.* The engage operation enables the subject to allocate attention to a location in response to a cue. Disengagement occurs when attention is "released" from the cued location and is freed to be allocated elsewhere. The move operation supports the shifting of the attention spotlight from one location to another.

In their investigation of patients with focal parietal lobe damage primarily due to stroke, Posner and his colleagues demonstrated a specific and selective disturbance of spatial attention that can be attributed to impairment of the disengage component (Posner et al., 1984). A typical patient with right parietal damage shows benefits from valid cues presented to the left or right side of space, which indicates that he is able to engage the cue and allocate attention to its location, even when attending to the left side of space is required. Furthermore, the effects of SOA on benefits to valid cues indicate that attention is allocated at a normal rate, which in turn indicates that the move operation is intact.

A selective, direction-specific deficit is revealed on invalid trials. When the left box is cued but the target appears on the right, the pattern of costs is normal. However, if attention is directed to the right box and the target occurs on the left, the response to the target is abnormally slow. According to Posner's model, the disengage operation is responsible for releasing attention from a cued location so that it can be allocated elsewhere. The problem for patients with right parietal damage seems to lie specifically in disengaging attention from the rightward location to reorient to the left. Left parietal patients show the opposite pattern, but the magnitude of the deficit is typically less robust (Posner, et al., 1984; Baynes et al., 1986; Morrow and Ratcliff, 1987). The unilateral disturbance of attention, known as neglect, that is common after right parietal damage may be due in part to damage of the mechanism responsible for disengaging attention in order to move left. With left neglect, attention becomes "anchored" on the right side of space. The directional specificity of attentional control by each hemisphere has also been shown in commissurotomy patients (Gazzaniga and Ladavas, 1987) and in normal subjects (Reuter-Lorenz et al., 1990).

Other evidence has linked the move and engage components to different neural structures. Problems with the move operation have been associated with damage to midbrain structures (Posner et al., 1982; Rafal et al., 1988). Patients with progressive supranuclear palsy are typically impaired in making voluntary eye movements in the vertical plane. With the attention-shifting task these patients also demonstrate selective impairment in moving their attention vertically. This is evidenced by an absence of reaction time benefits in response to *valid* cues unless the time interval between the cue and the target is relatively long. The presence of benefits only at longer SOAs indicates that the speed of attention shifting is affected by damage to midbrain structures. Using the Posner paradigm with monkeys, Petersen and colleagues (1987) found that pharmacologic manipulation of γ-amino-butyric acid (GABA) levels in the pulvinar influence the magnitude of the attentional response (i.e., costs and benefits) to the cue. This finding suggests that portions of the pulvinar may play a special role in the engage operation. Deficits in visual attention following unilateral thalamic hemorrhage in humans also suggest that this area is important to the engage component of visual attention (Rafal and Posner, 1987).

The interaction between cortical and subcortical components of the attention system is further supported by work with commissurotomy patients. Holtzman and colleagues (1981) have shown that the separated hemispheres can cooperate in control of spatial attention despite the inability to share information about the identity of a stimulus.

By studying the performance of these various patient groups using a relatively simple but well defined task, components of the attention-shifting process have been identified and associated with different neural structures. This work demonstrates how the cognitive neuropsychological approach can help to map out a functional system and reveal deficits in elementary mental operations that may underlie more general neurobehavioral symptoms.

FUNCTIONS REDEFINED

The neurocognitive and neurolinguistic approaches to studying brain-behavior relations have led to the redefinition of old functions in addition to the specification of new ones. This section highlights how the results from experimental investigations urge a revision of former models of structure-function relations.

The classic Wernicke-Geschwind model explains language comprehension and production by positing three basic processes that are localized in different regions of the brain (Wernicke, 1874/1910; Geschwind, 1965, 1968, 1970). (1) Wernicke's area, a region of auditory association cortex, is responsible for recognizing words arriving via the auditory channel. Through this area semantic associations are aroused and give meaning to the stream of auditory input. Comprehension of written and spoken language depends on Wernicke's area (Geschwind, 1970). (2) Broca's area, a region of motor association cortex, "contains the learned rules for translating a particular heard sound into a motor sequence" (Geschwind, 1968, p. 109). For the generation of meaningful speech, Broca's area receives input from Wernicke's area via the arcuate fasciculus. (3) The angular gyrus contains the rules for cross-modal associations. Word reading depends on the translation of visual input into an auditory code in the angular gyrus, which can then access meaning through Wernicke's area. According to this model, the dysfluent, telegraphic speech of Broca's or anterior aphasic patients results from disruption of speech output programs, leaving comprehension relatively intact. Posterior or Wernicke's aphasia, characterized by poor comprehension and fluent, grammatic, but semantically aberrant speech, results from dissolution of the semantic network representing word meanings.

Broca's Area Reassessed

The idea that Broca's area is responsible primarily for speech production has been called into question by evidence of comprehension deficits in aphasics with anterior left hemisphere damage. Prior to this evidence, it was generally accepted that telegraphic, agrammatic output economized on the effort needed during the laborious process of speech production (Lennenberg, 1973). However, the fact that a particular class of words, i.e., grammatic morphemes and functors (Goodglass, 1976), was affected more than other classes did not fit neatly into the motor sequencing account of the disorder (Geschwind, 1968). Since the mid-1970s a number of studies have demonstrated a receptive deficit in Broca's aphasics when comprehension depends on processing syntactic elements, such as semantically reversible, passive voice and center-embedded sentences (Caramazza and Zurif, 1976; Heilman and Scholes, 1976; Schwartz et al., 1980). Based on these findings it was proposed that a fundamental deficit in syntactical processing lies at the heart of the production and comprehension impairment of anterior aphasics (e.g., Berndt and Caramazza, 1980; Schwartz et al., 1980). Although evidence has suggested that some agrammatic patients retain particular syntactic abilities (Linebarger et al., 1983; Berndt, 1987; see also below), it is clear that aspects of comprehension depend on the integrity of anterior language areas. Although the precise characterization of the function of Broca's area awaits future research, these functions apparently extend beyond the domain of speech production.

Wernicke's Area Reassessed

The second aspect of the Wernicke-Geschwind model that has been influenced by neurolinguistic research is the characterization of the function of Wernicke's area. Early investigations of lexical organization in Wernicke's aphasics supported the idea that left posterior language areas are necessary for semantic processing. Wernicke's aphasics give aberrant responses on standard word association tasks (Howes, 1967). They are relatively unable to sort words or pictures on the basis of semantic features; and when judging whether two words are related, their responses are slow and inaccurate (Goodglass and Baker, 1976).

Yet evidence suggests that Wernicke's aphasics may have more information about semantic relations than was previously thought. Using a semantic priming task, Milberg and Blumstein (1981) found evidence that the lexical network in Wernicke's aphasics may be partially intact. When normal subjects have to judge whether a string of letters forms a word in the English language, their decisions are made faster when the string is preceded by a word that is semantically related than when preceded by unrelated or nonword strings (e.g., Posner and Snyder, 1975; Neely, 1977). Using this type of paradigm, Milberg and Blumstein (1981; Blumstein et al., 1982) found that Wernicke's aphasics were faster at making lexical decisions for semantically related pairs than for pairs that were unrelated. In another task where patients explicitly judged the semantic relatedness of the same pairs of items, Wernicke's aphasics showed little knowledge of semantic relations.

These findings and others (e.g., McCleary and Hirst, 1986) indicated that Wernicke's aphasics may be sensitive to certain aspects of word meanings. However, whether their knowledge can be demonstrated depends on the how it is measured. The fact that semantic associations can influence performance on at least some tasks suggests that the lexicon may be more intact than was previously thought. Poor performance may reflect impairment of the processes that operate on or access information from the semantic network rather than disruption of the network itself (see below). An access problem may have an attentional basis (Milberg and Blumstein, 1981) or involve disturbances in conscious processing (Schacter et al., 1988). In either case, experimental analysis suggests that Wernicke's area plays a critical role in operating on stored semantic associations but may not be the place where the associations are stored. Specifying the precise nature of the processing operations carried out by Wernicke's area is a challenge for future research.

PARADIGMATIC PRINCIPLES

Disconnection

The disconnection notion has been a mainstay of neurologic and neuropsychological explanations over the past 25 years. The disconnection notion originated around the turn of the century (e.g., Lichtheim, 1885) and was reintroduced to neuropsychology when it was fruitfully applied to the analyses of the behavioral consequences of neurosurgical interventions (Gazzaniga et al., 1962; Geschwind and Kaplan, 1962; Geschwind, 1965). The neurosurgical cases offered a prototype that guided the analysis of deficit in cases of cerebrovascular damage where the locus of damage is less certain.

In Geschwind's analysis (1965), disconnection syndromes generally involved the isolation or separation of an input modality from a particular response system. The isolation of modality-specific information from language areas figured prominently in Geschwind's analysis of human disconnection syndromes. According to this view the disconnection lesion is either a large lesion of the association area surrounding primary sensory cortex or a lesion of white matter projections arising from these association areas.

Disconnection hypotheses offer explanations at the neurologic and psychological levels. At the neurologic level they specify the structures and pathways involved in a particular cognitive function. At the psychological level they specify, in general terms, the sequential stages of information processing. As the synthesis of cognitive psychology and neuropsychology continues, the disconnection accounts may be revised or supplanted by alternative notions of how cognitive systems are instantiated in the brain. In this section we consider how the disconnection concept can currently be applied from the perspective of cognitive neuropsychology.

First, there may be certain core symptoms for which the disconnection analysis offers the best available account at both the neurologic and psychological levels. This point is illustrated later by discussing the relevance of the disconnection notion to understanding the visual agnosias. Second, there are other symptoms for which the anatomic evidence may be consistent with some version of the disconnection hypothesis, whereas at the psychological level the account may be insufficient. For example, some deficits may be more accurately described in terms of the disruption of specific cognitive operations rather than as isolation of sensory input from verbal processes. To illustrate this point the problem of pure alexia will be examined. Finally, the disconnection notion may be appropriate at the psychological level of analysis, although neurologic evidence for it may be absent. The notion of "functional disconnection" retains the flavor of the original disconnection notion but is motivated by cognitive models of task performance and makes no necessary assumptions about the type of lesion giving rise to the behavioral dissociations. The following sections examine each of these points in turn.

Core Disconnection Symptoms?

In this section it is argued that only certain core deficits fit relatively cleanly into the neuroanatomic and psychological framework entailed in the traditional disconnection account. The understanding of other deficits is limited if the accounts of these deficits are constrained by the disconnection model.

Visual agnosia is a modality-specific deficit of recognition. Geschwind (1965) acknowledged the multiple parallel routes supporting recognition and originally proposed that most forms of visual agnosia could be explained by visual-verbal disconnection in combination with the disruption of visual-tactile associations. This process, typically requires a large bilateral lesion of the occipitoparietal area. In the language-dominant hemisphere the lesion would interfere with the direct transfer of visual input to the speech areas. Splenial involvement would preclude the indirect transfer of visual input from right occipital cortex to speech areas. Bilateral lesions also disrupt visual-tactile associations, preventing visual input from reaching speech areas via integration with tactile information.

Visual recognition, however, is not a unitary process and can break down in a variety of ways. Lissauer (1890/1988) distinguished between apperceptive and associative agnosia. A third disorder of visual recognition, optic aphasia or optic anomia, was first reported in 1889 by Freund (cited by Beauvois, 1982). Patients with apperceptive agnosia cannot recognize items presented visually, nor can they copy or match visual forms or objects despite intact elementary visual functions. In associative agnosia patients can match and draw pictures of presented objects; however, they cannot name or describe the function of an object, or demonstrate its use (Bauer and Rubens, 1985; Damasio, 1985). Patients with optic anomia cannot name visually presented items; but unlike associative and apperceptive agnosics, they can demonstrate their use and in some cases select objects when given the name. Patients with optic anomia are relatively unimpaired at naming in response to nonvisual modes of presentation, which distinguishes them from anomic aphasics who are impaired for all modalities (Goodglass et al., 1968). The status of optic anomia as a subtype of visual agnosia has been questioned, in part because recognition of visually presented objects is intact apart from impaired naming. However, a strong case for the visual-verbal disconnection mechanism can be made on the basis of optic anomia (Lhermitte and Beauvois, 1973; Beauvois, 1982). There are good reasons to favor alternative mechanisms for apperceptive and associative agnosia.

Rubens (1979) and others have suggested that these three types of recognition impairment represent a continuum of deficit that varies in severity. Cases of apperceptive agnosia that have resolved into an associative agnosia (e.g., Larrabee et al., 1985) and cases of associative agnosia that resolved into optic anomia (Rubens, 1979) support this idea. If visual-verbal disconnection is at the heart of visual agnosia, it might be argued that greater recognition impairment is associated with greater severity of disconnection. The evidence, however, does not favor this proposal. Whereas recognition impairment is clearly more severe in associative agnosia than in optic anomia, optic anomia entails a more complete visual-verbal disconnection than does associative agnosia. For example, associative agnosia can occur without other disorders of visual naming, such as color anomia or impaired letter and word identification (e.g., Mack and Boller, 1977; Albert et al., 1979). On the other hand, optic anomia is strongly associated with general impairment of visual naming that includes color anomia and poor letter and word reading (Larrabee et al., 1985; Lindeboom and Swinkels, 1986; see also Poeck, 1984, for review).

As a general model for agnosias, visual-verbal disconnection can be questioned on neuroanatomic grounds because of the absence of splenial damage in some cases of associative agnosia (Albert et al., 1979; McCarthy and Warrington, 1986). This inconsistency has been explained by a revised disconnection hypothesis proposing that recognition impairment results from the isolation of visual input from limbic structures by bilateral lesions affecting the inferior longitudinal fasciculus (Albert et al., 1979). This account cannot explain associative agnosia in cases with unilateral damage without splenial involvement (McCarthy and Warrington, 1986). It should also be noted that this revision represents a fundamental departure from Geschwind's original hypothesis because it no longer emphasizes the isolation of sensory input from verbal processes.

In contrast, the original visual-verbal disconnection account remains tenable in cases of optic anomia for which the available neuroanatomic evidence is consistent with splenial involvement (e.g., Larrabee et al., 1985; Lindeboom and Swinkels, 1986). If visual-verbal disconnection underlies optic anomia, splenial damage without right hemianopia should produce the disorder exclusively in the left visual field (LVF). Evidence from a case study conforms with this prediction (Degos et al., 1987). This patient did not have a right hemianopia but had ischemic destruction of the splenium that was verified at autopsy. Behavioral investigation revealed significant impairment in object and letter naming only for LVF stimulus presentation. This finding raises the possibility that tachistoscopic examination of patients with posterior cerebral artery infarction may reveal that unilateral optic anomia is more common than is currently believed (DeRenzi et al., 1987). To our knowledge, no cases of unilateral associative agnosia have been reported. The existence of such patients would strengthen the case for visual-verbal disconnection as the basis for associative agnosia.

It is more likely that differences in severity among forms of agnosia are due to disruption at different stages of the recognition process (e.g., Lissauer, 1890/1988; Ratcliff and Newcombe, 1982; Humphreys and Riddoch, 1987). Current models of visual recognition specify different levels of transformation that a percept must undergo prior to semantic analysis and name retrieval (Warrington and Taylor, 1978; Marr, 1982; Ratcliff and Newcombe, 1982). With apperceptive agnosia, impairment at the early states of visual transformation precludes the ability to organize and integrate the formal or structural features of the percept. By this view, the deficit in apperceptive agnosia occurs prior to the stage of visual-verbal integration.

With associative agnosia, the formal characteristics of the stimulus are accurately specified and integrated, but the ability to analyze an object's meaning is impaired. In this case the deficit may lie at the level of input to the semantic system, or the semantic system itself may be damaged. If the problem involves accessing the semantic system and that system is verbal or linguistic, some form of the visual-verbal disconnection hypothesis may remain viable. Therefore the nature of the semantic system becomes a critical issue for the visual-verbal disconnection account of associative agnosia. There is currently a good deal of debate about the nature of the semantic system subserving visual recognition (e.g., Humphreys and Riddoch, 1988; Shallice, 1988), but most researchers agree that it is not simply a verbal or language-based system. Instead, evidence (Silveri and Gainotti, 1988; Farah et al., 1989) suggests that semantic memory is organized by modality as well as by category (e.g., living versus nonliving). On psychological grounds, then, the visual-verbal disconnection account of associative agnosia may have to be abandoned as the nature of the semantic system is clarified.

In contrast, the deficit in optic anomia appears to occur relatively late in the processing sequence, with stages up to and including semantic analysis remaining relatively intact. These features of optic anomia have been demonstrated in an extensive case study of a patient with bilateral infarctions affecting the left occipital cortex and the posterior limb of the right internal capsule (Coslett and Saffran, 1989b). In view of the available evidence, cases of optic anomia, like the LVF naming deficit that is typical of commissurotomy patients, may represent the clearest cases of visual-verbal disconnection. Explanations of the deficits found in apperceptive and associative agnosia require a more comprehensive account of the processes involved in visual object recognition.

Processing Alternative

Pure alexia or alexia without agraphia may occur as part of the constellation of symptoms of optic anomia. However, it can also occur as an isolated symptom with other forms of visual naming intact (e.g., Vincent et al., 1977; Damasio and Damasio, 1983). Pure alexia is considered a classic disconnection symptom; and like visual agnosia it was originally explained by visual-verbal disconnection (Dejerine, 1892; Geschwind, 1965).

In this section we argue that consideration of the processing operations involved in reading may offer a more satisfactory account of pure alexia than the classic disconnection hypothesis. At the heart of the disconnection account is the idea that comprehension of written language depends on the translation of words from a visual to auditory or phonologic code in the left angular gyrus. This account requires that the lesions in pure alexia isolate the angular gyrus from the visual input. The typical combination is a lesion of the left occipital cortex and splenial damage that blocks the transmission of input from the right visual cortex. However, because pure alexia can occur without other disorders of visual naming, such as optic anomia or color anomia (Greenblatt, 1973; Vincent et al., 1977), it has been proposed that splenial fibers carrying different types of visual input can be damaged selectively (Damasio and Damasio, 1983). Further modifications of the disconnection hypothesis have been necessary to account for cases of pure alexia without right hemianopia (Greenblatt, 1973) and cases without splenial involvement (Damasio and Damasio, 1983; McCarthy and Warrington, 1986). It has been proposed that the splenial lesion is not necessary if there is sufficient destruction of the pathways within the left hemisphere that carry visual input from both occipital cortices to the left angular gyrus. Although the neuroanatomic evidence has led to revisions of the original disconnection account, the current proposal retains the core element of visual-verbal disconnection. From the cognitive neuropsychological viewpoint, there are reasons to question this account.

First let us evaluate the strength of the idea that reading a word depends on its translation to an auditory code. Although this idea has intuitive appeal, there is strong experimental evidence from research on normal reading processes that phonologic recoding is not essential for semantic processing of written language (Carr and Pollatsek, 1985). Furthermore, a recent brain imaging study by Petersen and colleagues (1988) failed to support the recoding hypothesis. Positron emission tomography was used to determine which brain regions were active while subjects analyzed the meanings of words presented in either the visual or the auditory modality. They found that there was no posterior brain region that was activated by *both* modalities of stimulus presentation. As the authors noted, this finding calls into question the obligatory translation from a visual to an auditory word code (see also Henderson, 1986). If reading can proceed normally in the absence of auditory recoding, what then is the deficit in pure alexia? A number of mechanisms have been suggested (e.g., Kinsbourne and Warrington, 1962; Warrington and Shallice, 1980; Paterson and Kay, 1982). We focus on the proposal that for at least a subset of cases the deficit in pure alexia begins with impairment in processing letters. Letter processing is usually assessed by having the patient simply name or match a small sample of letters. Despite informal procedures and insensitive measures, some impairment is usually found. This fact leaves open the possibility that at least some of the reading difficulty in pure alexia is due to impaired letter processing. Current models of word reading include a level of cognitive processing that is concerned with the specification of the letter units of the input string (e.g., Adams, 1979; McClelland and Rumelhart, 1981; Carr and Pollatsek, 1985). According to these models, some degree of letter analysis precedes and interacts with subsequent stages of word identification.

An experimental evaluation of letter processing in a pure alexic was carried out in our laboratory (Reuter-Lorenz and Brunn, in press). The patient had a left occipital lesion due to surgical resection of an arteriovenous malformation, which resulted in a right homonomous hemianopia and a reading disability. There was no optic or color anomia and no indication of splenial involvement on magnetic resonance imaging (MRI) or CT scans (Tramo et al., 1989).

Under free-viewing conditions this patient had no apparent difficulties identifying letters and clearly used a letter-by-letter reading strategy as evidenced by longer reading times with increasing word length. Using an experimental paradigm developed by Posner and Mitchell (1967), letter perception was evaluated at two levels: the level of physical identity and name identity. For the physical identity condition, two letters are presented in the same case (e.g., A A) and the subject decides if they are the same or different letters. For the name identity condition, two letters of different case (e.g., A a) are presented, and the subject decides if they are the same or different letters. The former task can be done purely on the basis of physical features. The latter task requires that the letters are analyzed to a level of a supramodal code or abstract identity (Boles and Eveland, 1983; Coltheart, 1987). Normal subjects take about 80 msec longer to compare letters of different case than to compare letters of the same case. For our alexic patient, under conditions where physical matches were performed within normal limits, cross-case matches took more than three times longer than for normal subjects. The patient was also particularly impaired for either type of match when the members of the letter pairs were presented simultaneously rather than sequentially. This pattern is consistent with the idea that pure alexia involves a deficit in simultaneous processing (e.g., Kinsbourne and Warrington, 1962).

These findings raise the possibility of a deficit early in the analysis of visual language prior to the word-form level of analysis (Warrington and Shallice, 1980) and prior to the stage of visual-auditory integration entailed in the disconnection hypothesis. The disproportionate impairment in matching letters of different case suggests that pure alexia may involve specific impairment when determining the abstract identities of letters. The bottleneck that contributes to the letter-by-letter strategy is the determination of individual letter identities.

Our analysis is admittedly based on a small sample and may be relevant only for cases in which general hemispheric disconnection can be ruled out (i.e., when there is no evidence for optic anomia). However, a report by Bub and colleagues (1989) demonstrated impaired letter priming in a patient similar to ours. Although some version of the disconnection account may be viable on the neuroanatomic level, from the cognitive perspective it may be more relevant to describe the deficit in terms of impairment of specific visual processing operations.

Functional Disconnection

Some studies of pure alexia indicate that patients may be able to make semantic judgments about words that they cannot identify explicitly (Landis et al., 1980; Shallice and Saffran, 1986; Coslett and Saffran, 1989a; however, see Patterson and Kay, 1982). The presence of tacit knowledge about a word can be explained in a variety of ways depending on, for example, the mechanism hypothesized to underlie the pure alexic impairment and assumptions about right hemisphere reading ability (see Shallice and Saffran, 1986). Generally speaking, the finding of tacit lexical knowledge suggests that some components of the reading system have information that other components do not have.

The neuropsychological literature contains a number of examples of dissociations of this type: Patients are impaired on direct or explicit measures of a particular cognitive domain but show preserved abilities on tasks that measure knowledge indirectly (see Schacter et al., 1988, for review). The notion of functional disconnection or access failure may explain such dissociations. Functional disconnection differs from the original disconnection notion in that (1) it is not limited to the isolation of input from output processes, (2) the anatomic locus need not involve connecting pathways, and (3) mechanisms other than impaired information transmission may be responsible for the observed effects. For example, damage to an early processing component could degrade information sent to components upstream. Some components are able to operate on this information even in its degraded form, whereas others cannot. Those that cannot would be functionally disconnected from other components of the system. Functional disconnection could also result when control processes (e.g., attention) that manage the flow of information between various components of the system are damaged. Components that rely more heavily on these control processes are not able to operate properly, whereas other components may be unaffected.

As an account of impaired performance, access failure is fundamentally different from the idea that stored information has been lost and leads to different conclusions about what is localized (see the discussion of Wernicke's aphasia, above). Shallice (1987) has suggested some criteria for distinguishing between these types of account.

If, in fact, a functional disconnection can be established, determining which mechanism is responsible will be a considerable challenge.

Syndrome

In this final section we consider the notion of the "syndrome" or "symptom complex" from the vantage point of cognitive neuropsychology. The specification of a symptom complex has practical utility for the development of diagnostic taxonomies that can assist in lesion localization and treatment planning. Such taxonomies may also provide a valuable first level parse of a domain of behavioral disturbance that can guide the development of fine-grained descriptions of deficits. A symptom complex is of theoretical interest because it may offer insight into a "core deficit" or basic mental operation that is essential for the integrity of each affected behavior. However, the analytic problem entailed in delineating the nature of a single deficit is compounded when considering a constellation of symptoms. Under close scrutiny, each symptom may fractionate into finer symptoms, which in turn may dissociate or co-occur in a variety of complex ways. The search for a "core deficit" may be misguided if some other associated symptom has been overlooked. If and when a symptom complex is defined, the important problem of specifying the common basis for the component symptoms can be approached. Moreover, there is always the possibility that the symptom complex does not have a common functional basis but results instead from the anatomic proximity of component processes that are functionally unrelated.

These analytic and procedural issues have led cognitive neuropsychologists to question the value of the syndrome approach (Mehler et al., 1984; Schwartz, 1984; Ellis, 1987). We advocate a moderate position in which syndromes are considered "hypotheses" about the relations between symptoms. As such, they should be tested and their status as a syndrome determined empirically. For the syndrome approach to continue to be valuable in relating structure to function, consideration must be given to the problems syndromes entail. We see three problems, in particular, that are relevant to the agenda of cognitive neuropsychology.

Problem of Exclusion

The importance of certain associated deficits may go unrecognized if the framework through which a syndrome is analyzed does not attribute relevance to those deficits or if the tasks used to measure them are too gross. This situation may be called the *problem of exclusion.* This problem is illustrated in the changing characterization of Broca's aphasia. When dysfluent aphasia was conceptualized as a motor programming deficit, the associated problems in comprehension were not considered informative features of the symptom complex. Once the receptive features were included in the characterization of anterior aphasia, theoretical accounts of the disorder were revised, and ideas about the function of Broca's area shifted away from the motor programming and toward syntactic operations.

Pure alexia may offer another illustration of the problem of exclusion. Most accounts of the disorder, including the disconnection account, focus on impairment at the level of word processing. Yet, as noted above, the importance of associated problems with processing letters (and possibly numbers) (e.g., Henderson, 1987) may have been underestimated. If impairment at the letter-level proves to be a reliable sign, the neurologic and psychological theories of pure alexia may have to be revised to account for this symptom.

Problem of Overinclusion

A deficit that is considered part of a symptom complex may be defined too generally. Researchers may overlook the fact that the deficit can be fractionated into "subdeficits," some of which may be more closely associated with the complex than others.

Finger agnosia, right-left confusion, agraphia, and acalculia may comprise the classic example of a syndrome that has been defrocked. Gerstmann's syndrome (Gerstmann, 1930/1977) was originally believed to have value as a localizing sign and as a clue to some basic mental substrate. Prior to Benton's (1961) investigation, however, the elements of the syndrome had not been systematically measured or quantified. Benton tested a sample of 100 patients with varying lesion loci using a multiitem test battery to evaluate each symptom of the complex. For example, finger agnosia was assessed using an 80 item test battery that varied input modality and response mode. In addition to assessing the elements of the syndrome, constructional apraxia and visual memory were also evaluated. Benton found that the "syndrome" elements correlated no more highly with each other than with the other deficits measured.

Yet the rather high correlation among all of the measures raises the possibility that although the tests were objective and quantitative the assessment approach was not sensitive enough to discriminate between types of failure (Kinsbourne, 1971). The range of behaviors deemed relevant for assessing each symptom was not constrained by empirically or theoretically based models. Therefore the approach to evaluating Gerstmann's syndrome may have been overinclusive in that elements of the syndrome were too broadly defined. For example, although the analysis of these deficits is still in the early stages, the symptoms of agraphia (Roeltgen, 1985) and acalculia (Levin and Spears, 1985) clearly fractionate into subtypes. It is possible that only a particular subtype of each symptom reliably co-occurs with the other "syndrome" elements. Some version of Gerstmann's syndrome may be rediscovered when the elements of the syndrome are defined more precisely.

The problem of overinclusion is also evident in the research on anterior aphasia. The omission of grammatic morphemes is the cardinal feature of agrammatic speech (Goodglass, 1976). However, other features such as simplified sentence structure, short utterance length, and effortful articulation make up the general clinical picture of the agrammatic aphasic. In one study, Berndt (1987) asked the question: Must all of these features co-occur and if not which ones are related to agrammatic comprehension? Six dysfluent aphasics were subclassified on the basis of their speech with respect to dysfluency, morpheme omission, and structural simplicity. Two of the patients showed all three symptoms, two showed dysfluency and structural simplification but did not omit morphemes, and two were only dysfluent. Comprehension of syntax was also evaluated in these patients. Berndt found that only the four patients whose production was characterized by structural simplicity had an associated deficit in auditory sentence comprehension.

The observations indicate that the various elements that were grouped together as related signs of agrammatism are dissociable. Thus any attempt to identify and localize a unitary mechanism for the signs of agrammatism would have been misguided by inclusion of elements that may have a different functional basis.

Problem of Nontransparency

The nontransparency problem arises in the interpretation of "single" symptoms as well as syndromes and is related to the general difficulty of bridging levels of explanation or, in this case, mapping cognitive functions onto brain functions (Caramazza, 1984). Symptom clusters may have the greatest impact on neuropsychological theories if they reveal relations among behaviors or cognitive abilities that are not obvious from studying normal behavior. How do we specify and localize a unitary mechanism or common dysfunction on the basis of a reliable constellation of behavior deficits? In essence, this subject has been the theme of the entire chapter.

There are at least three factors that may be essential to a successful approach to this problem. First, a cognitive model or theory is needed that specifies the component operations underlying the relevant cognitive abilities and relates the various deficits to a common component or process. Second, the mental operations or computations that are ascribed to the components of the model should be sufficiently detailed and well specified that they could be relevant to neural systems. Constraints on such descriptions can come, for example, from neuroscientific evidence detailing the response properties and connectivity of cells in the relevant brain regions (Sejnowski and Churchland, 1989) and from computer models that attempt to simulate the cognitive functions. Third, there must be means of measuring whether the individual components specified by the model are functional. This point requires a task or series of tasks that are uniquely sensitive to different component operations.

Symptom clusters can be predicted on the basis of a well specified model. For example, it was illustrated in the first section of the chapter how Kosslyn's imagery model predicted that imagery deficits and visual recognition deficits should co-occur in some patients because of damage to long term visual memory, a component shared by imagery and perceptual systems (see above). This feature of the model is supported by the finding that these symptoms are associated (see Farah, 1984). Note also that a modeling approach can guard against the problem of overinclusion, discussed above, because it requires explicit delineation of the processing operations underlying a particular cognitive ability, and it offers theoretically motivated criteria for selecting the behaviors to be measured.

We illustrate further now how cognitive neuropsychology can approach the nontransparency problem by considering the syndrome of unilateral neglect. Unilateral neglect is the failure to attend or respond to stimuli arising from the side of space contralateral to the lesioned hemisphere. The disorder can manifest in a variety of ways and with varying degrees of severity. Some patients show neglect primarily at the level of sensory or input processes, whereas others have primarily motoric manifestations (Heilman et al., 1985). Patients can be affected in a single or in multiple sensory modalities, and neglect of mental imagery can also occur (Bisiach et al., 1979). The effort to characterize different subtypes or manifestations of neglect is still at the early stages (Bisiach et al., 1985; Heilman et al., 1985: Reuter-Lorenz and

Posner, 1990). Nevertheless, the question of a core deficit emerges when considering the mechanisms underlying the various phenomena of hemineglect.

A possible candidate for a basic dysfunctional component or "core deficit" of neglect is the disengagement deficit. In Posner's model (see above), the disengagement operation releases attention from one point of focus so that it can be shifted elsewhere. A direction-specific disengagement deficit was inferred from the performance of patients with parietal damage on the attention-shifting task. Although the suggestion is speculative, there are at least two good reasons that this component operation is a suitable candidate for a "core deficit" in neglect (see Roy et al., 1987, for further discussion). First, there is strong evidence from single cell recording in alert primates that cells in the parietooccipital area play an essential role in the attention-shifting operations that are reflected in the Posner paradigm (see Robinson and Petersen, 1986, for review). In humans, damage to this brain region is most likely to produce neglect (DeRenzi, 1982). Furthermore, reports have indicated that the severity of the disengagement deficit correlates with the severity of neglect, as reflected in other more standard measures of neglect, such as drawing and search tasks (Morrow and Ratcliff, 1987).

According to this proposal, behavioral features associated with neglect, such as directional hypokinesia, allesthesia, and deficits in imagery, co-occur because they share a common dysfunctional component. Patients for whom these symptoms predominate should show the performance pattern on Posner's task associated with a deficit in disengagement. Such a finding might suggest that the disengage operation is a component of a larger attentional network that contributes to the directional control of the limbs and imagery scanning, in addition to being part of the visual attention system. Those patients who do not show this pattern may constitute a subtype with a qualitatively different form of neglect. The important point is that on the basis of a well defined account of attention and model tasks that are sensitive to the relevant cognitive operations, we may identify a component deficit that is common to different symptoms and distinguish between mechanisms underlying different subtypes of attentional disturbance.

CONCLUDING REMARKS

Our optimism about the potential for localizing functions in the brain is due in part to the new insights that have emerged from the cognitive neuropsychological approach, some of which we have reviewed in this chapter. We are also encouraged by the significant progress being made in techniques for mapping the human brain that allow greater precision in defining the locus of damage (Gazzaniga, 1989; Jouandet et al., 1989) and by advances in brain imaging (Raichle, 1986; see also Chapter 4) that reveal functional lesions at sites removed from the structural lesion. In summary, a key factor in localizing functions in the brain is how those functions are defined. As cognitive neuropsychologists aim to be explicit and precise about the elementary operations that comprise cognitive abilities using modeling techniques and neuroscientific evidence to guide and constrain their ideas, the promise of a truly interdisciplinary brain science may be realized.

ACKNOWLEDGMENTS

The authors thank Kathleen Baynes, Robert Fendrich, and Mark Tramo for their comments on earlier drafts of this chapter. The preparation of this manuscript was supported by NIH 5PO1-NS17778 and Javits Award 1 RO1-NS22626.

REFERENCES

Adams, M.J. (1979). Models of word recognition. *Cogn. Psychol.* **11,** 133–176.

Albert, M.L., Soffer, D., Silverberg, R., and Reeches, A. (1979). The anatomic basis of visual agnosia. *Neurology,* **38,** 876–879.

Bauer, R.J., and Rubens, A.B. (1985). Agnosia. In: K.M. Heilman and E. Valenstein, eds., *Clinical Neuropsychology,* 2nd ed., pp. 187–241. New York: Oxford University Press.

Baynes, K., Holtzman, J.D., and Volpe, B.T. (1986). Components of visual attention: alteration in response pattern to visual stimuli following parietal lobe infarction. *Brain,* **109,** 99–114.

Beauvois, M.F. (1982). Optic aphasia: a process of interaction between vision and language. *Philos. Trans. R. Soc. Lond.,* **B298,** 35–47.

Benton, A.L. (1961). The fiction of the "Gerstmann syndrome." *J. Neurol. Neurosurg. Psychiatry,* **24,** 176–181.

Berndt, R.S. (1987). Symptom co-occurrence and dissociation in the interpretation of agrammatism. In: M. Coltheart, G. Sartori, and R. Job, eds., *The Cognitive Neuropsychology of Language,* pp. 221–233. Hillsdale, N.J.: Lawrence Erlbaum Associates.

Berndt, R.S., and Caramazza, A. (1980). A redefinition of Broca's aphasia: implications for a neuropsychological model of language. *Appl. Psycholing.* **1,** 225–278.

Bisiach, E., Berti, A., and Vallar, G. (1985). Analogical and logical disorders underlying unilateral neglect in space. In: M.I. Posner and O.S. Marin, eds., *Attention and Performance XI,* pp. 239–249. Hillsdale, N.J.: Lawrence Erlbaum Associates.

Bisiach, E., Luzzatti, C., and Perani, D. (1979). Unilateral neglect, representational schema and consciousness. *Brain,* **102,** 609–618.

Blumstein, S.E., Milberg, W., and Shrier, R. (1982). Semantic processing in aphasia: evidence from an auditory lexical decision task. *Brain Lang.,* **17,** 301–315.

Boles, D.B., and Eveland, D.C. (1983). Visual and phonetic codes and the process of generation in letter matching. *J. Exp. Psychol. [Hum. Percept.],* **9,** 657–673.

Brain, R.W. (1950). The cerebral basis of consciousness. *Brain,* **73,** 465–479.

Bub, D.N., Black, S., and Howell, J. (1989). Word recognition and orthographic context effects in a letter-by-letter reader. *Brain Cogn.,* **36,** 357–376.

Caramazza, A. (1984). The logic of neuropsychological research and the problem of patient classification in aphasia. *Brain Lang.,* **21,** 9–20.

Caramazza, A., and Zurif, E. (1976). Dissociation of algorithmic and heuristic processes in language comprehension: evidence from aphasia. *Brain Lang.,* **3,** 572–582.

Carr, T.H., and Pollatsek, A. (1985). Recognizing printed words: a look at current models. In: D. Besner, T.G. Waller, and G.E. MacKinnon, eds., *Reading Research: Advances in Theory and Practice,* Vol. 5, pp. 1–82. New York: Academic Press.

Coltheart, M. (1987). Functional architecture of the language system. In: M. Coltheart, G. Sartori, and R. Job, eds., *The Cognitive Neuropsychology of Language,* pp. 1–25. Hillsdale, N.J.: Lawrence Erlbaum Associates.

Coslett, H.B., and Saffran, E.M. (1989a). Preserved reading in pure alexia. *Brain,* **112,** 327–359.

Coslett, H.B., and Saffran, E.M. (1989b). Preserved object recognition and reading comprehension in optic aphasia. *Brain,* **112,** 1091–1110.

Damasio, A., and Damasio, H. (1983). The anatomic basis of pure alexia. *Neurology,* **33,** 1573–1583.

Damasio, A.R. (1985). Disorders of complex visual processing: agnosias, achromatopsia, Balint's syndrome and related difficulties of orientation and construction. In: M.M. Mesulum, ed., *Principles of Behavioral Neurology,* pp. 259–288. Philadelphia: Davis.

Degos, J.D., Gray, F., Louarn, F., Ansquer, J.C., Poirier, J., and Barbizet, J. (1987). Posterior callosal infarcts. *Brain,* **110,** 1155–1171.

Dejerine, J. (1892). Contribution a l'etude anatomo-pathologique et cliniques des differentes varietes de cecite verbale. *Mem. Soc. Biol.,* **44,** 61–90.

DeRenzi, E. (1982). *Disorders of Space Exploration and Cognition.* New York: Wiley.

DeRenzi, E., Zambolin, A., and Crisi, G. (1987). The neuropsychological impairment associated with left posterior cerebral artery infarcts. *Brain,* **110,** 1099–1116.

Ehrlichman, H., and Barret, J. (1983). Right hemispheric specialization for mental imagery: a review of the evidence. *Brain Cogn.,* **2,** 39–52.

Ellis, A.W. (1987). Intimations of modularity or the modularity of mind: doing neuropsychology without syndromes. In: M. Coltheart, G. Sartori, and R. Job, eds., *The Cognitive Neuropsychology of Language,* pp. 397–408. Hillsdale, N.J.: Lawrence Erlbaum Associates.

Farah, M.J. (1984). The neurological basis of mental imagery: a componential analysis. *Cognition,* **18,** 245–272.

Farah, M.J., Gazzaniga, M.S., Holtzman, J.D., and Kosslyn, S.M. (1985). A left hemisphere basis for visual imagery. *Neuropsychologia,* **23,** 115–118.

Farah, M.J., Hammond, K.M., Mehta, Z., and Ratcliff, G. (1989). Category-specificity and modality-specificity in semantic memory. *Neuropsychologia,* **27,** 193–200.

Gazzaniga, M.S. (1989). Organization of the human brain. *Science,* **245,** 947–952.

Gazzaniga, M.S., and Ladavas, E. (1987). Disturbances of spatial attention following lesion or disconnection of the right parietal lobe. In: M. Jeannerod, ed., *Neurophysiological and Neuropsychological Aspects of Neglect,* pp. 203–213. New York: North Holland.

Gazzaniga, M.S., Bogen, J.E., and Sperry, R.W. (1962). Some functional effects of sectioning the cerebral commissures in man. *Proc. Natl. Acad. Sci. USA,* **48,** 1765–1769.

Gerstmann, J. (1977). The symptoms produced by lesions of the transitional area between the inferior parietal and middle occipital gyri. In: D.A. Rottenberg and F.H. Hochberg, eds., *Neurological Classics in Modern Translation,* pp. 150–155. London: Hafner Press (originally published 1930).

Geschwind, N. (1965). Disconnection syndromes in animals and man. *Brain,* **88,** 237–294, 585–644.

Geschwind, N. (1968). Problems in the anatomical understanding of the aphasias. In: A.L. Benton, ed., *Contributions to Clinical Neuropsychology,* pp. 107–128. Chicago: Aldine Press.

Geschwind, N. (1970). The organization of language in the brain. *Science,* **170,** 940–944.

Geschwind, N., and Kaplan, E. (1962). A human cerebral deconnection syndrome. *Neurology,* **12,** 675–685.

Goodglass, H. (1976). Agrammatism. In: H. Whitaker and H.A. Whitaker, eds., *Studies in Neurolinguistics,* Vol. 1, pp. 237–259. Orlando: Academic Press.

Goodglass, H., and Baker, E. (1976). Semantic field, naming, and auditory comprehension in aphasia. *Brain Lang.,* **3,** 359–374.

Goodglass, H., Barton, M.I., and Kaplan, E.F. (1968). Sensory modality and object-naming in aphasia. *J. Speech Hearing Res.*, **11**, 488–496.

Greenblatt, S. (1973). Alexia without agraphia or hemianopia: anatomical analysis of an autopsied case. *Neurology*, **21**, 873–876.

Grossi, D., Orsini, A., Modafferi, A., and Liotti, M. (1986). Visuoimaginal construction apraxia: on a case of selective imagery deficit. *Brain Cogn.*, **5**, 255–268.

Head, H., and Holmes, H.G. (1911). Sensory disturbances from cerebral lesions. *Brain*, **34**, 102–254.

Heilman, K.M., and Scholes, R.J. (1976). The nature of the comprehension deficit in Broca's conduction and Wernicke's aphasia. *Cortex*, **12**, 258–265.

Heilman, K.M., Watson, R.T., and Valenstein, E. (1985). Neglect and related disorders. In: K.M. Heilman and E. Valenstein, eds., *Clinical Neuropsychology*, 2nd ed., pp. 243–293. New York: Oxford University Press.

Henderson, V.W. (1986). Anatomy of posterior pathways in reading: a reassessment. *Brain Lang.*, **29**, 119–133.

Henderson, V.W. (1987). Is number reading selectively spared in pure alexia? *J. Clin. Exp. Neuropsychol.*, **9**, 41.

Hernandez-Peon, R. (1964). Psychiatric implications of neurophysiological research. *Bull. Menninger Clin.*, **28**, 165–185.

Holtzman, J.D., Sidtis, J.J., Volpe, B.T., Wilson, D.H., and Gazzaniga, M.S. (1981). Dissociation of spatial information for stimulus localization and the control of attention. *Brain*, **104**, 861–872.

Howes, D. (1967). Some experimental investigations of langauge in aphasia. In: K. Salzinger and M. O'Connor, eds., *Research in Verbal Behavior and Some Neurophysiological Implications*. Orlando: Academic Press.

Humphrey, M.E., and Zangwill, O.L. (1951). Cessation of dreaming after brain injury. *J. Neurol. Neurosurg. Psychiatry*, **14**, 322–325.

Humphreys, G.W., and Riddoch, M.J. (1987). *To See But Not to See: A Case Study of Visual Agnosia*. London: Lawrence Erlbaum Associates.

Humphreys, G.W., and Riddoch, M.J. (1988). On the case for multiple semantic systems: a reply to Shallice. *Cogn. Neuropsychol.*, **5**, 143–150.

Jouandet, M.L., Tramo, M.J., Herron, D.M., Hermann, A., Loftus, W.C., Bazell, J., and Gazzaniga, M.S. (1989). Brainprints: computer generated two dimensional maps of the human cerebral cortex in vivo. *J. Cogn. Neurosci.*, **1**.

Kinsbourne, M. (1972). Cognitive deficit: experimental analysis. In: J.L. McGaugh, ed., *Psychobiology*, pp. 285–338. Orlando: Academic Press.

Kinsbourne, M., and Warrington, E.K. (1962). A disorder of simultaneous form perception. *Brain*, **85**, 461–486.

Kosslyn, S.M. (1980). *Image and Mind*. Cambridge: Harvard University Press.

Kosslyn, S. (1981). The medium and the message in mental imagery: a theory. *Psychol. Rev.*, **88**, 46–66.

Kosslyn, S.M., Holtzman, J.D., Farah, M.J., and Gazzaniga, M.S. (1985). A computational analysis of mental image generation: evidence from functional dissociations in split-brain patients. *J. Exp. Psychol.* [*Gen.*], **114**, 311–341.

Landis, T., Regard, M., and Serrant, A. (1980). Iconic reading in a case of alexia without agraphia caused by a brain tumor: a tachistoscopic study. *Brain Lang.*, **11**, 45–53.

Larrabee, G.J., Levin, H.S., Huff, F.J., Kay, M.C., and Guinto, F.C. (1985). Visual agnosia contrasted with visual-verbal disconnection. *Neuropsychologia*, **23**, 1–12.

Lennenberg, E.H. (1973). The neurology of language. *Daedalus*, **102**, 115–133.

Levin, H.S., and Spiers, P.A. (1985). Acalculia. In: K.M. Heilman and E. Valenstein, eds., *Clinical Neuropsychology*, 2nd ed., pp. 97–114. New York: Oxford University Press.

Levine, D.N., Warach, J., and Farah, M. (1985). Two visual systems in mental imagery: dissociation of "what" and "where" in imagery disorders due to bilateral posterior cerebral lesions. *Neurology,* **35,** 1010–1018.

Lhermitte, F., and Beauvois, M.F. (1973). A visual-speech disconnection syndrome: report of a case with optic aphasia, agnosia alexia and colour agnosia. *Brain,* **96,** 695–714.

Lichtheim, L. (1885). On aphasia. *Brain,* **7,** 432–484.

Lindeboom, J., and Swinkels, J.A. (1986). Interhemispheric communication in a case of total visuo-verbal disconnection. *Neuropsychologia,* **24,** 781–792.

Linebarger, M., Schwartz, M.F., and Saffran, E.M. (1983). Sensitivity to grammatical structure in so-called agrammatic aphasics. *Cognition,* **13,** 361–392.

Lissauer, H. (1988). A case of visual agnosia with a contribution to theory. *Cogn. Neuropsychol.,* **5,** 157–192 (originally published 1890).

Luria, A.R. (1966). *Higher Cortical Functions in Man.* New York: Basic Books.

Mack, J.L., and Boller, F. (1977). Associative agnosia and its related deficits: the role of the minor hemisphere in assigning meaning to visual perceptions. *Neuropsychologia,* **15,** 345–349.

Marr, D. (1982). *Vision.* San Francisco: W.H. Freeman.

Martin, R.C., and Caramazza, A. (1986). Theory and method in neurolinguistics: the case of acquired dyslexia. In: H.J. Hannay, ed., *Experimental Techniques in Human Neuropsychology,* pp. 363–385. New York: Oxford University Press.

McCarthy, R.A., and Warrington, E.K. (1986). Visual associative agnosia: a clinico-anatomical study of a single case. *J. Neurol. Neurosurg. Psychiatry,* **49,** 1233–1240.

McCleary, C., and Hirst, W. (1986). Semantic classification in aphasia: a study of basic superordinate and function relations. *Brain Lang.,* **27,** 199–209.

McClelland, J.L., and Rumelhart, D.E. (1981). An interactive activation model of context effects in letter perception. Part 1. An account of basic findings. *Psychol. Rev.,* **88,** 375–407.

Mehler, J., Morton, J., and Jusczyk, P.W. (1984). On reducing language to biology. *Cogn. Neuropychol.,* **1,** 83–116.

Milberg, W., and Blumstein, S. E. (1981). Lexical decision and aphasia: evidence for semantic processing. *Brain Lang.,* **14,** 371–385.

Morrow, L.A., and Ratcliff, G.G. (1987). Attentional mechanisms in clinical neglect. *J. Clin. Exp. Neuropsychol,.* **9,** 74.

Neely, J.H. (1977). Semantic priming and retrieval from lexical memory. *J. Exp. Psychol.* [*Gen.*], **106,** 226–254.

Nielsen, J.M. (1946). *Agnosia, Apraxia and Aphasia: Their Value in Cerebral Localization.* New York: Paul B. Hoeber.

Nielsen, J.M. (1955). Occipital lobes, dreams and psychosis. *J. Nerv. Ment. Dis.,* **121,** 30–32.

Patterson, K.E., and Kay, J. (1982). Letter-by-letter reading: psychological descriptions of a neurological syndrome. *Q. J. Exp. Psychol.,* **34a,** 411–441.

Petersen, S.E., Robinson, D.L., and Morris, J.D., (1987). Contributions of the pulvinar to visual spatial attention. *Neuropsychologia,* **25,** 97–105.

Petersen, S., Fox, P.T., Posner, M.I., Mintun, M., and Raichle, M.E. (1988). Positron emission tomographic studies of the cortical anatomy of single-word processing. *Nature,* **331,** 585–589.

Poeck, K. (1984). Neuropsychological demonstration of splenial interhemispheric disconnection in a case of "optic anomia." *Neuropsychologia,* **22,** 707–713.

Posner, M.I. (1980). Orienting of attention. *Q. J. Exp. Psychol.,* **32,** 3–25.

Posner, M.I., and Boies, S.J. (1971). Components of attention. *Psychol. Rev.,* **78,** 391–408.

Posner, M.I. Cohen, Y., and Rafal, R.D. (1982). Neural systems control over spatial orienting. *Phil. Trans. Royal Soc.* (Lond.) Series B, **2908,** 187–192.

Posner, M.I., and Mitchell, R.F. (1967). Chronometric analysis of classification. *Psychol. Rev.,* **74,** 392–409.

Posner, M.I., and Presti, D.E. (1987). Selective attention and cognitive control. *Trends Neurosci.,* **10,** 12–17.

Posner, M.I., and Snyder, C.R.R. (1975). Attention and cognitive control. In: R.C. Solso, ed., *Information Processing and Cognition: The Loyola Symposium.* Hillsdale, N.J.: Lawrence Erlbaum Associates.

Posner, M.I., Walker, J.A., Friedrich, F.F., and Rafal, R.D. (1984). Effects of parietal injury on covert orienting of attention. *J. Neurosci.,* **4,** 1863–1874.

Rafal, R.D., and Posner, M.I. (1987). Deficits in human visual spatial attention following thalamic lesions. *Proc. Natl. Acad. Sci. USA,* **84,** 7349–7353.

Rafal, R.D., Posner, M.I., Friedman, J.H., Inhoff, A.W., and Bernstein, E. (1988). Orienting of attention in progressive supranuclear palsy. *Brain,* **11,** 267–280.

Raichle, M.E. (1986). Neuroimaging. *Trends Neurosci.,* **9,** 525–529.

Ratcliff, G., and Newcombe, F. (1982). Object recognition: some deductions from clinical evidence. In: A.W. Ellis, ed., *Normality and Pathology of Cognitive Function,* pp. 147–171. Orlando: Academic Press.

Reuter-Lorenz, P.A., and Brunn, J.L. (1990). A pre-lexical basis for letter-by-letter reading: a case study. *Cogn. Neuropsychol.* **7,** 1–20.

Reuter-Lorenz, P.A., and Posner, M.I. (1990). Components of neglect from right hemisphere damage: an analysis of line bisection. *Neuropsychologia,* **28,** 327–333.

Reuter-Lorenz, P.A., Kinsbourne, M., and Moscovitch, M. (1990). Hemispheric control of spatial attention. *Brain Cogn.* **12,** 240–266.

Robinson, D.L., and Petersen, S.E. (1986). The neurobiology of attention. In: J. Ledoux and W. Hirst, eds., *Mind and Brain.* New York: Cambridge University Press.

Roeltgen, D. (1985). Agraphia. In: K.M. Heilman and E. Valenstein, eds., *Clinical Neuropsychology,* 2nd ed., pp. 75–96. New York: Oxford University Press.

Roy, E.A., Reuter-Lorenz, P.A., Roy, L.G., Copland, S., and Moscovitch, M. (1987). Unilateral attentions deficits and hemispheric asymmetries in the control of attention. In: M. Jeannerod, ed., *Neurophysiological and Neuropsychological Aspects of Neglect,* pp. 25–39. New York: North Holland.

Rubens, A.B. (1979). Agnosia. In: K.M. Heilman and E. Valenstein , eds., *Clinical Neuropsychology,* pp. 233–267. New York: Oxford University Press.

Schacter, D.L., McAndrews, M.P., and Moscovitch, M. (1988). Access to consciousness: dissociations between implicit and explicit knowledge in neuropsychological syndromes. In: L. Weiskrantz, ed., *Thought Without Language,* pp. 242–278. Oxford: Oxford University Press.

Schwartz, M.F. (1984). What the classical aphasia categories can and can't do for us. *Brain Lang.,* **21,** 3–8.

Schwartz, M.F., Saffran, E.M., and Marin, O.S.M. (1980). The word order problem in agrammatism. I. Comprehension. *Brain Lang.,* **10,** 249–262.

Sejnowski, T.J., and Churchland, P.S. (1989). Brain and cognition. In: M.I. Posner, ed., *Foundations of Cognitive Science,* pp. 301–356. Cambridge, MA: MIT Press.

Shallice, T. (1987). Impairments of semantic processing: multiple dissociations. In: M. Coltheart, G. Sartori, and R. Job, eds., *The Cognitive Neuropsychology of Language,* pp. 221–233. Hillsdale, N.J.: Lawrence Erlbaum Associates.

Shallice, T. (1988). Specializations within the semantic system. *Cogn. Neuropsychol.,* **5,** 133–142.

Shallice, T., and Saffran, E. (1986). Lexical processing in the absence of explicit word identification: evidence from a letter-by-letter reader. *Cogn. Neuropsychol.*, **3,** 429–458.

Silveri, M.C., and Gainotti, G. (1988). Interaction beween vision and language in category specific semantic impairment. *Cogn. Neuropsychol.*, **5,** 677–709.

Spalding, J.M.K., and Zangwill, O.L. (1950). Disturbances of number-form in a case of brain injury. *J. Neurol. Neurosurg. Psychiatry,* **13,** 24–29.

Taylor, A., and Warrington, E.K. (1971). Visual agnosia: a single case report. *Cortex,* **7,** 152–161.

Tramo, M.J., Reuter-Lorenz, P.A., and Gazzaniga, M.S. (1989). Pure alexia: cognitive and anatomic correlates. *Ann. Neurol.,* **26,** 126.

Vincent, F.W., Sadowsky, C.H., Saunders, R.L., and Reeves, A.G. (1977). Alexia without agraphia, hemianopia, or color-naming defect: a disconnection syndrome. *Neurology,* **27,** 689–691.

Wapner, W., Judd, T., and Gardner, H. (1978). Visual agnosia in an artist. *Cortex,* **14,** 343–364.

Warrington, E.K., and Shallice, T. (1980). Word-form dyslexia. *Brain,* **103,** 99–112.

Warrington, E.K. and Taylor, A. (1978). Two categorical stages of object recognition. *Perception,* **7,** 695–705.

Wernicke, C. (1910). The symptom-complex of aphasia. In: A Church, ed., *Modern Clinical Medicine: Diseases of the Nervous System.* New York: Appleton (originally published 1874).

III

Recovery and Treatment

14

Neuropsychological Recovery After Cerebral Infarction

MANFRED J. MEIER AND SILVIA E. STRAUMAN

A striking feature of the effects of acute cerebrovascular infarction is the wide range of individual differences in recovery course over the weeks and months following the episode. The importance of spontaneous recovery is underscored by the limited effectiveness demonstrated to date of cognitive remediation and rehabilitation procedures. If retraining and remediation procedures do not produce gains beyond spontaneous recovery, the effectiveness of rehabilitation procedures may ultimately be evaluated primarily on the basis of the degree to which acceleration of spontaneous recovery changes can be achieved. Despite the substantial attention to recovery in the animal experimental neuropsychological literature, relatively little clinical neuropsychological research has been done in the determinants of recovery after cerebrovascular infarction. Thus there is a need for clarification and understanding of the determinants of recovery. An obvious challenge for clinical neuropsychology is the prediction of outcome on the basis of quantitative and qualitative behavioral assessments. Clinical neurospychological measurements may ultimately help identify the boundaries within which specific behavioral treatment procedures may become effective. Hopefully, it would lead to more precise prediction of specific individual recovery, either spontaneously or with formal remedial intervention.

The purpose of this chapter is to examine some of the factors that have been shown to contribute to recovery and to review some of the interactions among these variables that may contribute to the wide range of individual differences observed on (dependent) outcome variables as assessed by means of neuropsychological tests. It is a widely held expectation that patterns of impaired and spared functions early in the recovery process are related, directly or indirectly, to outcome. In turn, initial and subsequent performance levels are affected by means of single and interactive effects of variables that are known to contribute to individual differences in life-span development. Facilitative or detrimental effects may be related to factors of a genetic, environmental, social, and biologic nature (Schaie and Schaie, 1977). The large numbers of possible interactions among these variables likely has an important role in the wide range of individual outcomes that characterize clinical recovery. With cerebrovascular disease the biologic determinants of outcome include the specific neuropathologic and pathophysiologic effects of the cerebrovascular infarction. These variables include the location and depth of the lesion, the extent or severity of neurologic involvement, and the preexisting status of the cerebral hemispheres and any affected deeper structures. Cerebral and subcortical status, in turn, may be affected by age, time since symptom onset, and variation in cerebral organization or dominance. In addition, factors that influence that bilateral representation of higher congitive functions may interact with premorbid environmental or life style factors, such as education, nutrition, vocational level, general systemic health, and psychological health. Furthermore, an extensive array of detrimental historical factors such as alcohol and drug abuse, prior exposure to industrial toxins, and chronic functional psychopathology would also be expected to introduce constraints on the ultimate level of recovery in individual cases.

This chapter does not review the vast basic and clinical literature on recovery of function. Numerous reviews are available, though the clinical recovery literature is more extensive for closed head injury than for cerebrovascular disease (Stein et al., 1974, 1983; Newcombe and Ratcliff, 1979; Newcombe, 1982; Brooks et al., 1984).

CENTRAL NERVOUS SYSTEM MECHANISMS OF RECOVERY

Since the early 1970s there has been an impressive conceptual and experimental analysis of recovery in animals. The appearance of the volume on plasticity and recovery of function in the central nervous system (CNS), edited by Stein and colleagues (1974), provided integration of the recovery literature to that date. The animal literature is remarkable in volume and sophistication. It warrants careful examination by anyone with clinical neurobehavioral interests and may be accessed readily (Luria, 1963; Rosner, 1970; Goldman, 1974; Teuber, 1975; Finger, 1978; Finger and Stein, 1982; Stein et al., 1983).

Central to these deliberations has been the concept of "plasticity," which has acquired various meanings and interpretations. As Stein et al. (1983) pointed out, this concept remains elusive to systematic analysis and investigation owing to the difficulties encountered in operational definitions at the level of anatomic, physiologic, and behavioral analysis. Limited to the description of response to injury, the concept seems to be well accepted (Geschwind, 1974). However, there appears to be a danger that the concept of "plasticity" may become reified in explanations of recovery phenomena and thus become meaningless. Nevertheless, search for the meaning of the concept has led to much productive work and to the identification of numerous possible mechanisms that intrinsically relate to the recovery process.

Diaschisis

One such mechanism, diaschisis, has received considerable attention in the literature and provides a point of departure for a summary of such recovery mechanisms. Others include the masking effects of cerebral edema during the acute phase of recovery, the resumption of flow after interruptions of cerebral blood flow, regeneration of neural elements, denervation supersensitivity, substitution of a structural nature, and substitution at the response or performance level. One or more of these mechanisms may be operating in a constantly changing temporal pattern and in interaction with covariates such as age, either singly or in combination. It seems unlikely that any single factor, extrinsic or intrinsic, accounts for all recovery changes seen in a particular patient. Assessment and intervention challenges for the neuropsychologist and other neurobehavioral specialists can then be seen as enormous. It is these challenges that appear to have heightened interest in seeking a more effective relation between these disciplines.

Introduced by von Monakow (1914/1969), diaschisis relates to the effects of a lesion or disease process on remote as well as proximal structures. It is most conspicuous during the immediate effects of a cerebrovascular accident in which there may be considerable swelling of brain (edema) as well as alterations in blood flow through patent vessels. Such acute effects may mask or distort functions in essentially intact regions of the brain. Dissipation of such effects may account for a substantial proportion of early recovery and for some of the dramatic recovery changes seen in selected patients with severe or profound initial neurologic and neuropsychological deficit. Several studies using xenon 133 cerebral blood flow measurement (Meyer et al., 1970; Fujishima et al., 1974; Lavy et al., 1975; Slater et al., 1977) have demonstrated decreased blood flow in the hemisphere contralateral to cerebral infarction. In addition, indirect evidence for diaschisis can be derived from observations on serially lesioned animals, for example, who evidence much milder impairments of briefer duration than do animals with comparable lesions introduced in one stage (Adametz, 1959). Even with more prolonged interoperative or postoperative intervals, recovery effects may be remarkable even after left hemispherectomy in man, for example, where recovery of language function seems almost paradoxical (Smith, 1977). The validity of the concept of diaschisis as an explanation for recovery of function remains questionable. However, most theoreticians in neuropsychology acknowledge that the underlying pathophysiologic components are likely to be identified in the future (Teuber, 1975). To distinguish it from other mechanisms, it is important to stress that diaschisis refers to the progressive reestablishment of function in neural systems that are transiently and incidentally disrupted by the lesion. Thus if valid, the concept may encompass redundancy of function in the CNS but would not account for any reorganization of neural systems into new configurations based on other mechanisms, such as modified neural growth and regeneration.

Regeneration of Neural Elements

There is increasing evidence of at least a potential for selective regeneration of neural elements during recovery (Finger and Stein, 1982). Regeneration is defined as any change in the morphologic organization of the nervous system that may occur in response to injury (Moore, 1974). Any growth of neuronal processes would then lead to the formation of new and presumably functional synaptic contact between surviving neurons. Whether such contact would facilitate, inhibit, or disrupt function remains an empiric question. Regenerative sprouting from transected axons and collateral sprouting from intact axons have been identified for some time (Stein et al., 1983). Axons of the central adrenergic neurons have been shown to be most capable of regenerative sprouting and growth following transection. However, it remains of doubtful functional significance in humans and does not appear to account for recovery. Collateral sprouting has been demonstrated to occur from intact neurons and results in some reorganization of the synaptic structure in a denervated area. The collateral sprouting seen in transected axons appears to maintain a relatively constant contact field so that any newly formed terminals, if they are to become functional, do so at the expense of other synaptic connections. Of perhaps even greater significance are developments in the basic neuroscience literature that demonstrate the potential for further neural growth in response to the presence of transplanted brain tissue (O'Connor and Cermak, 1987). To the extent that such neural growth can lead to the establishment of new functional systems and can be facilitated by other favorable determining factors, some true reorganization of function may be possible.

Denervation Supersensitivity

Some basis for redundancy of function in the CNS might be found in the phenomenon of denervation supersensitivity. Cannon and Rosenblueth (1949) referred to the increased sensitivity to neurotransmitter agonists and antagonists in denervated neurons. It appears to be due to an increase in the number of receptor sites and has been demonstrated in skeletal muscles, peripheral neurons of the autonomic ganglia, and spinal neurons. Recovery of function may be attributable in part to increased sensitivity to the remaining influence of areas of the brain that are partially denervated by the lesion, which might lead to the participation of a partially denervated region subserved by the affected region. The role of this mechanism in CNS recovery remains questionable and might in turn be facilitated or inhibited by collateral sprouting from both intact and denervated axons (Stein et al., 1983). If potentially capable of enhancing recovery, the phenomenon would add to the potential for reorganization of function. Such enhancing properties, of course, could also be offset by possible detrimental effects of partial denervation.

Structural Substitution or Vicariation

As applied to CNS structure, structural substitution (vicariation) has been invoked to account for locomotor recovery following unilateral lesion of the motor cortex (Kennard, 1938). This mechanism involves the postulation that an intact structure can assume the functions of an affected structure. Redundancy of discrete or primary sensory and motor functions is seen more frequently in animals than in humans, where recovery of such functions may sometimes be nil. Small lesions that affect the internal capsule may produce relatively permanent, profound hemiplegia, though exceptions have been noted in humans (Geschwind, 1974). There are known individual differences in the relative concentration of the pyramidal tract on either side so that some individuals may have substantial ipsilateral control of motor and somatosensory functions. Even an extensive lesion in one hemisphere would then not produce permanent contralateral effects in such individuals (Yakovlev, 1971). Redundancy of function may be more feasible when the function is independent of primary cortical or peripheral structures. Thus greater overlap of zones that subserve language, visuospatial, and abstract reasoning functions may account for the fact that some degree of recovery of such functions is seen in virtually all patients following cerebrovascular accidents or closed head injuries. It may be due in part to less discrete involvement of the brain in closed head injury, where both focal and nonfocal as well as multilevel effects may be present.

Structural substitution remains a somewhat nebulous concept and, like "plasticity," is subject to reification; that is, it may have no conceptual meaning beyond the descriptive behavioral features of recovery. Redundant representation may exist within a structural system, so that it may not be necessary to postulate substitution of systems to account for that portion of recovery that reflects redundancy (Rosner, 1970).

Behavioral Substitution

The animal and human clinical literature are replete with examples of response or behavioral substitution in which there is a marked increase in efficiency in achieving an end despite the persistence of a psychological deficit. It gives the misleading impression of intrinsic recovery of a function when it is not the function but, rather, the strategy used for applying intact functions toward achieving a goal that produces the change. Thus a problem that cannot be solved directly because the behavioral response may no longer be available can be solved by introducing new strategies or ways for reaching the goal (Stein et al., 1983). Valentino and Stein (1983) examined the relation between age and staging of lesions of the frontal cortex to produce differences in the ability to select and pursue effective strategies in goal-directed behavior. Young rats with single-stage lesions were more variable than controls but ultimately found and utilized an effective strategy. Young rats with two-staged lesions were virtually indistinguishable from normals in the way in which they adapted and utilized an effective strategy. A contrasting older group of rats, even with two-staged lesions, remained confused and unable to identify the effective strategy for solving the maze. For that matter, age was overwhelmingly the strongest determinant, as nonoperated controls were also impaired in this respect.

Most clinicians become keenly aware of the need to foster response substitution as a means of improving overall function. Neuropsychological test procedures have not been investigated extensively from this perspective. It is generally accepted that failure to identify a deficit by means of a neuropsychological test of known validity indicates that the individual is unimpaired for that function. On the other hand, rehabilitation personnel who have daily contact with that patient may report that there is a deficiency in the effective execution of that function in particular ecologic circumstances. An important area for future investigation is the assessment of preferred strategies and their effectiveness in arriving at particular solutions. As Finger (1978) has pointed out, strategy failures may be due simply to a shift in response preference; thus adaptive failures may not be due to a loss of function but, rather, to application of a faulty strategy. Eliciting repsonses by means of alternate but relevant cues should also favor generalization of function recovery to different environments. The neuropsychological literature is lacking in validation studies that emphasize ecologic criteria (but see McSweeney et al., 1985). This point seems especially important for work with older individuals, who may exhibit reduced ability to utilize new strategies or respond to novel stimuli, even in the absence of demonstrable neurologic disease.

Secondary Mechanisms in Cerebrovascular Infarction

Within days of onset of cerebrovascular infarction, considerable cerebral edema or brain swelling occurs as a function of the lesion size. It may produce distant effects due to compression of and displacement of brain tissue. With pharmacologic intervention and time, edema subsides and the infarct becomes progressively more identifiable as the tissue becomes necrotic. This factor is probably of minimal consequence except in studies where the baseline data are obtained very early. The factor is operative with other etiologies as well, such as closed head injury, especially in severe forms (Hardman, 1979). Both experimental animal and clinical studies have revealed prolonged bilateral reduction of cerebral blood flow for a period of at least several weeks following a cerebrovascular episode (Meyer et al., 1970; Fujishima et al., 1974). Cortical hypoperfusion has been demonstrated in reversible "subcortical" aphasia, suggesting that recovery of language function in such cases may be due to the resolution of transient cortical hypoperfusion (Olsen et al., 1986). This conclusion was derived from evidence of normal regional cerebral blood flow (rCBF) in ten patients with subcortical lesions who were not aphasic. Reperfusion of hypoperfused areas is assumed to underlie many early recovery changes due to the resumption of adequate function in compromised but uninfarcted surrounding tissue. Also, the availability of collateral circulation through patent vessels varies significantly across individuals and in different regions of the cerebral hemispheres. The exact circumstances involving collateral circulation are usually unknown except as inferred from clinical deficits or revealed by angiographic studies.

CODETERMINANTS OF RECOVERY

The determinants of the immediate and prolonged effects of stroke are determined by a number of neurologic and individual specific variables, such as the location of the lesion, extent or severity of neurologic involvement, the specific hemodynamic circumstances surrounding the occurrence of the infarct, age at onset, time since symptom onset when measurements are made, the relative rate of recovery of affected functions, variations related to cerebral dominance, and premorbid cerebral status as inferred from environmental, life style or direct neuropathologic assays.

Lesion Localization

Much of the early neuropsychological research on the localization of higher cortical functions is based on the effects of acute cerebrovascular infarction. This literature also involves assessment of the effects of removal of focal, static, and atrophic lesions, usually of early origin, that have produced focal seizure disorders. However, as noted by others in this volume, there may be some particular advantages to studying the effects of focal strokes. Infarction in the distribution of small branches of arterial territories may result in restricted lesions, which may provide the opportunity for studying neurobehavioral systems in which one focal component is compromised. In contrast, the lesion characteristics in other populations may create difficulties in the theoretical interpretation of results. For example, patients with seizure disorders with early onset may have abnormal patterns of development of hemispheric specialization. Therefore development of models of higher cognitive function based on such populations may not necessarily generalize to other groups without such ontogenetic influences.

Many of the studies of higher cognitive functions have emphasized the systematic analysis of the behavioral effects of focal and circumscribed lesions and, in some studies, the longitudinal course of some functions. It is beyond the scope of this chapter to provide detailed descriptions of the tests utilized in such studies. Useful references are available for such information (Milner, 1964, 1971; Teuber, 1975; Luria, 1980; Lezak, 1983; Meier and Thompson, 1983). Clinical syndrome descriptions have been derived primarily from patients immediately after stroke. The most extensive literature relates to the aphasias, apraxias, and neglect as reviewed by Geschwind (1965) and others (Goodglass and Kaplan, 1972; Luria, 1980; Heilman and Valenstein, 1985). In addition to syndrome delineation, it is also important to emphasize that patients with focal strokes have been useful for the development of models of brain function and organization (Posner, 1988; see also Chapter 13). The studies of neurobehavioral deficit and recovery of function have focused primarily on several areas of the association cortex. The areas that have been most frequently implicated in regard to higher cognitive function deficit in these studies includes the frontal/prefrontal, inferolateral/mesial temporal, and posterior temporoparietal association regions.

Frontal/Prefrontal Region

Quantitative neuropsychological studies of the effects of focal frontal and prefrontal lesions have demonstrated a wide range of impairments. These deficits include productivity or executive functions and may be nonspecific or specific (hemisphere-dependent). There may be a deficit in abstract reasoning and categorical thinking, especially where there is involvement of the lateral convexity. The tests most likely to demonstrate such a deficit include sorting procedures, such as the Wisconsin Card Sorting Test (Milner, 1964). Beyond the severe, nonfluent aphasia produced by a lesion in Broca's area, there may be less dramatic declines of expressive language functions such as selective changes in verbal associative fluency as measured by the Oral Word Association Test (Borkowski et al., 1967). Comparable changes in associative fluency have been demonstrated with right prefrontal involvement utilizing a figural production task such as generating forms that cannot be encoded verbally (Jones-Gotman and Milner, 1977). Some aspects of attentional dysfunction may appear and may be related to reduced exploratory visual functioning (Teuber, 1964). Impaired regulatory control of more complex psychomotor functions necessary for adequate goal-directed behavior may lead to gross declines in planning and foresight abilities as reflected in reduced maze-solving ability (Porteus, 1959). They may be compounded by disturbances in perceptual organization due to right hemisphere involvement (Critchley, 1953; Benton, 1979). There may be evidence of an abnormally brief response to personal failure experiences in addition to judgmental lapses, impulsivity, and euphoria associated with orbital-basal lesions (Teuber, 1964). Combined declines in planning, initiative, and elaborate volitional processes may be disabling even with relatively intact information processing and general intellectual functioning (Hebb and Penfield, 1940; Milner, 1964).

When information processing and general intellectual functions undergo significant recovery, the patient may give the impression of being more competent to engage in purposeful choice situations and exercise adequate judgment than may be possible. Executive functions have not been studied extensively in cerebrovascular recovery, though it can be assumed that these changes are among the last to recover. They are likely to be the most severe with bilateral frontal disease or with preexisting diffuse disease in an individual who sustained a cerebrovascular infarct. They may be less critical in the patient with a unilateral prefrontal lesion, but they can be demonstrated with unilateral disease of other etiologies, such as closed head injury or partial complex seizure disorders of anterior origin (Milner, 1971). Such deficits may account for the frequent failure of generalizability of recovery changes (as measured or as observed during rehabilitation) to natural environments.

Anterior Infero/Mesial Temporal Region

Involvement or removal of the anterior temporal lobe has been associated with material-specific learning and memory deficits but relatively intact planning and executive functioning. More acutely, such lateralized effects on learning and memory may be obscured by language or visual spatial disorders, depending on the site of the cerebrovascular infarction or atrophic lesion. Unilateral ablations result in reasonably good recovery, though subtle and persisting deficits in verbal learning and memory have been shown after left temporal lobectomy and nonverbal memory after right temporal lobectomy (Milner and Teuber, 1968; Milner, 1971). These conspicuous material-specific deficits in learning and recent memory functioning are directly related to the extent of hippocampal removal (Milner, 1964). Deficits in verbal and visuospatial processing are not excessive after unilateral ablation and tend to be of little consequence except with large ablations that may intrude on the posterior information-processing zones of the posterior and superior portion of the temporal lobes (Milner, 1964).

With unilateral cerebrovascular accidents, the lesions are rarely limited to the anterior temporal region, so that the immediate effects are more pronounced and characteristically produce a more posterior focal syndrome that involves either verbal or visuospatial processing deficits due to dysfunction of the posterior temporoparietal region. When an infarction produces a posterior syndrome, resolution with recovery might yield the misleading impression that other higher functions subserved by the posterior portions of the hemispheres are intact. Verbal and nonverbal learning and memory test procedures should be included in any battery in order to evaluate for such a possible outcome pattern and inferred residual anterior temporal lobe dysfunction, for example. Many of the personality disturbances seen in cerebrovascular disease may also be related to lesions in this region, as both affective and ideational disturbances have been observed with involvement of the anterior and mesial temporal regions, though evidence is equivocal (Stevens and Hermann, 1981). If a cerebrovascular lesion limited to this region were encountered, information processing and perceptual deficits would be expected to be minimal, though even in such cases in the epilepsy literature some evidence of complex visual discrimination and facial recognition deficits have been demonstrated (Meier and French, 1965; Milner, 1971). The immediate and widespread effects of a lesion in this region might well produce demonstrable language or visuospatial deficits acutely. Recovery would be expected to be relatively rapid; but with resolution of any presenting syndrome, memory deficits and personality changes might be present on a more prolonged basis.

Posterior Temporoparietal Region

Unlike anterior temporal and prefrontal lesions, posterior lesions are more likely to produce sizable discrepancies between verbal and visuospatial abilities on conventional intellectual tests and neuropsychological test batteries (Reitan, 1964; Meier, 1970). Verbal-visuospatial discrepancies may be present independently of somatosensory or motor deficits, as posterior lesions may spare such functions, although they frequently produce visual field defects (Benton, 1979). Lesions that invade the somatosensory cortex produce rather discrete changes that may be more focally represented in the left hemisphere than the right (Semmes et al., 1960; Semmes, 1968), although contradictory findings have been reported (Carmon, 1971). Nevertheless, posterior lesions produce the most consistent and predictable changes in neurologic and neuropsychological measures of any region within the cerebral hemispheres. For example, numerous information-processing deficits have been demonstrated including facial recognition (Warrington and James, 1967; Benton and Van Allen, 1971), visuospatial judgment (Benton et al., 1978); closure of incomplete figures, letters, and shapes (Kinsbourne and Warrington, 1963), rod and line-slope matching tasks (DeRenzi et al., 1971; Taylor and Warrington, 1973), and stylus maze performances (Milner, 1964; Ratcliff and Newcombe, 1973). The presence of visual field defects is associated with more severe deficits of visuospatial and visuoconstructional functioning, presumably because of larger and deeper lesions (DeRenzi et al., 1977). Personality changes appear to constitute a reaction to the more conspicuous deficits associated with posterior association lesions (Friedman, 1950). Although "denial" of neurologic involvement or deficit is an exception, it tends to be seen only in acutely involved individuals after cerebrovascular infarction whose body image distortions may be too severe to perceive the nature of the neuropsychological deficit (Critchley, 1953).

It should come as no surprise that small, circumscribed lesions produce less severe, briefer deficits (Kertesz and McCabe, 1977; Mazzochi and Vignolo, 1979). The advent of computed tomography (CT) and magnetic resonance imaging (MRI) has made it possible to measure the extent of the infarction more directly and precisely. Such indications of severity probably provide the single best neurologic predictor of outcome. For example, the severity of neglect was shown to increase with both the size of the lesion and the degree of premorbid diffuse cortical atrophy after right cerebral infarction (Levine et al., 1986). The severity of and recovery from left hemispatial neglect was dependent more on the integrity of the left cerebral hemisphere than on the extent of right cerebral hemisphere involvement. This study demonstrated the importance of estimating premorbid cerebral status by means of CT measurements and indirectly by means of covariates such as age, gender, educational level and dominance.

Age

The significance of age as a factor in recovery is more completely established for closed head injury, where persisting memory deficits, attentional dysfunction, confabulation, and secondary focal deficits in cognitive, psychomotor, and personality deficits are more severe in older individuals. Clinical experience suggests that younger stroke patients (below age 60) have a more favorable recovery course and a much higher likelihood of returning to at least a semiautonomous level of functioning in the community. Because head injuries occur with greater frequency in younger individuals, the age level for predicting a poor outcome may be much lower. When there is overlap in age between subgroups of stroke and head injury patients, the prognosis may vary as a function of age. The outlook appears to be much worse for a head-injured individual, for example, in the 50- to 60-year age group (assuming that other determining factors are equal in influence). However, a stroke patient in the same age group (again assuming that other factors are equal in influence) might carry a much better prognosis.

An essential methodologic issue when studying age differences during recovery relates to the difficulty of establishing functions during normal aging. As in disease states affecting the nervous system, "normal" aging may occur differently in different individuals. Facilitative factors may protect against age-related declines in visuospatial, visuoconstructional, and memory functioning with age (Benton, 1981; Bornstein and Suga, 1988). Individuals with high initial ability levels tend to survive longer and to achieve higher performance levels as they age (Schaie, 1970; Botwinick, 1977). Similarly, people of higher educational level may survive longer to achieve the same result.

The norms of neuropsychological tests are characteristically established on a cross-sectional basis, which introduces a higher likelihood of overestimating the degree of deficit that would occur normally with age. Such norms confound age and cohort-related effects and yield a gradient of earlier and steeper decline of function in people in their sixties and seventies (Schaie and Schaie, 1977). In normal aging studies, such declines are seen especially on speeded psychomotor and nonverbal functions, which are known to be affected by cerebral disease, including stroke. The life-span developmental psychology literature has identified the problems of measurement involved in establishing norms for tests in clinical use, including many standardized neuropsychological tests. Age norms should be established for each new test developed.

Valid age norms require that age (ontogenetic), cohort-related (generational), and historical (time of measurement) factors be separated in order to provide an accurate gradient of performance related to age. It will be necessary to identify age-related determinants of change and recovery in order to quantify neuropsychological deficits and to design appropriate intervention strategies to reverse, slow, or facilitate the development of compensatory strategies.

Studies of the relation between age and recovery in stroke have been inconsistent. Vignolo (1964) reported greater improvement in aphasics under age 40 years compared with a group 60 years of age or older. Similarly, Sands and colleagues (1969) reported greater language recovery in a subgroup under 50 years of age. Other reports, however, have failed to confirm these findings (Culton, 1969; Sarno and Levita, 1971; Kertesz and McCabe, 1977). There is some evidence of a higher incidence of Broca's aphasia than Wernicke's and global aphasias in younger stroke patients (Obler et al., 1978; Eslinger and Damasio, 1981; Kertesz and Shephard, 1981), although it may be related to different etiologies of stroke in younger and older patients. Schechter et al. (1985) reported an age difference at 4 to 5 months after onset but failed to find differences between these aphasic syndromes at 1 month post-stroke. They reported a higher correlation between the presence of auditory verbal comprehension deficits and age and concluded that there is a shift in the age–syndrome relation during the recovery period, which has negative implications for recovery in the older individual. Thus as the recovery process proceeds, a selective factor that predisposes the older individual to a clearer congruency with global or Wernicke's aphasia may appear; and it may reflect a differential pattern of recovery, with older patients obtaining less recovery of posterior and global language function. After failing to demonstrate an age effect in early studies, Wade and Langton Hewer (1986) conducted an analysis of covariance to identify the influence of age on initial function loss and cognitive and social function at 6 months. With a larger sample, they reported that the older stroke patients had greater initial disability (as measured by Barthel Activities of Daily Living scores), greater disability at 6 months, and lower social functioning at 6 months (Frenchay Activities Index). It is apparent that age does not operate in a unitary manner and interacts with other facilitative or detrimental factors associated with later development.

Gender

Gender differences in lateral specialization of function are somewhat controversial (McGlone, 1980; Inglis and Lawson, 1981; Bornstein, 1984; Herring and Reitan, 1986). When reported, these differences are reflected in relatively greater superiority of verbal processing abilities in women. Visuospatial integration and abstract nonverbal processes have been favored in men. However, there is considerable overlap in the distributions of these functions in large samples. In children, both males and females evidence lateralized asymmetries in hemisphere structure and function (Witelson and Pallie, 1973; Wada, 1976). The influence of gender on recovery is not well understood if in fact it plays a role at all. Like age, gender may interact with a variety of environmental factors, incremental and decremental, to influence the recovery course. Such interactions may be expressed as differences in aptitude, motivation, and strategy (McGlone, 1980). The methodologic difficulties associated with the definition of higher cortical functions become even more germane when determining sex-related differences with their multitude of cultural and biologic determinants (Caplan et al., 1985).

Longitudinal studies of recovery have not revealed striking sex differences. It has been argued that women have a wider representation of cerebral language functions than men, which accounts for a lower incidence of aphasia in women (McGlone, 1977). More recent studies, however, have not demonstrated gender differences in the incidence of aphasia. Thus when adjusting the incidence of aphasia in women for the relatively lower incidence of stroke, the male-female difference in the incidence of aphasia disappears (Kertesz and McCabe, 1977; Kertesz and Shepherd, 1981). There have been reports of a higher incidence of Broca's and global aphasias among men (Brust et al., 1976; Eslinger and Damasio, 1981). However, Vignolo et al. (1986) reported a striking double dissociation between anterior versus posterior lesions and gender in a group of global aphasics. In patients with circumscribed lesions, global aphasia was associated with anterior lesions in women and posterior lesions in men. When lesions were deep or less circumscribed, the gender difference did not appear. This discrepancy was regarded as consistent with a report by Kimura (1980) of a higher incidence of anterior lesions in female aphasics and posterior lesions in males. The latter study did not involve global aphasics but nevertheless adds to the basis for pursuing gender differences in localization and recovery.

Demographic Variables

Neuropsychological performance, irrespective of direct effects of lesions, is related to individual characteristics such as education, socioeconomic level, vocational choice, and ethnicity. Methodologic consideration of these and other determinants in clinical research and application are discussed elsewhere (Parsons and Prigatano, 1978; Meier and Thompson, 1983). These factors rarely represent primary determinants and may interact with the entire range of other determining conditions for characterizing the course of recovery. Highly overlearned and practiced functions may be represented more redundantly and, accordingly, may be subject to less initial impairment and more rapid recovery. Earlier longitudinal studies did not reveal a major effect of demographic variables. For example, Smith (1981) found no relation between educational level or occupational status and recovery after hemispherectomy. These variables, however, may help explain unexpected outcomes in terms of both the initial effects of the lesion and recovery. Demographic considerations may reflect underlying factors that may interact especially with age, as higher educational and socioeconomic levels have been associated with better maintenance of higher cortical functions in older individuals (Benton, 1981; Bornstein and Suga, 1988). Thus these variables may indirectly represent incremental or detrimental effects on neuropsychological functioning. Such factors might usefully be incorporated into clinical formulations as moderating variables as the literature increases our understanding of their effects, singly or in combination, on recovery patterns (Meier and Thompson, 1983). Although such variables probably operate with limited influence, their consideration is obviously necessary for understanding atypical or unexpected characteristics of the neuropsychological data and are particularly relevant for rehabilitation planning and decision making.

Cerebral Dominance

An important source of individual differences in the organization of function may be cerebral dominance. It is well accepted that most right-handers are left-cerebral dominant for language and right-cerebral dominant for visuospatial functioning. It is also increasingly accepted that these functional dichotomies are relative, rather than absolute. For example, a number of studies have identified right hemisphere capacities in language functions (Segalowitz, 1983). Despite the well lateralized nature of cerebral dominance in right-handers, there are exceptions among right-handers who occasionally are right-hemisphere-organized for speech. It is generally acknowledged that in left-handers patterns of hemispheric specialization tend to be more variable, suggesting that higher cortical functions may more often be bilaterally represented, though perhaps not symmetrically in this group. This point may well account for the reports of a more rapid and extensive recovery of language functioning in left-handed aphasics despite the greater incidence of language deficits with lesions in either hemisphere in this group (Sarno and Levita, 1971). Several studies have shown that left-handers as well as right-handers with a history of familial left-handedness show a greater degree and rate of recovery (Gloning et al., 1969; Subirana, 1969; Luria, 1970). Conflicting findings are not unexpected, as the effect of any single determining factor among these covariates could easily be overridden by the presence of an alternative factor at a higher level of expression.

QUANTITATIVE LONGITUDINAL ASSESSMENT OF NEUROPSYCHOLOGICAL RECOVERY

Several studies have contributed to the establishment of a conceptual base and for evaluating neuropsychological recovery (Bond and Brooks, 1976; Bach-y-Rita, 1981; Newcombe, 1982; Rothi and Horner, 1983; Long et al., 1984). Studies of recovery of function in humans have been either cross-sectional or longitudinal in design. Cross-sectional studies examine neuropsychological functioning at a single point in time following a specified time interval since symptom onset. Longitudinal studies evaluate change in a function or set of functions over time and from a baseline set of measurements obtained at a specified point in time following symptom onset and again at intervals extending over months and years. Cross-sectional studies do not yield a direct analysis of the inferred recovery process and relate more to an understanding of the effects of a given etiology when behavioral outcomes are contrasted with those of an appropriate control group. Longitudinal studies permit inferences about the recovery process but confound time (or developmental) effects with practice owing to repeated measurements. Both types of study yield useful information for predicting the natural course of recovery and for designing intervention strategies that may be adjusted for recovery changes as they evolve in the treatment process. Benton (1979) provided a summary of cross-sectional studies of the cognitive consequences of closed head injury. Similarly, Levin et al. (1982) reviewed the cross-sectional and longitudinal studies of memory, intellectual, language, perceptual, psychomotor, and psychosocial consequences of head injury. Excellent reviews exist for both basic and applied research on attentional deficits (Gummow et al., 1983) and for the entire range of neuropsychological functions after closed head injury (Newcombe, 1982). The corresponding literature on cerebral vascular disease is not as extensive, possibly owing to the less central place of behavioral research in funded programs. Nevertheless, some primary sources are available (Benton, 1968).

Quantitative studies of recovery of function are based on group data that may mask individual differences, particularly if the patient pool is heterogeneous with respect to the covariates underlying these differences, as is typically the case in clinical populations (Bond and Brooks, 1976). Newcombe and Ratcliff (1979) analyzed recovery curves for specific linguistic functions in individual head-injured patients and found that there was variability despite overall similarities in the recovery curves. Hiorns and Newcombe (1979) derived a recovery curve that could be described in simple mathematic terms but found that the formula oversimplified the entire recovery process, making the curves potentially misleading when applied to describing the longitudinal course of recovery in a particular patient. Studies of the natural history of neuropsychological recovery characteristically show that the mean recovery function reaches an asymptote after an accelerated rate of recovery during the early stages after an injury or cerebrovascular accident (Meier et al., 1982; Newcombe, 1982). The rate of gain slows at 6 months to 1 year; but, again, there are wide individual differences in the length of time following injury during which recovery changes are likely to occur. Although these group curves are relatively consistent and replicable, they do not encompass the late recovery changes that have been reported in some individuals. Late recovery changes appear to occur most frequently in the highest cognitive functions such as language (Geschwind, 1974). (Brooks et al., 1984) identified some general methodologic principles for interpreting sequential studies of neuropsychological recovery. Their guidelines embraced the derivation of follow-up schedules, the selection and definition of the function being measured, the selection of patient and control groups, the control of practice effects, and the optimal length of a follow-up study. Although their work was based largely on head injury, their guidelines apply equally to the design of sequential studies of recovery in stroke. Methodologic issues in single case and intervention design have not been addressed in stroke research. An extensive analysis of the methodologic issues in single case design are available in the head injury literature, however (Gordon, 1987).

Quantitative longitudinal studies of neuropsychological recovery after stroke were initially done in rehabilitation settings where the baseline testing for subsequent follow-up was established 6 months or more after symptom onset. Many of the spontaneous recovery changes, particularly in sensory and motor functions, have already occurred by that time. Nevertheless, some limited predictability of rehabilitation outcome was demonstrated late in the recovery period (Anderson et al., 1970; Ben-Yishay et al., 1970). The establishment of cerebrovascular research centers during the 1960s permitted investigation of the predictability of behavioral outcomes from baselines established early in the recovery period (Meier and Resch, 1967; Benton, 1968; Meier, 1970). Kertesz (1979) reviewed much of the behavioral neurologic and neuropsychological literature on recovery from aphasia in studies that included substantial numbers of patients with cerebrovascular disease. A small number of quantitative follow-up investigations involving neuropsychological test batteries have been reported since 1980.

Kinsella and Ford (1980) explored unilateral spatial neglect as a predictor of functional recovery. The procedures were not specified but were alleged to include quantitative measures of neglect, constructional, motor, planning, reasoning, learning, and memory functioning plus the Norwick Park Activities of Daily Living Index (Sheikh et al., 1979). The finding that unilateral spatial neglect at 4 weeks was predictive of poorer activities of daily living (ADL) outcomes at 12 weeks may have resulted from confounding lesion size with this clinical sign, as it tends to appear more frequently with larger lesions, particularly in the posterior parietal region. ADL and motor recovery changes exceeded those observed for the various cognitive abilities assessed in their (undescribed) battery. Follow-up interval was limited to 12 weeks and is probably not sufficient to determine the extent of cognitive recovery (Meier et al., 1982). The hypothesis that unilateral spatial neglect, independent of the primary hemisphere involved or other lesion variables, is predictive of a less adequate outcome remains to be confirmed.

In another longitudinal study of unilateral spatial neglect (Levine et al., 1986), the severity of neglect increased as a function of the size of the lesion and the degree of diffuse cortical atrophy as inferred from CT scans to have been present premorbidly. Neglect was assessed initially 2 to 4 weeks after right cerebral infarction and again 3 to 5 months post-stroke utilizing the copy trial of the Rey-Osterrieth Complex Figure (Lezak, 1983), a line crossing task (Albert, 1973), a horizontal line bisecting task, a paragraph reading task, and a writing to dictation task. Severe neglect persisted only in patients with marked cortical atrophy. Anatomic criteria were established for indexes of lateral ventricular size and lesion size derived from CT scans. Severity of neglect did not correlate with age, but older patients had smaller lesions. This study represents another instance of the interaction of subject characteristics and lesion variables complicating interpretation of the data. Nevertheless, the data clearly showed that persistent left neglect was a function of both lesion size and the relative integrity of the unaffected (left) cerebral hemisphere.

In a longitudinal investigation of a nonhemorrhagic, thrombotic stroke sample, Meier et al. (1982) confirmed the utility of a Porteus Maze Test Age of 8 for predicting psychomotor and cognitive recovery in 6 months. Early neurologic studies suggested that sensory and motor changes tend to reach an asymptote at about 6 weeks (Twitchell, 1951; van Buskirk, 1954). Repeated measures of fine manipulative dexterity, index finger tapping speed, ballistic arm tapping rates, and tactually guided form placements tended to confirm these earlier impressions, as substantial recovery changes, particularly in those patients who had evidenced a Porteus Test age of 8 or more within 1 week of the episode, occurred by the 2-month follow-up assessment on such functions. Isolated patients within the subsamples continued to show some improvement at the 6-month follow-up so that the variability tended to reduce the overall predictability of change. Of additional interest is the fact that this cutting score (Porteus Maze age score of 8), which had shown some validity in predicting rated neurologic outcome, was also able to predict the recovery of verbal comprehension (Token Test), language processing (Aphasia Screening Test), and visuoconstructional functioning in the same patients. Recovery of these higher order functions appeared substantially later, toward the end of the 6-month period. This study demonstrated that neuropsychological measures can be used as dependent variables to quantify and predict subsequent changes.

In a study that was limited to right hemisphere strokes (Hier et al., 1983) the relatively early recovery from unilateral spatial neglect was confirmed. However, an unexpectedly greater recovery rate of constructional apraxia, unilateral neglect, and motor impersistence was noted in the hemorrhagic stroke subgroup. This subgroup, however, was also shown to have smaller lesions and consisted of younger patients. It seems likely that hemorrhagic strokes in *surviving* patients are likely to be relatively more circumscribed and less debilitating over the long term unless there is some recurrence (as seen in multiinfarct dementia, for example). The study underscores the need to control the many covariates that may influence the recovery course. It also confirms the importance of establishing an early baseline for monitoring recovery.

Repeated follow-up assessments were carried out (five over 1 year) in a study (Meerwaldt, 1983) of patients with right posterior lesions. The study demonstrated that quickly administered tests of rod (DeRenzi et al., 1971) and line orientation (Benton et al., 1978) can yield a description of the recovery course that correlates with rated neurologic changes. Their findings of a relation between lesion size and recovery speed is consistent with other data. The rod orientation test was a better predictor of recovery and apparently was better correlated with lesion size. The study confirmed the characteristic course of recovery during the first 6 months after stroke.

The detrimental implications of age, extent of neurologic involvement, and degree of impairment of cognitive and memory abilities in predicting outcome was again demonstrated in an extensive study by Kotila et al. (1984). A characteristic negatively accelerated recovery curve that reached an asymptote at approximately 6 months to 1 year was observed for deficits in intellectual (WAIS), memory (Wechsler Memory Scale and Benton Visual Retention Test), and other "visuoperceptual" and "speech and language tasks." Like most studies in this area, the sample included a combination of hemorrhagic and thrombotic strokes. Because they covary with other variables, the neurologic and neuropsychological outcomes should be profiled separately. This study provided useful new information insofar as outcome was measured independently by means of ADL and return-to-work criteria. The hemorrhagic subgroup again showed a better recovery. However, when hemorrhagic patients were compared with age-matched thrombotic infarction patients, there were no differences in outcome. Despite the use of well known tests, specific quantitative information was not included in the report. This point is a common shortcoming in studies in this area. Nevertheless, the results are relatively consistent across these studies, suggesting that quantitative assessment approaches may yield valid predictors of the longitudinal course of recovery in individual patients, particularly when the many covariates that contribute to the determination of individual differences in outcome can be measured and incorporated into the predictive equations.

More recent research has focused on left cerebral infarctions and the recovery of language functions in aphasic patients. In an attempt to determine the relation between nonverbal IQ and language recovery, David and Skilbeck (1984) reported a negative relation between Ravens Colored Progressive Matrices performance and severity of aphasia as measured by the Functional Communication Profile (Sarno, 1969) and selected measures from the Minnesota Test for the Differential Diagnosis of Aphasia (Schuell, 1965). Baseline data were obtained at least 4 weeks post-stroke.

All patients were part of a controlled speech therapy trial, so that treatment was confounded with recovery effects. Milder aphasics had a more regular recovery curve and appeared to plateau earlier. However, after parceling out the effects of initial severity of aphasia, there was no relation between initial nonverbal IQ and recovery of functional communication skills. Similarly, there was no relation between nonverbal IQ and the Schuell scores. The results were considered inconsistent with previous reports (Bailey et al., 1981), but baselines were established much later, at approximately 5 months post-stroke in that study. IQ was related to the ability to walk independently at initial assessment and survival to at least 6 months. The Ravens IQ was interpreted to reflect stroke severity. It may also not constitute a pure measure of nonverbal intelligence, as the relation between Ravens IQ and lesion volume (Basso et al., 1987b) disappeared in this study when the effect of lesion volume was corrected for auditory verbal comprehension level. Many aphasics probably do not have the necessary auditory verbal comprehension to understand the instructions and the nature of the task and may fail for that reason. More specific nonverbal tasks were proposed to pursue a more direct test of the relation between nonverbal IQ and language recovery. Papanicolaou et al. (1988) provide evoked potential data to suggest right hemisphere involvement in recovery from aphasia.

Basso et al. (1987a) followed 26 patients, examined initially between 15 and 30 days after onset for a period of months. Patients with left hemisphere infarctions were selected for the presence of ideomotor apraxia (IMA) based on a 24-item test (DeRenzi et al., 1980) and automatic and intentional movements. The latter consisted of movements of the whole arm and hand or fingers, single or in sequence, meaningful or meaningless, which the patient had to imitate with the hand ipsilateral to the lesion. Patients were reassessed in 5 months and compared with a bilateral lesion group that performed the test with the left arm. On the basis of the Token Test score and the Standard Language Examination (Basso et al., 1979) patients were classified for severity, relative fluency, phrase length, rate of speech, articulation, and melodic line. The patients were also subdivided by lesion size on CT scan. An extended improvement course was observed but was not related to age, education, gender, type of aphasia, initial severity, or size of lesion. Recovery was greater with sparing of the posterior parietal and occipital regions, indicating that regions elsewhere within the left hemisphere and possibly also certain right hemisphere structures might participate in recovery. Type of aphasia (fluent or nonfluent) had no effect on recovery. Patients with anterior lesions tended to recover earlier, although the patients with posterior left hemisphere involvement (and more severe IMA) also evidenced substantial recovery. Recovery from IMA was correlated with recovery from oral apraxia to a greater extent than with the Token Test performance or Raven's IQ. The deficits in oral apraxia or IMA were not always present in combination, so they may be distinct deficits. However, they may be related to a common neural substrate or progressively disassociable effects of left anterior and posterior lesions, respectively. The focus of this study was on the conditions necessary for recovery to fail to occur. Although size of lesion did not predict the recovery course (some patients with large lesions eventually returned to normal levels), relations between IMA scores and other neuropsychological test variables (e.g., Porteus Maze, Tactual Performance Test) might conceivably yield greater predictability of IMA recovery.

Knopman et al. (1984) conducted a 6-month prospective study in 54 patients with left hemisphere stroke as part of a larger study of recovery of function (Rubens et al., 1984). The assessment included the confrontation naming subtest of the Boston Diagnostic Aphasia Examination (Goodglass and Kaplan, 1972), Token Test, single-word comprehension (Selnes et al., 1984), long-term memory (Risse et al., 1984), and fluency in spontaneous speech (Knopman et al., 1983). Baseline evaluations were done about 1 month post-stroke and revealed that almost all of the patients had moderate to severe dysnomia. Patients with large lesions (60 cm^3) were most likely to demonstrate persisting oral naming deficits at 6 months. As expected, more severe initial deficits were associated with poorer recovery. Some ability to name on confrontation at 1 month was associated with the best recovery. Essentially complete concordance between oral and written naming at 1 month was noted with the exception of one patient who reached a normal level of oral naming at 3 months despite severe initial deficits. Confrontation naming at 6 months tended toward a bimodal distribution, with about 30% continuing to demonstrate severe deficits. Oral and written naming remained highly correlated at 6 months. Adequate single-word comprehension at 1 month was associated with a more favorable recovery of oral naming. Early recovery of fluency by patients with impaired oral naming at 1 month was not predictive of recovery of oral naming at 6 months. This finding suggested dissociation of confrontation naming and fluency during the recovery process. The authors postulated the presence of multiple mechanisms (semantic and phonologic) associated with location of the lesion in either the posterior superior temporal region or the insula-putamen to account for this dissociation and for the types of error (retrieval failures versus linguistic errors in naming) in naming failure. Consistent with other studies of naming impairment (Kertesz and Benson, 1970; Cappa et al., 1981) lesions in the temporal lobe produced the most severe naming impairment, whereas nontemporal lobe lesions (insula and putamen) were related to naming impairments in some fluent patients. Knopman and colleagues concluded that phonologic errors are more related to involvement of the supramarginal gyrus, whereas semantic errors are more likely to result from lesions in the posterior superior temporal gyrus and the infrasylvian portion of the supramarginal gyrus. Deeper lesions also produced anomia, consistent with other reports (Damasio et al., 1982). Not surprisingly, the largest constraint on ultimate level of recovery was lesion size. Small lesions were related to milder initial deficits in confrontation naming, less initial impairment of word comprehension, and better recovery over 6 months.

One of the most extensive studies of the neurobehavioral recovery process following stroke was conducted by Rubens et al. (1984). The study attempted to elucidate the factors associated with return of language function. It included assessment of multimodal language, verbal/nonverbal memory and cognition, neurologic status, and CT scan as well as dichotic listening, cerebral blood flow, and the electroencephalogram. A group of 54 patients with left cerebrovascular accidents were examined at monthly intervals for several months. Overall, the mean percent change between month 1 and month 6 was about 20% across language modalities, which consisted in auditory comprehension, verbal expression, repetition, and word finding. The time course of recovery for all language variables was characterized by the observation that about 70% of the eventual improvement was attained by 3 months with word finding continuing to show improvement after the others had reached asymptote.

Although there were substantial individual differences in patterns of recovery, some generalizations could be drawn. Patients could be grouped into categories according to their characteristic patterns of change. For example, patients with initially severe deficits but good recovery on verbal expression also tended to show the same pattern in the areas of repetition and word finding. Examination of the relation between initial language measures and language scores at outcome (6 months later) revealed that "auditory comprehension" was consistently related to outcome measures both within and across major language modalities. In fact, auditory comprehension was deemed the best overall predictor of language outcome for all aphasia subtypes. Another general finding was that recovery could occur in auditory comprehension without a corresponding improvement in verbal expression, but the reverse was never true. Also, the prognosis for recovery of auditory comprehension was consistently better than that for verbal expression. Early performance on the various (verbal memory) tests in most cases did not appreciably add to the predictive utility of outcome beyond the month 1 language scores themselves. Also, without exception, patients with large lesions performed more poorly as a group on these verbal memory measures than those with small lesions (60 cm^3 or less).

On measures involving nonverbal cognition, it was consistently found that patients with severe early language impairment and comparably low scores on perceptual and "associative" tests (e.g., Spreen-Benton Embedded Figures or Sound Recognition) had a poor prognosis for recovery. In fact, Sound Recognition was among the few variables that added to the prediction at month 6 of language outcome beyond the information provided by month 1 language scores themselves.

All patients were impaired on nonverbal cognitive tests that required concept formation and logical deduction. Furthermore, nonverbal cognitive tests (at all levels of difficulty) correlated with language outcome if comparisons were being made within the low or high ends of the severity continuum. That is, patients scoring initially very low or very high on nonverbal cognitive tests tended to show comparable levels of performance across measures at 6 months. For patients falling within the moderate range of language performance acutely, the relations were less clear, and no predictive utility of initial nonverbal cognitive test scores was realized.

Visual field deficits and dense hemiparesis or hemiplegia correlated highly with lesion volumes and overall aphasia severity. The presence of severe visual field defect or severe buccofacial apraxia (on demonstration) were negative prognostic signs and contributed additionally to the prediction of outcome on language functioning and verbal expression, respectively. Response to verbal axial commands was a positive prognostic sign and added meaningfully to the prediction of outcome on auditory comprehension.

Lesion size strongly predicted language outcome. Grouping patients with lesion sizes below and above 60 cm^3 separated most patients with persistently severe verbal expression and auditory comprehension deficits at month 6 from those who attained higher levels. Finally, although lesion volume was important in determining the amount of overall recovery, it did not appear to be critically related to the rate of recovery.

CONCLUDING STATEMENT

The prediction of recovery based on quantitative neuropsychological tests constitutes a continuing challenge for clinical neuropsychologists and behavioral neurologists. The progress noted during the 1980s was substantial but fell short of providing predictors of high accuracy for projecting individual recovery course. The data clearly confirm earlier expectations that an individual differences model for predicting outcome in cerebrovascular disease requires control of the many covariates that contribute to outcome in addition to the more direct contributing factors such as lesion size, location, and premorbid cerebral status. Future research is expected to focus on combinations of determinants, the selection of which might be profitably guided by the robustness of a given variable as a potential predictor in research to date. These determinants may include subject characteristics (e.g., age, education) or disease-related variables such as a pathophysiologic mechanism (hemorrhagic versus thromboembolic). Certain studies have added significantly to the information base in this area of research, and application of this information should lead to further investigation. As predictors are identified, the moderating effects of cognitive remediation could then be determined. Identification of the boundary conditions within which recovery can occur would then be more feasible. Also, such predictors should be related to performance in different environments whose adaptive requirements can be specified in operational terms. Any indications of ecologic validity of neuropsychological predictors would enhance the role and effectiveness of clinical neuropsychologists in neurologic and rehabilitation settings.

REFERENCES

Adametz, J.H. (1959). Role of recovery of functioning in cats with rostal reticular lesions. *J. Neurosurg.,* **16,** 85–98.

Albert, M. (1973). A simple test of visual neglect. *Neurology,* **23,** 658–654.

Anderson, T.P., Boureston M., and Greenberg F.R., (1970). Rehabilitation Predictors in Completed Stroke: Final Report. Kenny Rehabilitation Institute, SRS Grant No. RD-1757-M-68-C3.

Bach-y-Rita, P. (1981). Central nervous system lesions; sprouting and unmasking in rehabilitation. *Arch. Phys. Med. Rehabil.,* **62,** 413–417.

Bailey, S., Powell, G.E., and Clark, E. (1981). A note on intelligence and recovery from aphasia: relationship between Raven's Matrices scores and change on the Schuell Aphasia Test. *Br. J. Disord. Commun.,* **16,** 193–203.

Basso, A., Capitani, E., and Vignolo, L.A. (1979). Influence of rehabilitation on language skills in aphasic patients: a controlled study. *Arch. Neurol.* 36, 190–196.

Basso, A., Capitani, E., Della Sala, S., Laiacona, M., and Spinnler, H. (1987a). Recovery from ideomotor apraxia: a study on acute stroke patients. *Brain,* **110,** 747–760.

Basso, A., Della-Sala S., and Farabola, M. (1987b). Aphasia arising from purely deep lesions. *Cortex,* **23,** 29–44.

Benton, A.L., ed. (1968). *Behavioral Change in Cerebrovascular Disease.* New York: Harper & Row.

Benton, A.L. (1979). Visuoperceptive, visuospatial and visuoconstructional disorders. In: K.M.

Heilman and E. Valenstein, eds., *Clinical Neuropsychology,* pp. 186–232. New York: Oxford University Press.

Benton, A.L. (1981). Aspects of the neuropsychology of aging. Invited Address, Division 40, American Psychological Association. Los Angeles.

Benton, A.L., and Van Allen, M.W. (1971). Prosapagnosia and facial discrimination. *J. Neurol. Sci.,* **15,** 167–172.

Benton, A.L., Varney N.R., and deS Hamsher, K. (1978). Visuospatial judgement. *Arch. Neurol.,* **35,** 364–367.

Ben-Yishay, Y., Gerstman, L., Diller, L., and Haas, A. (1970). Prediction of rehabilitation outcomes from psychometric parameters in left hemiplegics. *J. Consult. Clin. Psychol.,* **34,** 436–441.

Bond, M.R., and Brooks, D.N. (1976). Understanding the process of recovery as a basis for the investigation of rehabilitation for the brain injured. *Scand. J. Rehabil. Med.,* **8,** 127–133.

Bornstein, R.A. (1984). Unilateral lesions and the Wechsler Adult Intelligence Scale—Revised: no sex differences. *J. Consult. Clin. Psychol.,* **52,** 604–608.

Bornstein, R.A., and Suga, L.J. (1988). Educational level and neuropsychological performance in healthy elderly subjects. *Dev. Neuropsychol.* **4,** 17–22.

Borowski, J.G., Benton, A.L., and Spreen, O. (1967). Word fluency and brain damage. *Neuropsychologia,* **5,** 135–140.

Botwinick, J. (1977). Intellectual abilities. In: J.E. Birren and K.W. Schaie, eds., *Handbook of the Psychology of Aging,* pp. 580–605. New York: Van Nostrand Reinhold.

Brooks, D.N., Deelman, B.G., van Zomeren, A.H., van Dongen, H., van Harskamp, F., and Aughton, M.E. (1984). Problems in measuring cognitive recovery after acute brain injury. *J. Clin. Neuropsychol.,* **6,** 71–75.

Brust, J., Shafer, S., Richter, R., and Brunn, B. (1976). Aphasia in acute stroke. *Stroke,* **7,** 167–174.

Cannon, W.F., and Rosenblueth, A. (1949). *The Supersensitivity of Denervated Structures: A Law of Denervation.* New York: Macmillan.

Caplan, P.J., MacPherson, G.M., and Tobin, P. (1985). Do sex-related differences in spatial abilities exist? A multilevel critique with new data. *Am. Psychologist,* **40,** 786–799.

Cappa, A., Cavalotti, G., and Vignolo, L.A. (1981). Phonemic and lexical errors in fluent aphasia: correlation with lesion site. *Neuropsychologia,* **19,** 171–177.

Carmon, A. (1971). Disturbances in tactile sensitivity in patients with cerebral lesions. *Cortex,* **7,** 83–97.

Cattell, R.B. (1963). Theory of fluid and crystallized intelligence: an initial experiment. *J. Educ. Psychol.,* **105,** 105–111.

Critchley, M. (1953). *The Parietal Lobes.* London: Edward Arnold.

Culton, G.L. (1969). Spontaneous recovery from aphasia. *J. Speech Hear. Res.,* **12,** 825–832.

Damasio, A.R., Damasio, H., Rizzo, M., Varney, N., and Gersh, F. (1982). Aphasia with nonhemorrhagic lesions of the basal ganglia and internal capsule. *Arch. Neurol.,* **39,** 15–20.

David, R.M., and Skilbeck, C.E. (1984). Raven IQ and language recovery following stroke. *J. Clin. Neuropsychol.,* **6,** 302–308.

DeRenzi, E., Faglioni, P., and Scott, G. (1971). Judgment of spatial orientation in patients with focal brain damage. *J. Neurol. Neurosurg. Psychiatry,* **34,** 489–495.

DeRenzi, E., Faglioni, P., and Villa, P. (1977). Topographical amnesia. *J. Neurol. Neurosurg. Psychiatry,* **40,** 498–505.

DeRenzi, E., Motti, F., and Nichelli, P. (1980). Imitating gestures: a quantitative approach to ideomotor apraxia. *Arch. Neurol.,* **37,** 6–10.

Eslinger, P.J., and Damasio, A.R. (1981). Age and type of aphasia in patients with stroke. *J. Neurol. Neurosurg. Psychiatry,* **44,** 377–381.

Finger, S., ed. (1978). *Recovery from Brain Damage: Research and Theory.* New York: Plenum.

Finger, S., and Stein, D.G. (1982). *Brain Damage and Recovery.* Orlando: Academic Press.

Friedman, S.H. (1950). Psychometric effects of frontal and parietal lobe damage. Unpublished doctoral dissertation, University of Minnesota.

Fujishima, M., Tanaka, K., Takeya, Y., and Omae, T. (1974). Bilateral reduction of hemispheric blood flow in patients with unilateral cerebral infraction. *Stroke,* **5,** 648–653.

Geschwind, N. (1965). Disconnection syndromes in animals and man. *Brain,* **88,** 237–294, 584–644.

Geschwind, N. (1974). Late changes in the nervous system: an overview. In: D. Stein, J. Rosen, and N. Butters, eds., *Plasticity and Recovery of Function in the Central Nervous System,* pp. 467–508. Orlando: Academic Press.

Gloning, I., Gloning, K., Haub, G., and Quatember, R. (1969). Comparison of verbal behavior in right-handed and non-right-handed patients with anatomically verified lesions of one hemisphere. *Cortex,* **5,** 43–52.

Goldman, P.S. (1974). An alternative to developmental plasticity: heterology of CNS structures in infants and adults. In: D. Stern, J. Rosen, and N. Butters, eds., *Plasticity and Recovery of Function in the Central Nervous System.* pp. 149–174. Orlando: Academic Press.

Goodglass, H., and Kaplan, E. (1972). *Assessment of Aphasia and Related Disorders.* Philadelphia: Lea & Fibiger.

Gordon, W. (1987). Methodological considerations in cognitive remediation. In: M.J. Meier, A.L. Benton, and L. Diller, eds., *Neuropsychological Rehabilitation.* New York: Churchill Livingstone.

Gummow, L., Miller, P., and Dustman, R.E. (1983). Attention and brain injuiry: a case for cognitive rehabilitation of attentional deficits. *Clin. Psychol. Rev.,* **3,** 255–274.

Hardman, J.M. (1979). The pathology of traumatic brain injuries. *Adv. Neurol.,* **22,** 15–50.

Hebb, D.O., and Penfield, W. (1940). Human behavior after extensive bilateral removals from the frontal lobes. *Arch. Neurol. Psychiatry,* **44,** 421–438.

Heilman, K.M., and Valenstein, E. (1985). *Clinical Neuropsychology,* 2nd ed. New York: Oxford University Press.

Herring, S., and Reitan, R.M. (1986). Sex similarities in verbal and performance IQ deficits following unilateral cerebral lesions. *J. Consult. Clin. Psychol.,* **54,** 537–541.

Hier, D.B., Mondlock, J., and Caplan, C.R. (1983). Recovery of behavioral abnormalities after right hemisphere stroke. *Neurology,* **33,** 345–350.

Hiorns, O., and Newcombe, F. (1979). Recovery curves: uses and limitations. *Int. Rehabil. Med.,* **1,** 173–176.

Inglis, J., and Lawson, J.S. (1981). Sex differences in the effects of unilateral brain damage on intelligence. *Science,* **212,** 693–695.

Jones-Gotman, M., and Milner, B. (1977). Design fluency: the invention of nonsense drawings after focal cortical lesions. *Neuropsychologia,* **15,** 653–673.

Kennard, M. (1938). Reorganization of motor function in the cerebral cortex of monkeys deprived of motor and premotor areas in infancy. *J. Neurophysiol.,* **1,** 477–496.

Kertesz, A., and Benson, D.F. (1970). Neologistic jargon: a clinicopathological study. *Cortex,* **6,** 362–386.

Kertesz, A. (1979). Recovery and treatment. In: K.M. Heilman and E. Valenstein, eds., *Clinical Neuropsychology,* pp. 503–534, New York: Oxford University Press.

Kertesz, A., and McCabe, P. (1977). Recovery patterns and prognosis in aphasia. *Brain,* **100,** 1–18.

Kertesz, A., and Sheppard, A. (1981). The epidemiology of aphasic and cognitive impairment in stroke. *Brain,* **104,** 117–128.

Kimura, D. (1980). Sex differences in intra-hemispheric organization of speech. *Behav. Brain Sci.,* **3,** 240–241.

Kinsbourne, M., and Warrington, E.K. (1963). Localizing significance of limited simultaneous form perception. *Brain,* **86,** 699–702.

Kinsella, G., and Ford, B. (1980). Acute recovery patterns in stroke patients: neuropsychological factors. *Med. J. Aust.,* **2,** 663–666.

Knopman, D.S., Selnes, O.A., Niccum, N., and Rubens, A.B. (1983). A longitudinal study of speech fluency in aphasia: CT scan correlates of recovery and persistent nonfluency. *Neurology,* **33,** 1170–1178.

Knopman, D.S., Selnes, O.A., Niccum, N., and Rubens, A.B. (1984). Recovery of naming in aphasia: relationship to fluency, comprehension and CT findings. *Neurology,* **34,** 1461–1470.

Kotila, M., Waltimo, O., Niemi, M.L., Laaksonen, R., and Lempinen, M. (1984). The profile of recovery from stroke and factors influencing outcome. *Stroke,* **15,** 1039–1044.

Lavy, S., Melamed, E., and Portnoy, Z. (1975). The effect of cerebral infarction on the regional cerebral blood flow of the contralateral hemisphere. *Stroke,* **6,** 160–163.

Levin, H.S., Benton, A.L., and Grossman, R.G. (1982). *Neurobehavioral Consequences of Closed Head Injury.* New York: Oxford University Press.

Levine, D.N., Warach, J.D., Benowitz, L., and Calvanio, R. (1986). Left spatial neglect: effects of lesion size and premorbid brain atrophy on severity and recovery following right cerebral infarction. *Neurology,* **36,** 362–366.

Lezak, M.D. (1983). *Neuropsychological Assessment,* 2nd ed. New York: Oxford University Press.

Long, C.J., Gouvier, W.D., and Cole, J.C. (1984). A model of recovery for the total rehabilitation of individuals with head trauma. *J. Rehabil.,* **50,** 39–45.

Luria, A.R. (1963). *Restoration of Function After Brain Injury.* Oxford: Pergamon.

Luria, A.R. (1970). *Traumatic Aphasia.* The Hague: Mouton.

Luria, A.R. (1980). *Higher Cortical Functions in Man,* 2nd ed. New York: Basic Books.

Mazzocchi, F., and Vignolo, L.A. (1979). Localization of lesions in aphasia: clinical CT-scan correlations in stroke patients. *Cortex,* **15,** 627–654.

McGlone, J. (1977). Sex differences in the cerebral organization of verbal functions in patients with unilateral lesions. *Brain,* **100,** 775–793.

McGlone, J. (1980). Sex differences in human brain asymmetry: a critical review. *Behav. Brain Sci.,* **3,** 215–263.

McSweeney, A.J., Grant, I., Heaton, R.K., Prigatono, G.P., and Adams, K.M. (1985). Relationship of neuropsychological status to everyday functioning in healthy and chronically ill persons. *J. Clin. Exp. Neuropsychol.,* **7,** 281–291.

Meerwaldt, J.D. (1983). Spatial disorientation in right-hemisphere infarction: a study of the speed of recovery. *J. Neurol. Neurosurg. Psychiatry,* **46,** 426–429.

Meier, M.J. (1970). Objective behavioral assessment in diagnosis and prediction. In: A.L. Benton, ed., *Behavioral Change in Cerebrovascular Disease,* pp. 119–154. New York: Harper & Row.

Meier, M.J., and French, L.A. (1965). Changes in MMPI scale scores and an index of psychopathology following unilateral temporal lobectomy in epilepsy. *Epilepsia,* **6,** 263–273.

Meier, M.J., and Resch, J.A. (1967). Behavioral prediction of short-term neurologic change following acute onset of cerebrovascular symptoms. *Mayo Clin. Proc.,* **42,** 641–647.

Meier, M.J., and Thompson, W.G. (1983). Methodological issues in clinical studies of right cerebral hemisphere dysfunction. In: J.B. Hellige, ed., *Cerebral Hemisphere Asymmetry: Method, Theory, and Application,* pp. 46–94. New York: Praeger.

Meier, M.J., Ettinger, M.C., and Arthur, L. (1982). Recovery of neuropsychological functioning after cerebrovascular infarction. In: R. Malatesha and L. Hartlage, eds., *Neuropsychology and Cognition,* Vol. 2, pp. 552–564. NATO Advanced Study Series. The Hague: Martinus Nijhoff.

Meyer, J.S., Shinohara, Y., Kanda, T., Fukuuchi, Y., Ericsson, A.D., and Kok, N.K. (1970). Diaschisis resulting from acute unilateral cerebral infarction. *Arch. Neurol.,* **23,** 241–247.

Milner, B. (1964). Some effects of frontal lobectomy in man. In: J.M. Warren and K. Akert, eds., *The Frontal Granular Cortex and Behavior,* pp. 313–334. New York: McGraw-Hill.

Milner, B. (1971). Interhemispheric differences in localization of psychological processes in man. *Br. Med. Bull.,* **27,** 272–277.

Milner, B., and Teuber, H.-L. (1968). Alteration of perception and memory in man: reflections on methods. In: L. Weiskrantz, ed., *Analysis of Behavior Change,* pp. 268–375. New York: Harper & Row.

Moore, R.Y. (1974). Central regeneration and recovery of function: the problem of collateral reinnervation. In: D.G. Stein, J.J. Rosen, and N. Butters, eds., *Plasticity and Recovery of Function in the Central Nervous System,* pp. 111–128. New York: Academic Press.

Newcombe, F. (1982). The psychological consequences of closed head injury: assessment and rehabilitation. *Injury,* **14,** 111–136.

Newcombe, F., and Ratcliff, G. (1979). Long-term psychological consequences of cerebral lesions. In: M. Gazzaniga, ed., *Handbook of Behavioral Neurobiology,* Vol. 2, pp. 495–540. New York: Plenum Press.

Obler, L.K. Albert, M.L., Goodglass, H., and Benson, F.D. (1978). Aphasia type and aging. *Brain Lang.,* **6,** 318–322.

O'Connor, M., and Cermak, L. (1987). Rehabilitation of organic memory disorders. In: M.J. Meier, A.L. Benton, and L. Diller, eds., *Neuropsychological Rehabilitation.* New York: Churchill Livingstone.

Olsen, T.S., Bruhn, P., and Oberg, R.G. (1986). Cortical hypoperfusion as a possible cause of "subcortical aphasia." *Brain,* **109,** 393–410.

Papanicolaou, A.C., Moore, B.D., Deutsch, G., Levin, H.S., and Eisenberg, H.M. (1988). Evidence for right hemisphere involvement in recovery from aphasia. *Arch. Neurol.,* **45,** 1025–1029.

Parsons, O.A., and Prigatano, G.P. (1978). Methodological considerations in clinical and neuropsychological research. *J. Consult. Clin. Psychol.,* **46,** 609–619.

Porteus, S. (1959). *The Maze Test and Clinical Psychology.* Palo Alto: Pacific Books.

Posner, M.I. (1988). Structures and functions of selective attention. In: T. Boll and B.K. Bryant, eds., *Clinical Neuropsychology and Brain Function: Research, Measurement and Practice,* pp. 173–202. Washington, D.C.: American Psychological Association.

Ratcliff, G., and Newcombe, F. (1973). Spatial orientation in man: effects of left, right and bilateral posterior cerebral lesions. *J. Neurol. Neurosurg. Psychiatry,* **36,** 448–454.

Reitan, R.M. (1964). Psychological deficits resulting from cerebral lesions in man. In: J.M. Warren and K. Akert, eds., *The Frontal Granular Cortex and Behavior,* pp. 295–312. New York: McGraw-Hill.

Risse, G.L., Rubens, A.B., and Jordan, L.S. (1984). Disturbances of long-term memory in aphasic patients: a comparison of anterior and posterior lesions. *Brain,* **107,** 605–617.

Rosner, B.S. (1970). Brain functions. *Annu. Rev. Psychol.,* **21,** 555–594.

Rothi, L.J., and Horner, J. (1983). Restitution and substitution: two theories of recovery with application to neurobehavioral treatment. *J. Clin. Neuropsychol.,* **5,** 73–81.

Rubens, A., Selnes, O., Risse, G., Niccum, N., and Jordan, L. (1984). *A Comprehensive Study of Language Recovery Process in Adults with Aphasia Following a Cerebrovascular Accident.* Final Report. Bethesda: NINCDS (DH & HS), contract N01-NS-02378.

Sands, E., Sarno, M.T., and Shankweiler, D. (1969). Long-term assessment of language function in aphasia due to stroke. *Arch. Phys. Med. Rehabil.,* **50,** 202–207.

Sarno, M.T. (1969). *The Functional Communication Profile: Manual of Directions. Rehabilitation Monographs,* **42.** New York Institute of Rehabilitation Medicine.

Sarno, M.T., and Levita, E. (1971). Natural course of recovery in severe aphasia. *Arch. Phys. Med. Rehabil.,* **52,** 175–186.

Schaie, K.W. (1970). A reinterpretation of age-related changes in cognitive structure and functioning. In: C.R. Goulet and P.B. Baltes, eds., *Life-Span Developmental Psychology: Research and Theory,* pp. 485–507. Orlando: Academic Press.

Schaie, K.W., and Schaie, J.P. (1977). Clinical assessment and aging. In: J.E. Birren and K.W. Schaie, eds., *Handbook of the Psychology of Aging,* pp. 692–723. New York: Von Nostrand Reinhold.

Schechter, I., Schejter, J., Abarbanel, M., Grosswasser, Z., and Solzi, P. (1985). Age and aphasic syndromes. *Scand. J. Rehabil. Med.,* **12,** 60–63.

Schuell, H. (1965). *The Minnesota Test for the Differential Diagnosis of Aphasia.* Minneapolis: University of Minnesota Press.

Segalowitz, S.J., ed. (1983). *Language Functions and Brain Organization.* Orlando: Academic Press.

Selnes, O.A., Niccum, N., Knopman, D.S., and Rubens, A.B. (1984). Recovery of single word comprehension: CT-scan correlates. *Brain Lang.,* **21,** 72–84.

Semmes, J. (1968). Hemispheric specialization: a clue to mechanism. *Neuropsychologia,* **6,** 11–26.

Semmes, J., Weinsten, S., Ghent, L., and Teuber, H.L. (1960). *Somatosensory Changes After Penetrating Brain Wounds in Man.* Cambridge: Harvard University Press.

Sheikh, K., Smith, S., Meade, T., Goldenberg, E., Brennan, P., and Kinsella, G. (1979). Repeatability and validity of a modified activities of daily living (ADL) index in studies of chronic disability. *Int. J. Rehabil. Med.,* **1,** 51–58.

Slater, R., Reivich, M., Goldberg, H., Banka, R., and Greenberg, J. (1977). Diaschisis with cerebral infarction. *Stroke,* **8,** 684–690.

Smith, A. (1977). Dominant and nondominant hemispherectomy. In: M. Kinsbourne and W.L. Smith, eds., *Hemispheric Disconnection and Cerebral Function,* pp. 5–33. Springfield: Charles C Thomas.

Smith, A. (1981). Principles underlying human brain functions in neuropsychological sequelae of different neuropsychological processes. In: S.B. Filskov and T.J. Boll, eds., *Handbook of Clinical Neuropsychology,* pp. 175–226. New York: Wiley.

Stein, D.B., Rosen, J.J., and Buttles, N., eds. (1974). *Plasticity and Recovery of Function in the Nervous System.* Orlando: Academic Press.

Stein, D.G., Finger, S., and Hart, T. (1983). Brain damage and recovery: problems and perspectives. *Behav. Neural Biol.,* **37,** 185–222.

Stevens, J.R., and Hermann, B.P. (1981). Temporal lobe epilepsy, psychopathology and violence: the state of the evidence. *Neurology,* **31,**1127–1132.

Subirana, A. (1969). Handedness and cerebral dominance. In: P. Vinken and G. Bruyn, eds., *Handbook of Clinical Neurology,* Vol. 4, pp. 248–272. New York: Elsevier.

Taylor, A.M., and Warrington, E.K. (1973). Visual discrimination in patients with localized lesions. *Cortex,* **9,** 82–93.

Teuber, H.L. (1964). The riddle of frontal lobe function in man. In: J.M. Warrent and K. Akert, eds., *The Frontal Granular Cortex and Behavior,* pp. 410–444. New York: McGraw-Hill.

Teuber, H.L. (1975). *Recovery of Function After Brain Injury in Man,* pp. 159–190. Ciba Foundation Symposium 34. Amsterdam: North Holland Elsevier-Excerpta Medica.

Twitchell, T. (1951). The restoration of motor function following hemiplegia in man. *Brain,* **74,** 443–480.

Valentino, M.L., and Stein, D.G. (1983). Do rats have hypotheses? A developmental and means-ends approach to brain damage, recovery of function and aging. In: S. Scheff, ed., *Aging and Recovery of Function,* pp. 129–152. New York: Plenum Press.

Van Buskirk, C. (1954). Return of motor function in hemiplegia. *Neurology,* **4,** 919–928.

Vignolo, L.A. (1964). Evolution of aphasia and language rehabilitation: a retrospective exploratory study. *Cortex,* **1,** 344–367.

Vignolo, L.A., Boccardi, E., and Caverni, L. (1986). Unexpected CT-scan findings in global aphasia. *Cortex,* **22,** 55–59.

Von Monakow, C. (1969). Die lokalisation in grosshirn und der abbau der funktion durch korticale herde. In: K.H. Pribram, ed., *Mood States and Mind.* London: Penguin.

Wada, J. (1976). Cerebral anatomical asymmetry in infant brains: symposium on sex differences in brain asymmetry. Presented at the meeting of the International Neuropsychological Society, Toronto.

Wade, D.T., and Langton Hewer, R. (1986). Stroke: associations with age, sex, and side of weakness. *Arch. Phys. Med. Rehabil.,* **67,** 540–545.

Warrington, E.K., and James, M. (1967). An experimental investigation of facial recognition in patients with unilateral lesions. *Cortex,* **3,** 317–326.

Witelson, S.F., and Pallie, W. (1973). Left hemisphere specialization for language in the newborn: neuroanatomical evidence for asymmetry. *Brain,* **96,** 641–647.

Yakovlev, P.I. (1971). Neuroanatomical variants and neurological symptomatology. Invited address to the Department of Neurology, University of Minnesota Medical School.

15

Behavioral Correlates of Cerebral Revascularization

ANNE D. BAIRD

The chief aim of surgical revascularization procedures is to prevent a first or recurrent thromboembolic stroke, but questions also have arisen about behavioral benefits from these techniques. It is important but difficult to separate these two effects of surgery and to distinguish carefully between the heterogeneous revascularization procedures.

REVASCULARIZATION PROCEDURES

In the oldest of the cerebral revascularization procedures, carotid endarterectomy (CE), an incision is made in the extracranial portion of the internal carotid artery to remove an atherosclerotic blockage. In the neurologic and neurosurgical literature, there is continued discussion of the efficacy of this widely used procedure, particularly in view of surgical morbidity rates sometimes reported to be as high as 24% in the past (Patterson, 1987) and in view of the age and limitations of the large clinical trial done during the 1960s (Hachinski, 1987; Jonas, 1987).

Progress in neurosurgical technique has led to the development of other revascularization procedures, such as superficial temporal to middle cerebral artery (STA-MCA) bypass. Typically, STA-MCA bypass involves an intracranial anastomosis between a branch of the middle cerebral artery and the superficial temporal artery, a vessel that supplies the scalp. This procedure is used to provide additional cortical blood flow when one of three conditions exists: complete occlusion of the extracranial internal carotid artery, stenosis or occlusion of the intracranial portion of the internal carotid artery, and stenosis or occlusion of the middle cerebral artery.

Posterior fossa revascularization includes both extracranial procedures, chiefly vertebral endarterectomy and vertebral-to-carotid transposition, and intracranial bypasses, primarily anastomoses between the occipital artery and the superior cerebellar artery (SCA), the anterior inferior cerebellar artery (AICA), or the posterior inferior cerebellar artery (PICA). Surgical reports emphasize the difficulty of these procedures, which require long, tedious dissections of branch arteries deep in the brain stem and circumvention of the rich arterial plexus and the cranial nerves in the immediate area (Ausman et al., 1986a,b). The rich network of collateral vessels in the posterior fossa provides good protection against completed stroke when there are only isolated areas of stenosis. Because of the technical difficulty of these procedures and the protection afforded by collateral circulation, patients who undergo posterior fossa revascularization typically have experienced many, sometimes nearly continual, transient ischemic attacks (TIAs). Candidates for these procedures usually have multiple stenoses within the larger vessels of the vertebrobasilar arterial system, and have failed to obtain control of the symptoms with anticoagulant medications.

Neuropsychological studies of cerebral revascularization (Figure 15–1) candidates have shown that their preoperative level of behavioral impairment on average is mild, although the level of performance varies from normal to severely impaired (Dull et al., 1982). Most patients chosen for one or more of these procedures have had TIAs; a smaller number have had reversible ischemic neurologic deficits (RINDs) and minor strokes. Few patients who have had major strokes undergo cerebral revascularization, as it is presumed that there is little remaining viable brain tissue in the affected arterial territory. Histologic study has indicated that the transition between necrotic and normal areas is abrupt in patients with large, chronic infarcts, whereas a border zone including nonfunctional but viable neurons is thought to exist in patients with milder ischemic insults (Wedergaard et al., 1985). Among patients who subsequently undergo cerebral revascularization, neurobehavioral summary scores (e.g., average impairment ratings) and general screening measures (e.g., the WAIS Digit Symbol subtest score) correlate significantly with the duration of the longest ischemic episode before surgery (Dull et al., 1982) and with the severity and dissemination of atherosclerosis on the cerebral angiogram (Baird et al., 1985). However, one study suggested an absence of clear-cut differences between cerebral revascularization candidates with symptoms and angiographic findings primarily referable to the carotid arterial system versus candidates whose histories and radiographic results showed pathology predominantly in the vertebrobasilar arterial system (Baird et al., 1984).

REVIEW OF THE LITERATURE

Carotid Endarterectomy

Before 1980, some neuropsychological follow-up studies of CE patients showed gains in psychological test scores after surgery (Duke et al., 1968; Horne and Royle, 1974; Perry et al., 1975; Haynes et al., 1976; King et al., 1977). Most authors reported considerable variability in gains among patients, and several studies did not include unoperated groups or other assessment of practice effects. Moreover, in three studies

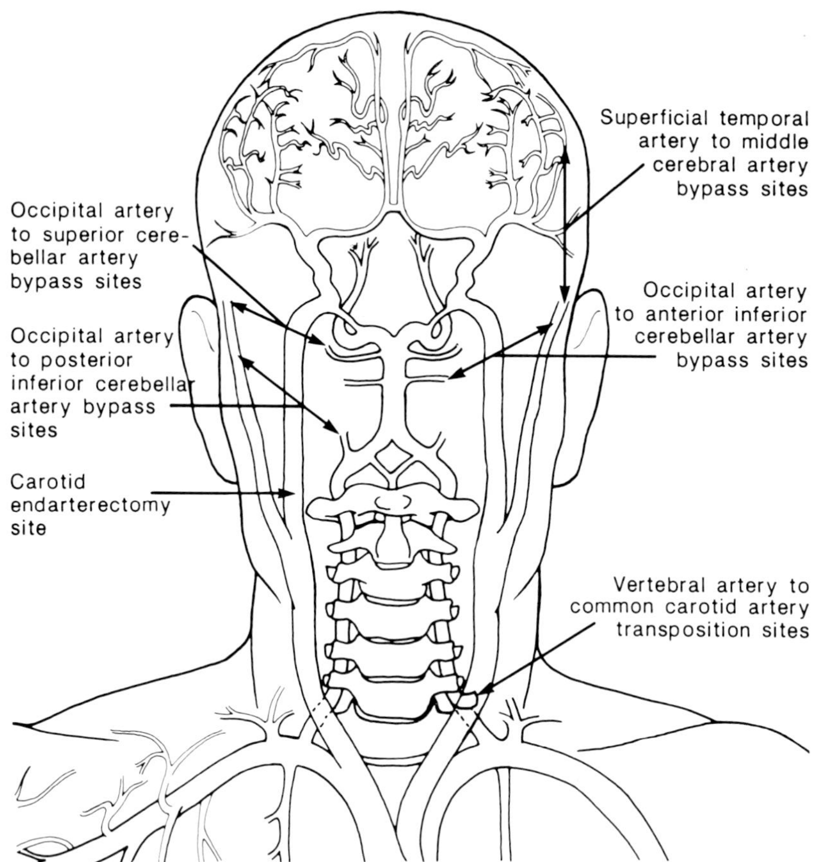

Figure 15–1 Common sites of cerebral revascularization. (Reproduced with permission of the Henry Ford Neurosurgical Institute, 1988.)

the authors interpreted small postoperative gains as most likely reflecting practice effects (Goldstein et al., 1970; Matarazzo et al., 1979) or relief from preoperative anxiety (Williams and McGee, 1964).

During the 1980s most studies of CE patients continue to show either no change (Boeke, 1981; Parker et al., 1983; Diener et al., 1984; Casey, 1989), or positive gains after surgery (Kelly et al., 1980; Bornstein et al., 1981a; Hemmingsen et al., 1982, 1986; Jacobs et al., 1983). Several authors have observed mild neuropsychological decrements in subsets of CE patients tested at 1 week or less after surgery (Owens et al., 1980; Brinkman et al., 1984; Cushman et al., 1984). These neuropsychological decrements correlated with small infarcts on computed tomography (CT) scans in the study by Owens et al. (1980) and with reduced cortical somatosensory evoked potentials in reports by Cushman et al. (1984) and Brinkman et al. (1984).

A number of studies have identified factors that correlate with behavioral status after CE. Unfortunately, the factors identified vary from study to study. In some cases multiple factors have been emphasized in one or more reports from the same center. Bornstein et al. (1981a) suggested that patients undergoing right CE improved more than those with left or bilateral CE; but the right CE group also contained more stroke patients, who had larger postoperative gains than TIA patients. In a different report, Bornstein and colleagues (1981b) suggested that serum glucose, serum cholesterol, hematocrit, and diastolic blood pressure correlated with postoperative gains, whereas hemoglobin did not correlate with improvement but did correlate with preoperative impairment. Jacobs et al. (1983) suggested that patients with hemodynamically significant lesions were more likely to show postsurgical gains than patients not fitting the criteria for low flow-endangered brain. In a more recent report from the same center, the authors emphasized that side of surgery was a determinant of postsurgical neuropsychological improvement (Greiffenstein et al., 1988). Relative to patients whose endarterectomies were postponed or canceled and those undergoing left CE, patients with right CE showed gains on a composite score derived from performance on tests deemed sensitive to attention and speed, i.e., the finger tapping, trail making, and digit-symbol substitution tests. Hemmingsen and coworkers (1982), using a different method to determine hemodynamic significance, did not find that it was a variable that significantly moderated postoperative recovery.

In a retrospective study, Trudel and colleagues (1984) found a modest negative correlation between the presence of medical risk factors preoperatively and global functional impairment 6 to 8 years after surgery. The medical factors included were severe obesity, chronic obstructive pulmonary disease, congestive heart failure, severe hypertension, and angina pectoris or myocardial infarction within the past 6 months. Unlike Bornstein et al. (1981b), Trudel's group (1984) did not address the issue of postoperative change nor did they describe their subjects' quality of life before surgery. However, together these studies suggest that medical risk factors, whether determined by laboratory test values or clinical diagnosis, probably have a negative relation with the level of adaptive functioning after CE.

Whereas most studies have focused on patients with lateralized ischemic episodes before surgery, Stark and Wodak (1983) described symptomatic relief in four patients who underwent CE for transient global changes in mental status as a result of orthostatic hypotension and carotid stenosis or occlusion. In addition to intermittent confusion and various other symptoms that occurred with standing, two of the four patients reported a chronic intellectual decline before surgery. Unfortunately, the authors failed to present psychological test data.

Several authors found evidence of lateralized improvement within the postsurgical test profiles of CE patients. Owens et al. (1980) found postoperative improvement in finger-tapping only on the side contralateral to surgery. Hemmingsen and his coworkers (1982) did not use the sensorimotor tests usually deemed most sensitive to lateralization, but they still found evidence of more gains in functions thought to be primarily subserved by the hemisphere that underwent operation. Specifically, patients who had left CEs improved on word pairs, trail making, and story recall, whereas patients with right CEs tended to show gains on visual gestalt, block design, and digit span subtests. A more recent study by the same group (Hemmingsen et al., 1986) also found general improvement in CE patients compared to age-matched patients with peripheral vascular disease, but gains were larger on measures judged to tap functions in the hemisphere ipsilateral to the operated carotid artery.

Four negative studies have included extensive neuropsychological batteries. Three of the four studies included comparison groups to control for age, education, practice, and other variables. Boeke's (1981) study involved cholecystectomy patients as a comparison group; the endarterectomy group included only TIA patients. The CE patients were less impaired and admitted to less emotional stress preoperatively than the cholecystectomy group. On one of eight measures, a verbal fluency test, Boeke found a significant interaction between groups and occasions, but he concluded that there was no overall selective improvement of the CE group 1 month postoperatively. Five patients who were retested 4.5 months after surgery showed no further gains on inspection of scores.

Parker and his associates (1983) studied CE patients and a separate group who either refused surgery or were inappropriate for surgery in other ways. The authors claimed there were no differences between the operated and nonoperated groups in terms of the incidence of fixed neurologic deficits and severe carotid narrowing, as well as age, education, and preoperative Full Scale IQ. A third control group underwent surgery not related to cerebrovascular disease. At 6-month follow-up, improvement on most test variables was observed across groups, but there was no group by trials interaction on any of 22 neuropsychological variables or on the Profile of Mood States and the Sickness Impact Profile, a life quality index. A report extending the follow-up to 2 years yielded essentially the same results (Parker et al., 1986).

A study by Casey and colleagues (1989) found no differential gains in TIA patients who underwent right or left CE compared to controls who also presented with TIAs but did not show the pattern or degree of carotid stenosis indicative of potential benefit from surgery. The researchers achieved unusually good control of several relevant dimensions. Equal numbers of right CE, left CE, and control patients were enrolled as subjects. The three groups were similar in age and education and on baseline intelligence test scores. To reduce the possibility that natural recovery might contribute to improvement over the follow-up interval, Casey et al. excluded potential subjects with abnormal neurologic examination results or with focal CT scan findings. During follow-up, the three groups improved equally on five intellectual, memory, attentional, sensory, and motor test scores, whereas no significant changes occurred on ten other measures. The authors concluded that practice effect was the most feasible explanation for the gains observed.

In a study of 23 patients seen before and 10 months after CE, Diener and coworkers (1984) concluded that, on average, surgery did not result in behavioral improvement. Although they did note gains on an intelligence task, performance on a memory test deteriorated, and scores on ten other measures were unchanged.

In several series of studies performed at the same centers, initial findings of postoperative improvement in CE patients have not held up with further study involving a longer follow-up period, a larger sample, or additional measures. A preliminary report by Fraser and colleagues (1983) reported early improvement in CE patients that was not sustained by those patients seen at a later follow-up date. Although the authors reported gains in intelligence and memory test scores in 35 patients seen 6 months after CE, these gains were erased in 15 patients followed to 18 months after surgery. Whereas studies by Hemmingsen, Boysen, and their colleagues consistently have reported cognitive gains after CE, the most recent study found a lack of correspondence between improvement on neuropsychological tests and evidence of physiologic recovery on CT scans and regional cerebral blood flow (Hemmingsen et al., 1982, 1986; Boysen et al., 1983). Finally, an initial study of 28 patients from the

Wadsworth Veterans Administration Medical Center reported a trend toward improvement 3 to 6 months after CE in 24 patients, even though five of these patients had silent infarcts 3 to 7 days after surgery and showed deterioration when tested at that time (Owens et al., 1980). Of these 24 patients 23 had preoperative carotid stenoses of more than 50% on the side of surgery. A later study of 45 patients without prior strokes but with at least 75% stenosis of the carotid on the side of surgery reported that a trend toward neuropsychological improvement during the perioperative period was followed by a return to the presurgical level of performance 3 months after surgery (Bennion et al., 1985). No significant postoperative changes were found in a group of 18 patients who had strokes before surgery.

STA-MCA Bypass

Although the first STA-MCA bypass procedures were done in 1967 by Yasargil (Tanahashi et al., 1985), the first psychological studies of changes following extracranial-intracranial arterial bypass (EIAB) did not appear until 1976 when Ferguson and Peerless published an abstract summarizing four case histories, and Evans and Austin (1976) reported on a series of 14 patients.

Ferguson and Peerless (1976) claimed significant intellectual improvement in three of four patients with multiple extracranial occlusions who underwent STA-MCA bypass. The test battery, scores, follow-up period, and enrollment procedure were not specified. All four patients were said to have dementia preoperatively, but the abstract did not specify how these patients were selected from their total sample of bypass patients. The authors termed the improvement as "modest" for one subject, "moderate" for another, and "dramatic" for a third. The fourth patient, said to be "vegetative" preoperatively, did not change appreciably after surgery. Psychological improvement obviously correlated with increased adaptive functioning: One patient regained the ability to walk.

Other reports of series of cases also suggested improvement in preoperative neurologic deficits and in quality of life (Peerless et al., 1977; Lee et al., 1980). In a report published in 1977, Peerless et al. indicated that one-half of their patients with "dementia" before undergoing STA-MCA bypass showed improvement after surgery.

Published case studies of STA-MCA bypass candidates have documented dramatic postoperative reversal of fixed neurologic deficits, including aphasia (Jacques and Garner, 1976), hemiplegia (Macon and Rice, 1985), and visual field deficits (Roski et al., 1978; Benzel and Mirfarkhraee, 1987). In the only report that presented extensive quantitative psychological test data, Hart and colleagues (1985) described a remarkable clearing of transcortical sensory aphasia from administration of the Boston Diagnostic Aphasia Examination 4 days before surgery to retesting 2 days after bypass. Because the patient's deficits had been stable or worsening for 3 months before operation, the authors reasoned that practice effects or natural recovery were unlikely explanations for these gains.

Early group studies of STA-MCA bypass patients were positive. Evans and Austin (1976) studied 14 patients a few days prior to operation and 2 to 5 weeks after surgery. All patients had experienced two or more TIAs. All patients had intracranial blockage on angiography and more than 20% "depression of cerebral blood flow" (p.

320). Preoperative–postoperative changes in scores were positive for 86% of WAIS scores, 45% of Bender-Gestalt scores, 58% of Draw a Man scores, and 75% of Proverb scores. Twelve patients showed improvement on a composite score derived from the test battery. However, no comparison group was employed, nor were alternate test forms utilized. Moreover, the authors did not specify how they measured cerebral blood flow, how they utilized blood flow measurement for surgical decision-making, and how they selected patients for this report. Still, the samples of Bender-Gestalt reproductions revealed pathognomonic preoperative constructional deficits that contrasted with accurate postoperative drawings. Because all patients had TIAs rather than strokes, natural recovery was an unlikely explanation for the observed gains. Hence this study, despite methodologic shortcomings, fostered hope that some patients might experience behavioral improvement after surgery.

In 1979 Greenhalgh and colleagues reported on nine patients with a history of completed stroke 1.5 to 12.0 months prior to STA-MCA bypass. The psychological test battery consisted of an intelligence test, a verbal and visual memory test, a verbal fluency test, and a visual perception test. The authors reported that patients with left-sided bypass improved on verbal fluency and intelligence, and right-sided bypass patients improved on visual perception. Remarkably, two-thirds of the patients showed marked lessening of motor deficits following surgery, presumably on the side of surgery. The authors verified bypass patency and reportedly observed increased oxygen utilization and cerebral blood flow after surgery, although they did not include values for specific physiologic parameters.

These gains must be balanced against the limitations of this study. The specific tests utilized, the manner in which patients were selected for this report, and the test-retest interval were not discussed. In the table of patient scores, individual change scores were small, inconsistent, and well within the area that could be explained by practice results. Although the authors reported that spontaneous recovery was an unlikely explanation for the results because subjects underwent operation an average of 6 months after stroke, inspection of the table indicates that only two of the four patients with stroke 6 to 12 months after surgery showed motoric improvement, and the patient with the most dramatic recovery, from total monoplegia to full function, had the shortest duration of symptoms (1.5 months).

Later studies of groups of bypass patients have failed to demonstrate large behavioral gains after bypass. Unlike earlier studies, more recent research typically has included a comparison group. For example, Binder and coworkers (1982) failed to find significant differential improvement in 12 STA-MCA bypass patients compared to 7 patients undergoing medical treatment for TIA and stroke. Despite ten or more univariate F-tests, only one significant interaction between time of testing and treatment was observed. This single finding favored the medical treatment group, who improved more on Symbol Digit Modalities, a psychomotor speed measure, than did the surgical group. Binder and his colleagues (1982) believed that the greater improvement in the medical group might be the result of a slightly higher educational level in the medical group and a trend for the medical group to obtain higher scores on the first testing, or simply to a random effect.

Drinkwater and colleagues (1984) studied 38 STA-MCA bypass candidates before surgery and 6 to 9 months later. The authors found no postoperative change on their two summary measures, although small but significant gains (all less than 5 T)

were noted in 6 of the 16 individual measures on which the composite scores were based.

The lack of a direct statistical comparison between the change from preoperative to postoperative testing in three groups limited the significance of a study of 33 STA-MCA bypass patients by Nielsen and colleagues (1986). The authors compared the preoperative and postoperative neuropsychological test scores of right STA-MCA bypass patients, left STA-MCA bypass patients, and medical controls; but they measured change over time only within groups. Such an approach, of course, does not allow one to control for practice effects as a source of gains over time. The authors also failed to give information regarding the time of the ischemic events in the bypass candidates. Their data suggested that any postoperative gains attributable to surgery were probably only small to moderate in size. Nielsen et al. emphasized the mildness of behavioral impairment of subjects preoperatively, despite the history of RIND or completed stroke in all patients and despite evidence of infarction on CT scans in 30 of 33 subjects.

Preoperatively, ten right STA-MCA bypass candidates had poorer scores on 14 of 15 psychological tests than did 12 patients who underwent minor surgery unrelated to brain function; but none of these differences were statistically significant (Nielsen et al., 1986). After STA-MCA bypass, these patients improved significantly relative to their own preoperative standing on 2 of 15 measures; but once again their postoperative test scores failed to differ significantly from those of the control group.

The larger group of 23 left STA-MCA bypass candidates scored significantly lower than the control group before surgery on 4 of 15 measures, although on an absolute basis mean scores were lower on all 15 measures (Nielsen et al., 1986). Relative to their own preoperative scores, left STA-MCA bypass patients improved on 5 of 15 measures. At the postoperative testing, left STA-MCA bypass patients scored significantly lower than controls on only one measure.

As in the CE literature (Hemmingsen et al., 1986) more recent work has failed to demonstrate consistent correlations between behavioral and physiologic improvement after STA-MCA bypass. In three preliminary studies without a control group, a multidisciplinary group at the University of Pennsylvania found significant cognitive gains 9 months after STA-MCA bypass surgery (Hungerbuhler et al., 1981; Gur et al., 1983; Younkin et al., 1985). However, in the most recent and thorough study (Younkin et al., 1985), the authors found that natural recovery was a viable explanation for these postoperative gains. The authors subdivided their total sample into patients with TIAs only, patients with strokes less than 3 months before surgery, and patients with older strokes. Only the subgroup with recent strokes obtained a significantly lower impairment rating 9 months after surgery. More discouragingly, the authors were unable to predict clinical gains with preoperative neurologic examination scores, neuropsychological summary scores, and regional cerebral blood flow measurements.

A study that reported positron emission tomography (PET) scan results on six STA-MCA bypass patients briefly discussed neuropsychological test results from three patients (Leblanc et al., 1987). Although the neuropsychological assessment apparently was thorough and included alternate forms where appropriate, only limited quantitative data were presented. Two of these three patients were said to have improved on neuropsychological testing performed 2 weeks before and after operation and again 3 months after operation. However, one of these patients, said to show dramatic reversal of a chronic preoperative dementia, improved only to about the level of performance 12 weeks before surgery; the authors did not report the frequency or duration of symptoms that occurred between assessments 12 and 2 weeks before surgery. Presumably, symptomatic episodes were limited to TIAs, but the patient was described as having hemiparesis, dementia, and bilateral lacunae before surgery. Hence it is conceivable that natural recovery is an explanation for postoperative recovery. This patient showed marked improvement on both cerebral blood flow and oxygen metabolism measures after surgery. In the other patient who showed gains, one can infer that improvement was limited to a 30-point gain in the Wechsler Memory Quotient, from the normal range to the very superior range. Again, symptom data are sparse. This patient also showed improvement in oxygen metabolism, but regional cerebral blood flow actually fell nonsignificantly postoperatively. No quantitative data were presented for the third patient, but he is reported to have shown no postoperative improvement on neuropsychological test scores. His postoperative cerebral blood flow and oxygen utilization measurements showed significant decreases from the preoperative level. The authors emphasized the variability in the hemodynamic changes seen in their six subjects postoperatively, though all subjects experienced relief from recurrent ischemic episodes. The detailed report of physiologic measurements makes this report important despite the small number of subjects and limited presentation of neuropsychological data.

The only randomized study to date, the multicenter Extracranial-Intracranial Bypass (EIAB) Trial, suggested transient deterioration in STA-MCA bypass patients relative to medically treated patients (Haynes et al., 1987) on a measure of functional status, a modification of the Katz Activities of Daily Living Scale. Neurologists rated subjects randomized to medical or surgical treatment before entry into the study, 6 weeks after entry, and at 3-month intervals thereafter until death or the end of the trial. Interrater agreement in a subsample of subjects was 0.90. Before entry into the study, both groups of subjects were of equivalent functional status. Six weeks after entry into the study, the surgical group manifested more impairment in six of the ten basic activities on the Katz scale: toileting, speech fluency, getting in and out of bed, cutting food and pouring beverages, dressing and undressing, and sitting down and standing up. By 4.5 months after entry into the study, the surgical patients were significantly inferior to the medically treated patients only in toileting activities, and at the 6-month follow-up and thereafter medically and surgically treated patients again were of equivalent functional status. Thus whereas the two treatment groups did not differ on stroke and death, the main dependent variables of this large study, the surgical group showed more dysfunction in daily life. Although this difference was transient, it was not limited to the immediate perioperative period.

Critics of the international EIAB trial have argued strongly that the subjects were not representative of the population of patients expected to benefit from surgery (Ausman and Diaz, 1986; Day et al., 1986; Goldring et al., 1987; Sundt, 1987). Raters of functional status apparently were not blind to patients' treatment group assignments at follow-up. Despite these drawbacks, the study seems rigorous enough to conclude that there probably is no major group-wide behavioral benefit from STA-MCA bypass when patients are selected only on the basis of neurologic examination, history, and cerebral angiography.

Posterior Fossa Revascularization

The neurobehavioral effects of this newer group of procedures are largely unexplored. In many candidates for posterior revascularization, the frequency and severity of TIAs may interfere significantly with day-to-day functioning, even if they never develop a fixed neurologic deficit. Neurologic and neurosurgical case studies and series reports generally have emphasized postoperative relief from TIAs. However, these reports also have described some patients with strokes before surgery as "improved" following surgery. Thus far, the nature of the improvement and the time of the strokes has usually gone unspecified (Hadley et al., 1985; Hopkins et al., 1987; Spetzler et al., 1987). A small group of patients undergoing a heterogeneous set of vertebrobasilar revascularization procedures has been followed as part of a larger study of multiple revascularization procedures (Adams et al., 1984; Baird et al., 1988).

Comparison of Revascularization Procedures

Two studies compared directly the neuropsychological effects of different cerebral revascularization procedures and reached somewhat divergent conclusions (Drinkwater et al., 1984; Baird et al., 1988). The study by Drinkwater and colleagues (1984) did not include unoperated comparison groups but featured one of the largest samples of STA-MCA bypass patients yet reported in the literature. The study by Baird and associates (1988) focused on four small groups of revascularization candidates and two groups of patients who did not undergo cerebral revascularization.

Drinkwater and colleagues (1984) compared the performance of 38 STA-MCA bypass candidates tested before surgery and 6 to 9 months later with that of 20 CE candidates described in an earlier study (Perry et al., 1975). Summary scores from the Halstead-Reitan neuropsychological battery did not show postoperative changes in the STA-MCA bypass group, although there were small, statistically significant changes on 4 of 15 scores from individual tests. The authors noted that 15 bypass patients had strokes before surgery and concluded that these small gains probably were best attributed to natural recovery. Although comparisons were apparently by inspection of group profiles of *T* scores and not by statistical analysis, Drinkwater stated that STA-MCA groups may show less behavioral improvement after surgery than CE patients. In the earlier study by Perry and coworkers (1975), CE patients had shown significant postoperative gains on the summary score and on two of eight individual test scores. Drinkwater and his colleagues (1984) indicated that the larger number of preoperative strokes in the bypass group may have been responsible for the differences in postoperative improvement.

Although an earlier report suggested the possibility of modest gains in most patients after STA-MCA bypass, with more dramatic improvement in isolated cases (Adams et al., 1984), a later study (Baird et al., 1988) found that behavioral changes in bypass candidates and in patients who underwent other types of revascularization procedures were not significantly greater than in two comparison groups retested at approximately the same interval. Specifically, this study included 14 CE patients, 16 STA-MCA bypass patients, 10 vertebrobasilar revascularization patients, and 8 patients who underwent multiple revascularization procedures, such as bilateral STA-MCA bypass procedures or CE and contralateral STA-MCA bypass. Eleven patients who had experienced recent severe spinal complaints comprised one comparison group. Seventeen patients who were considered for revascularization but did not undergo surgery during an 18-month follow-up period made up a second comparison group similar to that used by Parker et al. (1986). The cerebrovascular comparison group matched the revascularization groups in terms of severity and time of the ischemic symptoms as well as the age, education, and estimated premorbid intelligence of the patient.

Whether compared in sum or separately with each of the comparison groups, the four revascularization groups failed to show greater gains on a mean impairment rating based on eight tests than the two quasicontrol groups followed at the same interval, approximately 6 months (Baird et al., 1988). Whether contrasted as a combined group or singly with the unoperated cerebrovascular comparison group, the revascularization groups also did not show greater gains on a self-report life quality measure, the Sickness Impact Profile. Of the four revascularization groups, the vertebrobasilar group came closest to demonstrating significantly greater gains in self-reported life quality than the unoperated cerebrovascular comparison group. The authors concluded that the small gains seen in all six groups at follow-up could be attributed to practice effects but cautioned that the small number of subjects, the variability within revascularization groups, and the lack of a true control group might have hidden small to moderate benefits from surgery in some patients.

CONCLUSIONS

Over the long run, surgical revascularization procedures appear to have a relatively benign effect on neurobehavioral functions when the few patients who experience major postoperative stroke or death are excluded. There are short-term declines in some patients undergoing CE or STA-MCA bypass; there are some external intraoperative and postoperative measures that correlate well with these transient declines. However, to date no one has predicted which patients will experience this transient behavioral dysfunction before surgery.

At present, the literature does not strongly support the hypothesis that CE and STA-MCA bypass produce significant behavioral gains. The evidence suggests that CE and STA-MCA bypass yield clinically significant behavioral gains in only a small percentage of patients currently undergoing such surgery. In many studies reporting positive results, natural recovery is a viable alternative explanation for the improvement noted. There are four lines of evidence that support this conclusion.

First, to date, neuropsychological studies have not given convincing evidence of consistent moderate to large gains in small or moderate-sized groups compared to patients who did not undergo surgery but had symptoms associated with cerebrovascular disease and to those experiencing nonneurologic disorders. It is possible that there are large changes in a few patients or modest changes in large groups of patients that could be detected with randomized studies using a large sample and multiple neuropsychological measures.

Second, although there have been some dramatic reports of improvement after STA-MCA bypass, it has not been possible to predict which patients would improve before surgery or even to produce a general post hoc description of these patients. It is noteworthy that dramatic case reports typically involve patients with major stroke or RIND before surgery, whereas most candidates for CE and STA-MCA bypass are only mildly impaired before surgery. The mildness of impairment in most patients probably has not been emphasized sufficiently. The heterogeneity of impairment among surgical candidates and the mildness of impairment in most patients certainly make it more difficult to detect any behavioral gains after surgery and reduce the practical importance of psychological improvement as a possible benefit of revascularization.

Third, it has been difficult to link behavioral gains with expected physiologic changes after surgery. It is of course possible that measurement error in the physiologic measures available to date and the lack of more direct measures of neuronal function are responsible for the lack of correlation observed. Moreover, differences in subject selection strategies across studies may have obscured patterns of postoperative behavioral gains.

Fourth, several studies of CE and STA-MCA bypass patients have shown that initial postoperative improvement was not sustained. Blood flow studies have paralleled these findings (Yonekura et al., 1982; Younkin et al., 1985). The reasons for the reversal of early postoperative improvements in psychological test performance and in rCBF are not yet clear and deserve further study.

The behavioral effects of revascularization in the posterior fossa region are much less well studied than those of CE and STA-MCA bypass. Due to the frequency of TIAs experienced by posterior fossa revascularization candidates, it may be particularly important to emphasize the quality of day-to-day functioning during the follow-up of these patients. There may be a need to employ other, less traditional measures that are sensitive to the dysfunction and discomfort produced by recurrent or unremitting vertebrobasilar symptoms such as ataxia, vertigo, and diplopia.

In studies performed thus far, patients have been selected for the same revascularization procedure in varying ways. For example, in some studies, a particular pattern of results on rCBF studies was required for selection for STA-MCA bypass, whereas in others angiographic results and clinical symptoms sufficed for selection.

There are a number of possible mechanisms for behavioral gains after cerebral revascularization: increased rCBF throughout the distribution of the artery receiving increased blood supply, increased rCBF in regions with reversible neuronal dysfunction, prevention of continual microembolic events (Boysen et al., 1983), reversal of steal of blood from one region of the brain to another, formation of new collateral channels through a neovascularization process, heterogeneous unforeseen hemodynamic changes, and natural recovery. When neuropsychological test scores are used as the criterion for behavioral gains, practice effects may contribute to positive changes; when self-report life quality measures are employed, the Hawthorne effect may produce apparent postoperative improvement in functioning. Like the lack of consensus on the means of selecting revascularization candidates, the absence of clear-cut empiric support for a mechanism of improvement after revascularization leads one to view positive reports more cautiously.

SUGGESTIONS FOR FURTHER NEUROPSYCHOLOGICAL RESEARCH

Developments in surgical techniques, understanding of the coupling between brain metabolism and blood flow, and measurement of neuronal function are expanding rapidly. It seems important to avoid overgeneralizing from the largely negative results obtained thus far lest discouragement prevent us from recognizing future behavioral benefits from revised or more selective surgical treatment of patients with cerebrovascular occlusive disease.

If further controlled studies are planned, neuropsychological and life quality measurements, rather than merely functional ratings and stroke frequency, should be included as outcome measures. Because the main intent of surgery is stroke prevention rather than behavioral improvement, it is highly unlikely that a multicenter randomized trial could be conducted strictly to look at the neuropsychological effects of surgery. However, theoretically and practically, the question of reversibility of behavioral deficits through surgery is an important one. Looking simply at incidence of stroke after surgery, return to work, ambulatory status, or all three, may lead to neglect of some potential benefits from these surgical procedures. For example, it is possible that relief from TIAs and the inconvenience and side effects of taking oral anticoagulants are important outcomes of some cerebral revascularization procedures.

As in the past, future exclusively neuropsychological studies of cerebral revascularization patients are likely to lack randomized assignment to medical or surgical treatment. At present, it is questionable whether additional studies of CE and STA-MCA bypass patients in intact groups will be fruitful; but uncontrolled behavioral studies of posterior fossa revascularization may yield some direction for further work. Investigators should consider using multiple-baseline designs to evaluate the behavioral effects of cerebral revascularization. This method might help to illuminate the role of practice effects, natural recovery, and placebo effects in mediating changes over time in patients undergoing cerebral revascularization.

Behavioral studies of cerebral revascularization should utilize batteries with measures sensitive to both global and focal cerebral dysfunction, as some previous studies have reported changes correlated with the site of surgery, whereas others have focused on changes in general intellectual, memory, or perceptual-motor performance. Particularly in studies with a small number of subjects, use of the same measures or alternate forms before and after surgery is important. Studies also should include both reactive life-quality measures (e.g., self-report questionnaires) and nonreactive measures (e.g., a count of the number of medications needed before and after surgery).

More long-term behavioral studies of natural recovery from stroke and TIA should be carried out. By providing us with estimates of length and variability of natural recovery, we would be able to judge better the significance of case studies that report dramatic improvement after cerebral revascularization and the gains reported in some group studies.

SUMMARY

Thus far, we lack strong evidence that most patients manifest behavioral improvement after surgery. We have not identified consistent similarities among the few patients who have shown behavioral improvement after the procedures, much less formulated a strategy for identifying these patients before surgery. However, limitations in study designs available thus far and continuing technical advances by neurosurgeons and neurophysiologists suggest the need for restraint in drawing final conclusions about the possible behavioral benefits of cerebral revascularization in more precisely selected patient populations.

REFERENCES

Adams, K.M., Brown, G.G., Shatz, M.W., Baird, A.D., Diaz, F., and Ausman, J.I. (1984). In: R.R. Smith, ed., *Stroke and the Extracranial Vessels,* pp. 285–293. New York: Raven Press.

Ausman, J.I., and Diaz, F.G. (1986). Critique of the extracranial-intracranial bypass study. *Surg. Neurol.,* **26,** 218–221.

Ausman, J.I., Caplan, L.R., and Diaz, F.G. (1986a). Surgically created posterior circulation vascular shunts. *Clin. Neurosurg.,* **33,** 327–330.

Ausman, J.I., Diaz, F.G., and Dujovny, M. (1986b). Posterior circulation revascularization. *Clin. Neurosurg.,* **33,** 331–343.

Baird, A.D., Adams, K.M., Shatz, M.W., Brown, G.G., Diaz, F., and Ausman, J.I. (1984). Can neuropsychological tests detect the sites of cerebrovascular stenoses and occlusions? *Neurosurgery,* **14,** 416–423.

Baird, A.D., Boulos, R., Mehta, B., Adams, K.M., Shatz, M.W., Ausman, J.I., Diaz, F.G., and Dujovny, M. (1985). Cerebral angiography and neuropsychological measurement: the twain may meet. *Surg. Neurol.,* **23,** 641–650.

Baird, A.D., Adams, K.M., Shatz, M.W., Ausman, J.I., Diaz, F.G., and Dujovny, M. (1988). Neurobehavioral and life quality changes after cerebral revascularization. *J. Consult. Clin. Psychol.,* **56,** 148–151.

Bennion, R.S., Owens, M.L., and Wilson, S.E. (1985). The effect of unilateral carotid endarterectomy on neuropsychological test performance in 53 patients. *J. Cardiovasc. Surg.,* **26,** 21–26.

Benzel, E.C., and Mirfarkhraee, M. (1987). Complete homonymous hemianopsia: reversal with arterial bypass. *South. Med. J.,* **80,** 249–251.

Binder, L.M., Tanabe, C.T., Waller, F.T., and Wooster, N.E. (1982). Behavioral effects of superficial temporal artery to middle cerebral artery bypass surgery: preliminary report. *Neurology,* **32,** 422–424.

Boeke, S. (1981). The effect of carotid endarterectomy on mental functioning. *Clin. Neurol. Neurosurg.,* **83,** 209–217.

Bornstein, R.A., Benoit, B.G., and Trites, R.L. (1981a). Neuropsychological changes following carotid endarterectomy. *Can. J. Neurol. Sci.,* **8,** 127–132.

Bornstein, R., Trites, R., and Benoit, B. (1981b). Effects of medical risk factors on extent of improvement following carotid endarterectomy. Presented to the annual meeting of the International Neuropsychological Society, Atlanta, 1981.

Boysen, G., Hemmingsen, R., Mejsholm, B., Vorstrup, S., Lassen, N.A., Lester, J., and Engell, H.C. (1983). Cerebral blood flow and intellectual function before and after carotid endarterectomy. *J. Cereb. Blood Flow Metab.*, **3,** suppl. 1, S272–S273.

Brinkman, S.D., Braun, P., Ganji, S., Morrell, R.M., and Jacobs, L.A. (1984). Neuropsychological performance one week after carotid endarterectomy reflects intraoperative ischemia. *Stroke,* **15,** 497–503.

Casey, J.E., Ferguson, G.G., Kimura, D., and Hachinski, V.C. (1989). Neuropsychological improvement versus practice effect following unilateral carotid endarterectomy in patients without stroke. *J. Clin. Exp. Neuropsychol.* **11,** 461–470.

Cushman, L., Brinkman, S.D., Ganji, S., and Jacobs, L.A. (1984). Neuropsychological impairment after carotid endarterectomy correlates with intraoperative ischemia. *Cortex,* **20,** 403–412.

Day, A.L., Rhoton, A.L., and Little, J.R. (1986). The extracranial-intracranial bypass study. *Surg. Neurol.,* **26,** 222–226.

Diener, H.C., Hamster, W., and Seboldt, H. (1984). Neuropsychological functions after carotid endarterectomy. *Eur. Arch. Psychiatry Neurol. Sci.,* **234,** 74–77.

Drinkwater, J.E., Thompson, S.K., and Lumley, J.S.P. (1984). Cerebral function before and after extra-intracranial carotid bypass. *J. Neurol. Neurosurg. Psychiatry,* **47,** 1041–1043.

Duke, R.B., Bloor, B.M., Nugent, G.R., and Majzoub, H.S. (1968). Changes in performance on WAIS, Trail Making Test, and Finger Tapping Test associated with carotid artery surgery. *Percept. Motor Skills,* **26,** 399–404.

Dull, R.A., Brown, G.G., Adams, K.M., Shatz, M.W., Diaz, F.G., and Ausman, J.I. (1982). Preoperative neurobehavioral impairment in cerebral revascularization candidates. *J. Clin. Neuropsychol.,* **4,** 151–165.

Evans, R.B., and Austin, G. (1976). Psychological evaluation of patients undergoing microneurosurgical anastomoses for cerebral ischemia. In: G.M. Austin, ed., *Microneurosurgical Anastomoses for Cerebral Ischemia,* pp. 320–326. Springfield: Charles C Thomas.

Ferguson, G.G., and Peerless, S.J. (1976). Extracranial-intracranial arterial bypass in the treatment of dementia and multiple extracranial arterial occlusion. *Stroke,* **7,** 13 (abstract).

Fraser, P., Lane, B., Knight, D.K., and Walker, M.G. (1983). Cognitive function after carotid endarterectomy. *Br. J. Surg.,* **70,** (abstract), 388.

Goldring, S., Zervas, N., and Langfitt, T. (1987). The extracranial-intracranial bypass study: a report of the committee appointed by the American Association of Neurological Surgeons to examine the study. *N. Engl. J. Med.,* **316,** 817–820.

Goldstein, S.G., Kleinknecht, R.A., and Gallo, A.E. (1970). Neuropsychological changes associated with carotid endarterectomy. *Cortex,* **6,** 308–322.

Greenhalgh, R.M., Illingworth, R.D., McFie, J., Mills, S.P., Perkin, G.D., and Rose, F.C. (1979). Extracranial to intracranial microrevascularisation for the treatment of completed ischaemic stroke. *Br. Med. J.,* **2,** 18–19.

Greiffenstein, M.F., Brinkman, S., Jacobs, L., and Braun, P. (1988). Neuropsychological improvement following endarterectomy as a function of outcome measure and reconstructed vessel. *Cortex,* **24,** 223–230.

Gur, R.C., Gur, R.E., and Reivich, M. (1983). Neuropsychological consequences of superficial temporal to middle cerebral artery (STA-MCA) bypass surgery. Presented to the annual conference of the American Academy of Neurology, San Diego, 1983.

Hachinski, V. (1987). Carotid endarterectomy. *Arch. Neurol.,* **44,** 654.

Hadley, M.N., Masferrer, R., Zabramski, J.M., and Spetzler, R.F. (1985). Management of vertebrobasilar insufficiency. In: R.F. Spetzler, L.P. Carter, W.R. Selman, and N.A. Martin, eds., *Cerebral Revascularization for Stroke.* New York: Thieme-Stratton.

Hart, R.P., Rosner, M.J., and Muizelaar, P. (1985). Recovery from aphasia following extracranial-intracranial bypass surgery: case report. *J. Clin. Exp. Neuropsychol.,* **7,** 224–230.

Haynes, C.D., Gideon, D.A., King, G.D., and Dempsey, R.L. (1976). The improvement of cognition and personality after carotid endarterectomy. *Surgery,* **80,** 699–704.

Haynes, R.B., Mukherjee, J., Sackett, D.L., Taylor, W., Barnett, H.J.M., and Peerless, S.J. (1987). Functional status changes following medical or surgical treatment for cerebral ischemia. *J.A.M.A.,* **257,** 2043–2046.

Hemmingsen, R., Mejsholm, B., Boysen, G., and Engell, H.C. (1982). Intellectual function in patients with transient ischaemic attacks (TIA) or minor stroke. *Acta Neurol. Scand.,* **66,** 145–169.

Hemmingsen, R., Mejsholm, B., Vorstrup, S., Lester, J., Engell, H.C., and Boysen, G. (1986). Carotid surgery, cognitive function, and cerebral blood flow in patients with transient ischemic attacks. *Ann. Neurol.,* **20,** 13–19.

Hopkins, L.N., Martin, N.A., Hadley, M.N., Spetzler, R.F., Budny, J., and Carter, L.P. (1987). Vertebrobasilar insufficiency. Part 2. Microsurgical treatment of intracranial vertebrobasilar disease. *J. Neurosurg.,* **66,** 662–674.

Horne, D.J., and Royle, J.P. (1974). Cognitive changes after carotid endarterectomy. *Med. J. Aust.,* **1,** 316–318.

Hungerbuhler, J.P., Younkin, D., Reivich, M., Obrist, W.D., O'Connor, M., Goldberg, H., Gordon, J., Gur, R., Hurtig, H., and Amarnek, W. (1981). The effect of STA-MCA anastomosis on rCBF, neurologic and neuropsychologic function in patients with completed stroke. In: T.S. Meyer, H. Lechner, M. Reivich, E.O. Ott, and A. Aranibar, eds., *Cerebral Vascular Disease,* Vol. 3, pp. 73–75. Amsterdam: Excerpta Medica.

Jacobs, L.A., Ganji, S., Shirley, J.G., Morrell, R.M., and Brinkman, S.D. (1983). Cognitive improvement after extracranial reconstruction for the low flow-endangered brain. *Surgery,* **93,** 683–687.

Jacques, S., and Garner, J.T. (1976). Reversal of aphasia with superficial temporal artery to middle cerebral artery anastomosis. *Surg. Neurol.,* **5,** 143–145.

Jonas, S. (1987). Can carotid endarterectomy be justified? No. *Arch. Neurol.,* **44,** 652–654.

Kelly, M.P., Garron, D.C., and Javid, H. (1980). Carotid artery disease, carotid endarterectomy, and behavior. *Arch. Neurol.,* **37,** 743–748.

King, G.D., Gideon, D.A., Haynes, C.D., Dempsey, R.L., and Jenkins, C.W. (1977). Intellectual and personality changes associated with carotid endarterectomy. *J. Clin. Psychol.,* **33,** 218–220.

LeBlanc, R., Tyler, J.L., Mohr, G., Meyer, E., Diksic, M., Yamamoto, L., Taylor, L., Gauthier, S., and Hakim, A. (1987). Hemodynamic and metabolic effects of cerebral revascularization. *J. Neurosurg.,* **66,** 529–535.

Lee, M.C., Ausman, J.I., Diaz, F.G., Klassen, A.C., and Latchaw, R.E. (1980). In S.J. Peerless and C.W. McCormick, eds., *Microsurgery for Cerebral Ischemia,* pp. 357–361. New York: Springer-Verlag.

Macon, J.B., and Rice, J.F. (1985). Reversal of fixed hemiplegia due to middle cerebral artery occlusion by delayed superficial temporal to middle cerebral artery bypass graft: case report. In: R.F. Spetzler, L.P. Carter, W.R. Selman, and N.A. Martin, eds., *Cerebral Revascularization for Stroke,* pp. 470–474. New York: Thieme-Stratton.

Matarazzo, R.G., Matarazzo, J.D., Gallo, A.E., and Wiens, A.N. (1979). IQ and neuropsychological changes following carotid endarterectomy. *J. Clin. Neuropsychol.,* **1,** 97–116.

Nielsen, H., Hojer-Pederson, E., Gulliksen, G., Haase, J., and Enevoldsen, E. (1986). Reversible ischemic neurological deficit and minor strokes before and after EC/IC bypass surgery: a neuropsychological study. *Acta Neurol. Scand.,* **73,** 615–618.

Owens, M., Pressman, M., Edwards, A.E., Tourtellotte, W., Rose, J.G., Stern, D., Peters, G., Stabile, B.E., and Wilson, S.E. (1980). The effect of small infarcts and carotid endarterectomy on postoperative psychologic test performance. *J. Surg. Res.*, **28,** 209–216.

Parker, J.C., Granberg, B.W., Nichols, W.K., Jones, J.G., and Hewett, J.E. (1983). Mental status outcomes following carotid endarterectomy: a six-month analysis. *J. Clin. Neuropsychol.*, **5,** 345–353.

Parker, J.C., Smarr, K.L., Granberg, B.W., Nichols, W.K., and Hewett, J.E. (1986). Neuropsychological parameters of carotid endarterectomy: a two-year prospective analysis. *J. Consult. Clin. Psychol.*, **54,** 676–681.

Patterson, R.H. (1987). Can carotid endarterectomy be justified? Yes. *Arch. Neurol.*, **44,** 651–652.

Peerless, S.J., Chater, N.L., and Ferguson, G.F. (1977). Multiple-vessel occlusions in cerebrovascular disease—a further followup of the effects of microvascular bypass on the quality of life and the incidence of stroke. In: P. Schmiedek, ed., *Microsurgery for Stroke*, pp. 251–259. New York: Springer-Verlag.

Perry, P.M., Drinkwater, J.E., and Taylor, G.W. (1975). Cerebral function before and after carotid endarterectomy. *Br. Med. J.*, **4,** 215–216.

Roski, R., Spetzler, R.F., Owen, M., Chandar, K., Sholl, J.G., and Nulsen, F.E. (1978). Reversal of seven-year old visual field defect with extracranial-intracranial arterial anastomosis. *Surg. Neurol.*, **10**, 267–268.

Spetzler, R.F., Hadley, M.N., Martin, N.A., Hopkins, L.N., Carter, L.P., and Budny, J. (1987). Vertebrobasilar insufficiency. Part 1: Microsurgical treatment of extracranial vertebrobasilar disease. *J. Neurosurg.*, **66,** 648–661.

Stark, R.J., and Wodak, J. (1983). Primary orthostatic cerebral ischemia. *J. Neurol. Neurosurg. Psychiatry,* **46,** 883–891.

Sundt, T.M. (1987). Was the international randomized trial of extracranial-intracranial arterial bypass representative of the population at risk? *N. Engl. J. Med.*, **316,** 814–816.

Tanahashi, N., Meyer, J.S., Rogers, R.L., Kitagawa, Y., Mortel, K.F., Kandula, P., Levinthal, R., and Rose, J. (1985). Long-term assessment of cerebral perfusion following STA-MCA by-pass in patients. *Stroke,* **16,** 85–91.

Trudel, L., Fabia, J., and Bouchard, J.-P. (1984). Quality of life of 50 carotid endarterectomy survivors: a long-term follow-up study. *Arch. Phys. Med. Rehabil.*, **65,** 310–312.

Wedergaard, M., Astrup, J., and Klinken, L. (1985). Border of large chronic infarcts in the MCA territory in man. In: R.F. Spetzler, L.P. Carter, W.R. Selman, and N.A. Martin, eds., *Cerebral Revascularization for Stroke,* pp. 217–222. New York: Thieme-Stratton.

Williams, M., and McGee, T.F. (1964). Psychological study of carotid occlusion and endarterectomy. *Arch. Neurol.*, **10**, 293–297.

Yonekura, M., Austin, G., and Hayward, W. (1982). Long-term evaluation of cerebral blood flow, transient ischemic attacks, and stroke after STA-MCA anastomosis. *Surg. Neurol.*, **18,** 123–130.

Younkin, D., Hungerbuhler, J.P., O'Connor, M., Goldberg, H., Burke, A., Kushner, M., Hurtig, H., Obrist, W., Gordon, J., Gur, R., and Reivich, M. (1985). Superficial temporal-middle cerebral artery anastomosis: effects on vascular, neurologic, and neuropsychological functions. *Neurology,* **35,** 462–469.

16

Management of Aphasia

MARTHA TAYLOR SARNO

It is my intent in this chapter to describe a philosophy of aphasia rehabilitation based on an extended experience in a speech-language pathology program in the department of rehabilitation medicine of a major teaching hospital. Traditionally, aphasia therapy concentrates on linguistic performance in response to specified techniques. The model presented here considers the social-psychological dimensions of aphasia primary and a function of the chronicity of the disorder. That is, the linguistic aspect, more often than not, is overshadowed by psychosocial issues that become the major treatment concern in the post-stroke course. From this model a broad therapeutic program has evolved over the years that includes social and psychological services in addition to traditional language training. From this perspective, the process of recovery and rehabilitation is best understood in terms of the psychology of disability and loss. It is this therapeutic philosophy that suggests the term *management* rather than the usual "treatment" or "retraining." Rehabilitation medicine programs are ideally suited for managing aphasic patients, since they can provide the wide variety of services necessary to meet their needs.

Historically, the treatment of aphasia has exclusively attended to linguistic performance. In this regard, the contribution of neurolinguistics has been of great importance. A neurolinguistic approach has provided a rationale for pedagogic practices (drill and repetition) and for the development of a variety of novel techniques (e.g., Melodic Intonation Therapy) that are of both theoretical and practical importance. Contemporary research efforts addressing the neurolinguistic/cognitive processes subserving language use should continue to enhance the available repertoire of therapeutic techniques and their effectiveness, as well as provide a basis for an informed choice of therapeutic interventions.

Neurolinguists have also provided a basis for the description and interpretation of linguistic symptoms that is essential for the speech-language pathologist's work with patients. Aphasiology will undoubtedly continue to attract neurolinguists because of their interest in language pathology in general and in the development of theories of normal language processing through the study of language in dissolution. The application of neurolinguistics to aphasia rehabilitation practice, however, has been insufficient. Because of its interest in the phenomenology of aphasia, the discipline of neurolinguistics has become highly developed in recent years. Similar developments in the study of the psychosocial consequences (of aphasia) and their amelioration have not yet occurred.

Once the patient has stabilized, the chronic nature of aphasia requires that management be viewed in the broadest sense. In part, it is because management is influenced by the patient's ability to adjust to and compensate for limitations imposed by the language disability. In addition, the type and severity of the aphasic deficit, associated physical disabilities, premorbid personality, time since onset, cultural and educational background, associated neuropsychological deficits, and general physical condition are frequently cited as factors that contribute to the recovery process (Wepman, 1951; Schuell et al., 1964; Darley, 1970, 1972, 1975; Eisenson, 1973; Benson, 1979; Reinvang and Engvol, 1980; Sarno, 1980).

The material that follows reviews current practices, issues, and dilemmas but does not elaborate localization, classification, or assessment. It is assumed that the reader is familiar with the literature in these areas, which is reviewed in Albert and Helm-Estabrooks (1988), Goodglass and Kaplan (1972), Kertesz (1979), Sarno (1981), and Sarno and Hook (1980). The clinical skills and experience required to manage patients with aphasia are discussed and described in the course of the chapter. For material on specific techniques and approaches, the reader is referred to Halper and Burns (1988), Chapey (1986), Davis and Wilcox (1985), and Holland (1984).

HISTORICAL PERSPECTIVE

Despite Hippocrates' dim view of the benefits of treating apoplectic patients (Licht, 1975), there is no doubt that in early times many informal and undocumented attempts were made to "cure" individual aphasic patients. A number of innovative attempts to "cure" aphasia were reported before this century but none of these approximate contemporary aphasia rehabilitation practices. In Mettler's (1947) classic text, *History of Medicine,* for example, Avicenna is cited as recommending cashew (anacardium) "for virtually all psychiatric and neurological afflictions, especially aphasia." Undoubtedly, cautery, cupping, alchemy, and leeching were also tried before the seventeenth century.

The earliest reference to aphasia rehabilitation was a report in 1673 by a German physician named Johann Schmidt, who described working with two apoplectic patients with aphasia and alexia. Schmidt made note of the difference in the two patients regarding their response to retraining, observing that one of the patients recovered letter recognition whereas the other showed no improvement (Benton and Joynt, 1960). In the well known account of his own aphasia in 1783, Samuel Johnson attributed the beginning of his speech recovery to the fact that his doctor had pressed blisters into his back and from his ear to his throat (Critchley, 1970). Goodglass (1985) cited an 1879 paper that described a 40-year-old aphasic patient who was treated repeatedly by applying a strong current to his skin with an electric brush.

Dr. Thomas Hun (1847), at the Albany Medical College in New York, may have been the first to recommend systematic exercises in spelling, writing, and reading. Dr. Hun suggested these exercises be administered by the wife of a 35-year-old post-stroke aphasic patient, and he credited her with his recovery. Paul Broca was one of the first to discuss the feasibility of retraining in aphasia. Broca (1885) related some anecdotal experiences with retraining and theorized that aphasics could be taught language in the same way that children learn language skills, taking advantage of inherent left hemisphere language capacities.

Mills and Broadbent (Broadbent, 1879; Mills, 1880, 1904) reported the successful retraining of a post-stroke aphasic patient. They employed training methods that were similar to those of Hun (1847), including the systematic repetition of letters, words, and phrases, reading aloud, imitation, and graded exercises to improve grammar and vocabulary. Mills borrowed many rehabilitation techniques from Guitzmann (1894), Goldscheider (1902), and Dana (1904). Sometime later Henry Head commended Mills' work because it was not based on the rather artificial methods of training then widely advocated. In contrast to Broca, Head suggested that, because of prior experience and an established functional brain organization, the aphasic patient presented a challenge different from that of deficient language acquistion in children (Head, 1926).

Mills' report was notable in that it discussed some of the methods used with aphasic patients at the turn of the century and showed concern with some of the nonlinguistic aspects of aphasia rehabilitation (i.e., emotional factors, premorbid intelligence, and education). He even raised the possible differential influences of semantic, lexical, and cognitive factors in recovery and suggested that different methods are appropriate for different patients and syndromes. Like Schmidt two centuries earlier, Mills observed that not all patients benefit to the same degree from retraining and acknowledged that spontaneous recovery may influence the course and extent of recovery. Some of Mills' observations and approaches to aphasia rehabilitation are remarkably similar to those of current practice and thought.

The first large scale reports on aphasia rehabilitation appeared during the early part of the twentieth century and primarily represent the work of Emil Froeschels (cited in Schuell et al., 1964), Kurt Goldstein (1948), and Henry Head (1926). Head published a two-volume treatise based on his experience in the treatment of 26 victims of gunshot wounds during World War I. In Vienna, Froeschels treated hundreds of patients between 1916 and 1925, and in Frankfurt Goldstein published detailed descriptions of the systematic treatment of approximately 2000 patients who suffered brain damage in both world wars. Many of these patients were followed for 10 years.

The brain-damaged victims of World War II stimulated the proliferation of a host of treatment programs in military and civilian hospitals. In the United States a small aphasia rehabilitation literature began to emerge from the work done at several army hospitals established during the war. Reports of the treatment of post-stroke aphasic civilians receiving treatment were rare before World War II. Notable among them was a detailed description (Singer and Low, 1933) of a 39-year-old woman who suffered a stroke following a full-term delivery. Two years after onset she was unable to read or write, and her only verbal responses were reiterative stereotypies. Nevertheless, she showed continued language improvement with consistent training over a 10-year period and is reported to have used a vocabulary of 500 words freely and intelligibly. An autopsy 25 years later revealed complete absence of the posterior parts of the second and third frontal convolutions of the left hemisphere.

Many factors contributed to the marked increase in aphasia rehabilitation activity that began after World War II, including the seminal work of Luria (1948), Schuell et al. (1964), and Wepman (1951); the establishment of U.S. Army aphasia rehabilitation programs that evolved into today's Veterans Administration Hospital programs; the growth of the speech-language pathology profession; the emergence of rehabilitation medicine as a medical specialty; the mass media explosion; and a climate of increased expectations in an age of technology. These and other factors contributed to the development of aphasia therapy as an important component of the practice of rehabilitation medicine, especially for those with aphasia due to stroke or head trauma.

Since the early 1970s the volume of clinical and research activity in aphasia rehabilitation has expanded greatly. Furthermore, increases in the size of the general population, life-span expectancies, and the percentage of patients surviving stroke have led to a greater number of patients with aphasia. The increased rate of survival from head trauma due to technologic advances has also added to the pool of individuals with aphasia. It is estimated that there are one million individuals with acquired aphasia in the United States (National Institute of Neurological and Communicative Disorders and Stroke, 1979) with approximately 84,000 new cases each year (Brust et al., 1976). Because the most common cause of aphasia is stroke, the mean age of the aphasic population is generally near retirement age (Hooper and Dunckle, 1984). As the survival rates of those with aphasia secondary to head trauma increase, the average age of those with aphasia will probably decrease. The increasing prevalence of younger patients who will live long periods of time with aphasia underscores the social and economic importance of aphasia management and rehabilitation.

It is not known what proportion of the aphasic population has received language rehabilitation services, but there is a consensus that the availability, intensity, comprehensiveness, and duration of services fail to meet the needs of most patients (Sarno, 1986). Services to aphasics are generally provided in medical settings, especially rehabilitation medicine programs, as well as in free-standing speech/language pathology clinics, nursing homes, university speech pathology clinics, and, increasingly, speech/language pathology private practices. Unfortunately, the need for services in this important field currently far exceeds available resources. Partially in response to the increasing awareness of the problems of patients with aphasia, the National Aphasia Association was founded in 1987 to advocate for those with aphasia, educate the public regarding the nature of aphasia, and encourage the development of local support groups.

RATIONALE FOR TRADITIONAL APHASIA THERAPY

Approaches to aphasia therapy have generally followed one of two models: *a substitute skill model* or a *direct treatment model,* both of which are based on the assumption that the processes that subserve normal performance need to be understood (Goodglass, 1987) if rehabilitation is to succeed. The theoretical concepts of *competence* and *performance* generally applied to the study of normal language are often considered useful for accounting for the nature of language use in aphasia. In a study that followed aphasic patients for the first 3 months post-stroke, no changes were noted in language competence, but there were improvements observed in language performance (Ludlow, 1977). Competence refers to a speaker's "knowledge" of his own language, i.e., its rules. This theoretical psycholinguistic construct suggests that brain damage causes a deficit in language competence in contrast to impairment in language performance (i.e., the observable use of language.)

In practice, however, much of aphasia therapy addresses the "performance" aspects of language in which repeated practice and "teaching" strategies are assumed to help restore impaired skills through a "task oriented" approach (i.e., naming practice). One commonly used technique involves self-cuing and repetition exercises that manipulate components of grammar and vocabulary. Another approach involves "stimulating" the patient to use residual language by encouraging conversation and free association in a permissive setting where a patient's responses are accepted and topics are of personal interest.

Much of what has been done in recent decades stems, at least indirectly, from the earlier models of Wepman (1951), Wepman and Morency (1963), and Schuell et al. (1964). Although their approaches to aphasia therapy differed, both Wepman (1951) and Schuell et al. (1964) were the primary proponents of the stimulation models that have been followed by most speech-language pathologists since World War II. Wepman suggested that the manner of stimulus presentation was of paramount importance, and that it was not the role of the therapist to teach vocabulary or syntax. He chose film strips as one mode of stimulation after observing their effectiveness as stimuli during testing, particularly for patients with semantic or syntactic aphasia (Wepman and Morency, 1963).

A different stimulation approach was developed by Schuell and her associates (Schuell et al., 1964) who thought that the clinician's role was that of a facilitator rather than of a teacher. This approach deemphasized the therapists's role in teaching the patient to talk, read, write, or learn sounds or rules for combining words. Schuell's therapeutic approach was based on the premise that auditory processing impairments underlie aphasia. She stressed adequate stimulation carefully controlled for length, rate, and loudness; and she advocated individual rather than group therapy because of individual differences among patients and their deficits. Within her framework, one language modality is used to stimulate another in a program carefully graded for complexity. She stressed the importance of repetition and overt responses from patients with a minimum of correcting or explaining by the therapist. In addition, she considered the treatment atmosphere important in its ability to contribute to increasing the patient's self-esteem (Schuell et al., 1964).

It was Wepman's view that there were no specific formulas to be followed during aphasia therapy and that efforts should be stimulating, indirect, and not focused on specific behaviors. He suggested that, "Topics known to be of interest to the patient from his pre-morbid history should be elaborated largely through an increased focus on visualization." Stimulation was the core of therapy with ideas presented both verbally and nonverbally. Whatever the patients produced was accepted as their best possible response at the moment (Wepman, 1972). In later writings Wepman proposed the thesis that "language is inseparably related to thought but not identical with it . . . that it is the product of thought and the maidservant of man's highest mental processing." He saw the process of stimulation in speech therapy as an "embellishment of thought" and a vehicle for tapping residual language competence. He advocated removing the implied criticism of corrective therapy, accepting the patient's utterances as they occurred and never asking for or trying in any way to elicit verbal expression (Wepman, 1976).

Wepman's "indirect" stimulation approach was the natural result of his views on the nature of the disorder. He placed a premium on therapists' innovativeness, ingenuity, and individual creativity. In contrast, he saw direct, structured, performance-oriented attacks on the aphasic manifestation as most likely to become rigid language approaches. Wepman acknowledged, as have virtually all who work with cortical dysarthria (apraxia of speech) patients, that direct methods of articulation therapy along traditional lines based primarily on imitation practice with visual and kinesthetic cues is the appropriate approach.

In contrast to the loosely structured stimulation approach of Schuell et al. (1964) and Wepman's indirect protocols (1951), Luria (1970) proposed a direct, more controlled, step-by-step approach that is presumed to reconstruct the organization of language (i.e., processing). His model of aphasia rehabilitation proposed that language functions rely on complex neuronal networks he called complex functional systems, and that disruption of one part of the system impairs the entire system.

The renowned linguist Roman Jakobson (1968) considered aphasia a regressive phenomenon and suggested that intervention be based on an understanding of the stages of language development in normal children in all linguistic dimensions (i.e., phonologic, semantic, syntactic). To some extent Wepman (1964) also held to a regression theory by identifying five recovery stages as five types of aphasia: (1) global (prelanguage/absence of speech); (2) jargon; (3) pragmatic (increased acquisition of comprehension and oral production but limited in meaning and comprehension); (4) semantic (beginning of substantive propositional language); and (5) syntactic (the use of syntax/grammar in oral expression).

Lenneberg (1967), Schuell et al. (1964), and Weigl and Bierwisch (1970) maintained that although there is a disruption of performance in aphasia, linguistic competence is preserved. Lesser (1978) emphasized the wide range of language knowledge and skill among individuals as a function of age, education, culture, and social-intellectual factors. Lesser believed that linguistic competence in aphasia should not be compared with an ideal standard of linguistic behavior but with each individual's linguistic competence before the onset of aphasia.

One of the difficulties of designing a model of aphasia rehabilitation is that it is nearly impossible to do justice to the interaction of the cognitive, linguistic, and functional (pragmatic) components of communication behavior. The inadequacy of unidimensional models of the repertoire of behaviors that comprise communication is clear to those who have had the experience of observing large numbers of individuals with aphasia during the course of recovery. Wepman highlighted the need for combining "component" and "pragmatic" models as a basis for understanding recovery and rehabilitation by defining aphasia as "an impairment of the acquired capacity to comprehend and use verbal symbols for interpersonal communication" (Martin, 1986, p. 145).

In view of studies demonstrating the complexity of narrative discourse, particularly the need to make inferences, one can understand how speech therapy based on a stimulus-response model would be inadequate. Many investigators have begun to study narrative discourse in aphasia because most human communication takes place at this level.

RELEVANCE OF DIAGNOSIS AND CLASSIFICATION

Regardless of the theoretical model followed, the rationale for aphasia rehabilitation requires an understanding of the processes involved in normal communication, knowledge of classic aphasia syndromes, and careful analysis of a patient's linguistic deficits, residuals, and compensatory skills (Goodglass, 1987). The speech-language pathologist who has specialized in language disorders is uniquely equipped to assess both normal and pathologic speech and language performance, and to exercise the clinical judgment necessary to differentiate aphasia from other disorders. Differential diagnostic considerations may include cortical dysarthria (apraxia of speech), motor speech disorders, the speech and language of the healthy elderly, and the language disorders associated with dementia, Alzheimer's disease, or schizophrenia. Knowledge of normal speech-language behavior, speech science, neurolinguistics, the motor speech system, aphasia theory, the psychology of disability, and personality theory are essential to the differential diagnosis and assessment of rehabilitation candidacy. A differential diagnosis and aphasia classification are not simply of academic interest but are imperative, as they dictate the kind of rehabilitation management that is appropriate.

FUNCTIONAL COMMUNICATION IN APHASIA

Language use in natural situations differs significantly from language obtained from responses to structured tests (Gardner in Blumstein and Zurif, 1988; see also Taylor Sarno, 1965; Sarno, 1969, 1988). This point has been observed empirically and documented by the results of research. Our understanding of the characteristics of natural language behavior has been greatly enhanced by the considerable literature on the subject. During the 1980s studies of discourse analysis and pragmatics were particularly enlightening (Prutting and Kirchner, 1983). Although pragmatics, defined as the study of "the rules governing the use of language in context" (Bates, 1976), has been addressed by several investigators (Davis and Wilcox, 1981; Williams and Canter, 1982; Prutting and Kirchner, 1983; Hupet et al., 1986). The extent to which aphasics have a preserved knowledge of pragmatic functions and how it relates to functional communication behavior is in need of study.

Conversational speech does not resemble edited speech or any other form of structured speech. Natural conversation contains false starts, hesitations, word elongations, pauses, turn-taking, contextual cues, and many overlapping utterances in a complex interaction of speech and social behaviors comprising natural communication behaviors (Sarno, 1969, 1984; Sarno et al., 1971; Prutting and Kirchner, 1983; Davis and Wilcox, 1985; Lubinski, 1986). Natural language is influenced by the time and place of its occurrence, the purpose of the interaction, the individuals involved in the interaction, and a host of other contextual/environmental variables including certain nonverbal aspects of communication. Yet there appears to be some orderliness to natural speech, and it has been proposed that current studies might lead to a "grammar" of natural conversation.

The observation that an aphasic patient often performs differently on a formal language test than in a natural context is a common clinical report and has appeared frequently in the aphasia literature (Osgood and Miron, 1963; Sarno, 1969; Sarno et al., 1971; Wepman, in Garrett and Levine, 1973; Holland, 1982). For example, a patient who does poorly on a formal test of auditory comprehension may respond appropriately when asked a question casually. Another patient may show little difficulty understanding his wife when conversing about family matters but may not understand a paragraph that is read to him about the textile industry.

Psychological-situational factors may be important variables affecting functional communication in aphasia (Lesser, 1978). For example, patients and their families frequently report that the patient speaks best when using the telephone. This observation might relate to a higher anxiety level being associated with a face-to-face conversation. Furthermore, telephone language tends to be redundant and restricted with respect to its lexical-syntactic repertoire. Because communication is essentially a social behavior, a functional assessment of language must take into account the patient's family setting and living situation, vocational needs, premorbid personality, and life style. The uniqueness of the individual language user was well described by Critchley when he wrote "each person's manner of using language is something individual and personal, which he never altogether shares with the rest of the community; and it is something which reflects his total personality, in the same way as his handwriting or bodily mannerisms" (Critchley, 1952).

Compensatory strategies must also be accounted for in the assessment of functional communication effectiveness (Lomas and Kertesz, 1978). The same type and degree of impairment can manifest in different degrees of disability from one individual to the next. In other words, the degree of disability in a given patient need not be directly related to the amount of pathology. Green (1969) described a case in which the patient made himself understood by means of circumlocution, using "psychological" verbs and indefinite noun phrases. Green suggested that the person with anomic speech may order his language in such a fashion that he can elicit the words he needs from others. Earlier, Goldstein (1948) noted that one can sometimes be "deceived" by a patient's compensatory behavior.

Nonlinguistic factors also have an effect on the extent of functional communication disability. With severe aphasia, for example, the use of gestures, pantomime, alertness, awareness, activation, and the presence of a consistent and reliable yes–no response system may provide a degree of functional communication effectiveness despite a devastating language impairment. By contrast, if the ability to initiate is impaired and activational level is decreased, a patient may show functional impairment in the face of preserved vocabulary and syntax.

A functional frame of reference helps to define recovery by continually reminding us that the primary purpose of aphasia rehabilitation is to increase a person's ability to communicate in everyday life. In this regard, investigators have pointed out that (1) context is an important factor underlying language processing, and (2) aphasics perform best when dealing with personally relevant materials (Williams and Canter, 1982; Goodglass, 1987; Glosser et al., 1988).

Communication effectiveness (i.e., functional communication adequacy), then, is the sum total of the myriad linguistic and extralinguistic factors that contribute to the transmission of information, evaluated with respect to individual patients' life situations, reported premorbid personalities, levels of achievement, and other variables that contribute to their uniqueness as language users. The effects of verbal impairment on interpersonal interactions, use of verbal activities for leisure (e.g., watching television), ability to resume employment, overall impact on the quality of life, and ability to compensate or circumvent the deficits play a part in the patient's effectiveness as a communicator.

The current adoption of a functional frame of reference in much aphasia rehabilitation appears to represent an important shift from a simplistic, mechanistic, deficit-oriented conceptualization to a more context-, situation-, and person-dependent model. The change also reflects a more person-oriented view of the process and suggests that no single, specific technique can adequately meet the wide range of assets, liabilities, and needs manifest in each individual person with aphasia. Yet belief in the existence of single factor panaceas persists and can pose difficulty for patients and their families. Faced with complex, chronic medical conditions, they are accustomed to a medical model of health care in which there are often single, direct solutions to acute problems (e.g., surgery or drugs). When aphasic patients or their families hear of a successful clinical trial of a technique or approach, they not only want to try it immediately but the hope of a breakthrough compels them to seek the intervention regardless of cost.

ASSESSMENT OF FUNCTIONAL COMMUNICATION IN APHASIA

Traditional aphasia tests do not take into account the fact that aphasic patients may (1) use gestures, (2) respond accurately though inconsistently, or (3) have intact vocabulary and syntax but require greater time to respond orally. Until recently the measurement of verbal impairment in aphasia has been concerned with identifying deficits without particular regard to the effectiveness with which the damaged individual communicates in daily life. It bewilders many medical professionals whose most important concern is practical, functional efficiency in the face of disability. In their view the important consideration in aphasia rehabilitation is not the extent of pathology but, rather, the extent of its disabling effects on the individual.

Generally, in disciplines concerned with neuropathology, measures of aphasia have been primarily concerned with specific linguistic phenomena. Traditionally, aphasia assessment instruments are based on a stimulus–response behavioral model in which the patient is required to respond to specific stimuli/cues, and responses are scored on a correct/incorrect basis. In some tests the scoring system takes the type of error into account. Aphasia batteries generally sample a broad range of language behaviors in several modalities (e.g., speech production, auditory comprehension, written expression) at different levels of complexity. The available instruments represent a wide range of purposes, practicality, design, and standardization.

Most aphasia tests depend on brief samplings in many areas, resulting in a profile of strengths and weaknesses. They assess language skills within a constricted period under relatively artificial conditions (Sarno, 1980) and rely on the technique of "commanding" an aphasic patient to speak in order to obtain a language sample. This assessment method makes it highly unlikely that the performance approximates language use in a natural context. A study that addressed this issue compared findings on the Neurosensory Center Comprehensive Examination for Aphasia (NCCEA) and the Functional Communication Profile (FCP) in a group of patients who were administered the same battery of tests at each of four testing sessions 1, 3, 6, and 12 months post-stroke. The study results revealed a discrepancy in performance between structured language tests (NCCEA) and functional ratings (FCP) (Sarno and Levita, 1979).

Although traditional aphasia tests serve a purpose by identifying deficits for diagnostic classification and help in the determination of severity level and profile of impairment, they do not address the fundamentally important dimension of functional communication. In fact, preoccupation with the phenomenology of aphasia tends to draw attention away from the individual's use of residual and compensatory communication skills.

Functional Communication Profile

The first attempt to assess functional communication in aphasia appeared in 1965 (Taylor-Sarno, 1965) in a paper that introduced the concept. The report described the Functional Communication Profile (FCP), a rating scale that had been in use since 1955 at the Howard A. Rusk Institute of Rehabilitation Medicine of the New York University Medical Center. Later, Reinvang developed a Norwegian adaptation of the FCP called the Functional Aphasia Scale (Reinvang, 1969) The Communicative Abilities of Daily Living (CADL) is a more recent functional assessment tool (Holland, 1980). Functional measurement in aphasia is now an integral component of aphasia assessment on intake, during the course of recovery, and at discharge (Taylor Sarno, 1965; M.T. Sarno, 1969, 1980; J.E. Sarno et al., 1971).

On the FCP, weighted scores are converted into percentages in each of five modalities: Movement, Speaking, Understanding, Reading, and an Other category that includes writing and calculation. An overall score reflects the sum of the weighted scores and can be used as a single measure of an individual's functional communication effectiveness. The FCP was not intended to substitute for neurolinguistic measures of assessment but to complement them by providing a measure of the functional dimension of communication behavior.

Communicative Abilities in Daily Living

The CADL (Holland, 1977, 1982) is administered in the form of an interview that follows a script that attempts to incorporate natural language activities. The interview includes structured conversation and role-playing situations (i.e., pretending to be in a doctor's office).

NONVERBAL COMMUNICATION

The potential for using nonverbal means of communication in aphasia, especially in the severely impaired (sometimes globally aphasic) person has become a subject of interest. The presence of nonverbal communication impairments reflected in gestural deficits in aphasia is well known but not yet well understood. Some studies have supported a correlation between the degree of verbal deficit and impaired gesture and pantomime (Glosser et al., 1986; Coelho and Duffy, 1987). Despite this fact, the possibility that nonverbal channels might be available and functional in the context of aphasia continues to be a compelling area of methodologic and technologic development.

Studies in this area have been encouraging (Glass et al., 1975; Johanssen-Horback et al., 1985). Gardner and his team trained global aphasics to use a symbolic language called VIC, implemented with an index card system (Gardner et al., 1976); a computerized version called C-VIC (Weinrich, 1987); and Visual Action Therapy (VAT) designed to train patients to use representational gestures for communication (Helm-Estabrooks, 1982). These efforts have given impetus to the notion that alternative systems of communication might be available and functional for selected aphasic patients. However, the issue of candidacy for these approaches needs further study, as it is still not clear, even in a general sense, what configuration of pathophysiology, personality, aphasia type, severity, time since onset, and other variables characterizes the best candidates for nonverbal communication systems. It is also unclear what the most desirable time schedule for intervention might be. Should nonverbal communication systems be introduced after all traditional approaches have been explored? Is critical time lost if such systems are not introduced early or concomitantly with traditional approaches?

PSYCHOSOCIAL DIMENSION

Concern for the psychosocial dimensions of aphasia recovery and rehabilitation has increased in terms of the effects of psychosocial variables on both the recovery course and the quality of life. Aphasiologists generally agree that the basic personality of the person with aphasia does not change, but that premorbid personality patterns tend to be exaggerated (Horenstein, 1970; Benson, 1980; Martin, 1986). It is not surprising that the most commonly reported psychosocial symptom associated with aphasia is depression (Horenstein, 1970; Eisenson, 1973, Benson, 1980; Sarno, 1981; Borenstein al., 1987a, b; Wahrborg, 1988) since depression is a natural consequence of catastrophic illness. When a patient who depended on verbal skill for vocational and social fulfillment is severely depressed and keenly aware of his or her deficit, there may be some suicidal risk (Benson, 1980). Whether depression constitutes a reaction to the devastating reality of aphasia and its negative impact on most aspects of the individual's life or is the direct result of pathology to the dominant hemisphere has been questioned (Robinson and Szetala, 1981; Wahrborg and Borenstein, 1986; see also Chap. 8).

Depression is associated more frequently with Broca's aphasia (nonfluent aphasia that is generally the result of anterior lesions) than with Wernicke's aphasia (fluent aphasia that is usually secondary to posterior lesions) (Robinson and Szetala, 1981). This association has been attributed to the hypothesis that those with Broca's aphasia are more aware of their communication deficits, and their difficulty speaking makes their reaction to aphasia seem more appropriate than that seen in those with Wernicke's aphasia (Benson, 1980). However, the lack of awareness combined with impaired auditory comprehension may result in paranoia and impulsivity in patients with Wernicke's aphasia. These patients tend to blame others for their difficulty communicating and may also manifest anosognosia (Horenstein, 1970; Benson, 1980). A differential diagnosis between Wernicke's aphasia and psychiatric conditions is often difficult, especially if the patient uses jargon. In fact, most patients with aphasia who require psychiatric hospitalization are those with deficits in awareness, paranoia, and impulsive behavior (Benson, 1979, 1980).

Families of aphasic patients may also experience depression and react with overprotectiveness, hostility, anger, unrealistic expectations, and denial (Turnblom and Myers, 1952; Malone, 1969; Kinsella and Duffy, 1979; Code and Muller, 1983). Many of the emotional reactions displayed by patients and their families are influenced by the premorbid family structure. The advent of aphasia often precipitates a reversal of roles and changes in both levels of dependency and the family's economic situation. Family members may avoid the depressed aphasic patient and interpret depression as a sign of the patient "giving up," which may lead them to be angry and punitive. There is a common tendency for rehabilitation staff to feel helpless in the face of a depressed aphasic patient.

The depression associated with aphasia has been interpreted as a grief reaction, based on the idea that an acquired language loss must be mourned because it is the "loss" of a vital human function. Both real and symbolic loss can result from acquired communication deficits. In some ways the aphasic person grieves over a loss of the "self" that is closely identified with one's communicative effectiveness.

Maslow (1968) conceived of successful rehabilitation as a process of shifting from mere survival to self-actualization. Yet it has been noted that the disabled often show a reduced drive for self-actualization, which, if unrecognized when formulating rehabilitation goals, may lead to failure. Maslow stressed the fundamental relation between self-concept and the rehabilitation process, as self-actualization depends on the individual's becoming what he is "capable of becoming." For many disabled patients it means redefining the quality of life in an altered state.

Philosophically, for the disabled person there is a new "self," as the activities that contributed to the previous definition of that person are changed or no longer there. The person undergoing rehabilitation is a "dynamically evolving self" with a new relationship—to himself and to his world. In a sense, rehabilitation is a process of helping the patient think about and accept the new self—the self as it is now. Both patient and family need to evolve a new conception of self (Donnelley, 1988).

The techniques used for rehabilitation that meet the needs of patients with aphasia are to some degree based on approaches derived from psychotherapy, especially the principles underlying the psychology of disability and loss. One of the most effective management tools in aphasia is the selective and discriminating use of speech therapy to stimulate, support, and work through the various stages of recovery

(Brumfitt and Clarke, 1980; Sarno, 1980; Starkstein and Tanner, 1980). A therapeutic program is frequently a practical means of reducing depression (Horenstein, 1970; Benson, 1980; Sarno, 1981). While working on specific deficits, the patient is simultaneously adjusting psychologically. Speech therapy serves different purposes at different points in the recovery course. Sometimes it allows patients to "borrow time" (Baretz and Stephenson, 1976) and may help them arrive at a realistic assessment of language capacity.

With aphasia comes a "loss" of role in the family, community, and larger society (Starkstein and Tanner, 1980). The depressed aphasic patient often complains of chronic fatigue, passivity, lack of initiative, and a surrender to helplessness. When patients use denial as a defense against the reality of their situation, they may make unrealistic plans based on complete recovery, set deadline dates for recovery, or otherwise try to regain a sense of control over their lives while the depression resolves. Health professionals are generally unaccepting of these behaviors and tend to express anger at the patient's "unrealistic attitude," reflecting their own biases and fears of lack of success. This response can pose serious obstacles in the management process.

Grief is not a single reaction but a complex progression involving many emotions and attempts to adjust to and cope with loss. The now classic model proposed by Kubler-Ross (1969) of the stages that characterize the adjustment to death and dying is sometimes invoked to help explain the many reactions of grief and mourning observed in aphasics. Note that the difference between grief and depressive illness is as yet not clearly understood (Lindemann, 1944). Although specification of the order, duration, and progression of the stages of grieving varies from author to author, a progression of emotions and coping efforts is consistently reflected. Some personal accounts of aphasia support the conceptualization of the person with aphasia evolving through stages that culminate in adaptation (Wint, 1967). Some patients, of course, never come to terms with the loss and remain severely depressed (Espmark, 1973).

In an investigation of the nature of psychological regression in aphasia, Friedman (1961) concluded that, in addition to the communication difficulties posed by aphasia, a group of aphasic patients who met weekly to "discuss problems arising from language impairment" remained psychologically isolated. They did not develop and maintain a consistent level of group participation and expressed intense feelings that they were different from the others. They complained of these same behaviors in others; thus withdrawal and projection were also apparent. Friedman's study also suggested that aphasia can result in regressive behavior with impaired reality testing. Patients made defensive use of dependence, manifested in recurring demands that they be given more help by the therapist, preferably in smaller groups where greater individualized attention would be provided.

Observing that the variability of psychological reaction is rarely determined by the type or location of the lesion but is an expression of the whole life experience of the person who has had a stroke, Ullman (1962) wrote:

> [There is] need to focus not on an abstract appraisal of psychopathological matters but on understanding the current life situation and the consequent meaning of the stroke to the patient at this particular moment in his life. Repeatedly one gets the feeling in talking with these patients, that had the stroke occurred a year or two earlier or a year or two later, their reactions would have been quite different. At times it climaxes a process of resigna-

> tion and surrender set in motion years before; at other times it initiates such a process. In some patients it touches off a last-ditch stand dedicated to the pursuit of unattained life goals and ambitions. Occasionally it opens up new vistas for the elaboration of secondary gain from illness. Unrealistic strivings for independence and unrealistic dependency are perhaps the two main channels into which irrational modes of adaptation flow.

The work of Ullman (1962) and of Friedman has provided insights into the magnitude and complexity of the psychological and social consequences of stroke. Responding to this realization, individual psychotherapy and family counseling have been employed to alleviate aspects of the problem (Malone, 1969; Linell and Steg, 1980; Sarno and Sarno, 1981; Rollin, 1984; Hartman and Landau, 1987).

Two studies conducted in Goteborg, Sweden addressed the psychosocial consequences of aphasia. In one of the investigations, 11 clients with aphasia ranging in time since onset from 6 months to 7 years and seven family members were involved in a 5-day intensive residential program, with the goals of increasing information about aphasia and working on personal/interpersonal problems. One year later, nine of the patients met again, and great improvement was noted in their awareness and ability to deal with day-to-day difficulties. This innovative intervention had many positive effects on the participants' ability to cope with chronic aphasia (Borenstein et al., 1987a).

A second study investigated the effects of an educational program in a high school where eight young adults with chronic aphasia, whose mean time since onset was 3 years, were integrated into a normal curriculum. The patients were studied during a 30-week school semester while taking courses. All improved in verbal performance on language tests and showed a decrease in depression (Borenstein et al., 1987b).

In addition to depression, most patients with aphasia experience marked social isolation and are generally inadequately informed about the nature of aphasia. They feel imprisoned, irrevocably altered, and excluded from the mainstream of society. In 1987 the National Aphasia Association (NAA) conducted a national survey to identify the needs of the aphasic population. The respondents represented a cross section of age, time since onset, and social, educational, and economic status. Two thousand questionnaires were circulated, and responses were received from 10.5% of those polled. To the question, "What percentage of the general population do you think knows what aphasia is?" most (88%) responded "0 to 25%." Fifty percent reported that they did not have adequate information about aphasia. The most striking figure was related to feelings of isolation. Eighty-seven percent of the respondents indicated that they felt socially isolated.

The problem of social isolation, which stems directly from difficulty in communication, has a profound impact on those with aphasia. The extent to which they are able to come to terms with the diminished frequency and lack of intensity of social interactions and to carry on the everyday struggle with aphasia appears to have a great deal to do with each individual's premorbid personality and coping skills. For example, in those with type A personality, excessive work had often been used as a coping strategy (Pittner and Houston, 1980).

In the NAA survey, 68% responded that they had not returned to work (National Aphasia Association, 1988). This figure reflects a skewed sample, as those responding probably represent the mild end of the severity range. There is a great tendency to encourage aphasic patients to return to work, particularly if verbal deficits are mild.

If the patient's work depends on cognitive and verbal skills, even at fairly low levels, great caution should be exercised, as it is impossible to evaluate a patient's performance correctly except on the job. Premature attempts to return to work can be psychologically devastating. It is generally advisable to postpone such plans for as long as possible.

Assessing a patient's vocational potential and finding acceptable vocational alternatives where indicated is difficult, time-consuming, and often unsuccessful. A professional rehabilitation counselor is best equipped to help the patient work through the reality of his or her vocational limitations as well as to evaluate work performance and job requirements for those for whom an alternative vocation is a possibility.

Because aphasia is an impairment of communication, individuals feel altered in ways that affect their identity as people—their autonomy and self-determination. The aphasic patient may be perceived as having suffered a decline in intelligence. Those with aphasia, especially if it is severe, experience a profound sense of social deprivation. To some extent the feeling of isolation from the community and society at large seems partly related to society's prevailing negative attitudes toward, and low level of tolerance for, disability.

For professionals there is the danger of becoming so immersed in the details of a patient's communication disorder and linguistic recovery that the reality of the individual as a person is lost. The patients with their families need to be provided accurate, adequate information to help them allay fears, correct misconceptions, and help define the reality of aphasia. Patients also need to be allowed to be somewhat unrealistic during the time when they need to "borrow time" as a defense against the reality of the condition. It is essential to listen to the patient, particularly to expressions of loss; commiseration is usually more comforting than optimistic prognostic statements. The focus should be on function rather than recovery, and the patient needs to be given some sense of control and success.

In some of the larger programs where comprehensive services are offered, many types of therapeutic formats are provided. Group therapy designed to address various dimensions of rehabilitation management can be an effective method. Some groups focus on a particular modality for practice (e.g., reading), whereas others may concentrate on educating the patient about aphasia or on providing a setting for social conversation. In some programs functional activities have been introduced as part of the group therapy "curriculum" (i.e., ordering from menus or going shopping at a nearby store). Some patients reject group therapy, not wanting to identify as members of the disabled community.

Despite the quality and quantity of work in aphasia rehabilitation and an extensive world literature, many questions and dilemmas remain. Most have to do with the reality of aphasia as a chronic disability. A vivid illustration of the reaction of society to the individual aphasic was reported by a moderately impaired aphasic outpatient in his early thirties. The patient is a personable young man, 1 year poststroke, who commutes by train to our program several times a week. Recently he has begun to tell fellow train passengers that he is Swedish. This decision was the result of his realizing after several trips that if he tells people he is aphasic they tend to withdraw and avoid interacting with him. As a foreign visitor using English as a second language, strangers go out of their way to help him communicate. This anecdote not only highlights most people's reaction to the individual aphasic patient but also illustrates one patient's innovative way of dealing with the everyday struggle that characterizes aphasia.

RECOVERY: TIMETABLE AND EVOLUTION

The clinical judgment and skills required to manage the long-term aphasic can come only from first-hand knowledge of the natural history of aphasia. Individual variability across patients in both their profile of linguistic impairment and their reaction and adaptation to aphasia requires that therapists have direct experience with a large sample of patients systematically observed for a period of several years. Knowledge of the classic aphasia syndromes and their formal assessment alone is not adequate to meet the therapeutic needs of patients with chronic aphasia.

Patients' interpretations of recovery cover a wide range. Most do not consider themselves "recovered" unless they have returned fully to previous levels of language performance (Yarnell et al., 1976). On the other hand, patients with considerable impairment may adapt sufficiently to feel "recovered." If complete recovery is to occur, it usually happens spontaneously within hours or days of onset. Once aphasia has persisted for weeks and months, a complete return to a premorbid state is unusual (Kertesz, 1979).

It is desirable to distinguish between two recovery dimensions. One is totally objective and attempts to identify, as far as it is possible, whether and to what degree the patients have regained their previous language abilities. The second dimension assesses the degree of functional recovery and adaptation. Few if any investigators have considered this relevant dimension of the patient's perceptions of their "recovery" (Sarno et al., 1971).

Patients with aphasia improve over a long period (Kertesz, 1979; Sarno and Levita, 1979; Benson, 1980). An analogy can be found in the report of Brooks (1984), who pointed out that in the closed head injured patient there is significant improvement in functional performance that extends beyond the first year after injury. Changes after the first year post-stroke were noted by Marks et al. (1957) and Sands et al. (1969). Various investigators have reported different patterns of recovery that are probably a function of both the sample studied and the measures used. A number of studies have concluded that the greatest improvement occurs on imitative tasks, and that auditory comprehension improves more than expressive language in nonfluent aphasia (Vignolo, 1964; Kenin and Swisher, 1972; Lebrun, 1976; Prins et al., 1978). Lomas and Kertesz (1978) found equal improvement on all language tasks for patients with good comprehension, and more selective improvement largely in comprehension and imitative tasks, for patients with severely impaired auditory comprehension. In a small group of treated global aphasics the greatest improvement was noted in auditory comprehension and the least change in propositional speech at 3 months post-stroke (Sarno and Levita, 1981). Anomic aphasia is a common end-stage of evolution in addition to being a common aphasic syndrome (Goodglass and Kaplan, 1972; Kertesz, 1979).

In a study of 34 treated aphasic patients who were evenly distributed among fluent, nonfluent, and global aphasic categories, Sarno and Levita (1979) found that fluent and nonfluent groups were similar in performance and essentially equidistant from normal performance levels at 12 weeks post-stroke. Differential improvement was noted according to aphasia type across the first year. During the 3- to 6-month period post-stroke, fluent aphasic patients made the greatest gains, and the global group made almost no changes. During the 6- to 12-month period the greatest magnitude of improvement was noted on the Token Test for the global group. Nonfluent patients made steady gains over the first post-stroke year, never reaching the levels attained by the fluent aphasics. Ludlow (1977) found no difference between fluent and nonfluent patients in the sequence of recovery. Kertesz reported that initial severity, rather than type of aphasia, was the most important factor determining the recovery outcome and evolution of aphasia (Kertesz, 1979).

Those aphasiologists who have followed large samples of aphasic patients for long periods generally agree that linguistic changes become stabilized somewhere in the 12- to 18-month post-stroke period. The process of adjustment, adaptation, and compensatory behavior, however, continues for the remainder of the patient's life, though changes become more subtle as time passes. Occasionally, depression lifts after speech therapy has been initiated, reflecting the supportive and nurturing quality of the therapeutic relationship rather than an objective improvement in speech (Ullman, 1962). It is counterproductive to pressure patients into working hard on language tasks (Benson, 1979). Rather, speech therapy serves to expedite passage through the stages of aphasia rehabilitation, from grief reaction to adaptation, in addition to providing essential compensatory communication strategies.

ETHICAL PERSPECTIVE

Many issues and ethical-moral dilemmas face those who are managing aphasic patients. In some instances their resolution requires new knowledge if we are to make informed decisions. Rehabilitation medicine services are not a right or entitlement; they are provided on a selective basis to patients believed to have the potential to "benefit" (Caplan Haas et al., 1987; Haas, 1988). The practice of selecting patients for aphasia rehabilitation has been cited for the ethical-moral dilemmas it raises, as the factors that contribute to successful rehabilitation outcome are not clearly understood. The interactions of age, time since onset, personality, type and severity of aphasia, intervention techniques, and other variables are not yet clear, making it questionable if it is possible to select patients who can "benefit" (Sarno, 1986; Haas et al., 1988; Sarno in Haas et al., 1988).

Patients who receive aphasia rehabilitation services are generally selected on the basis of criteria determined by individual hospital committees, health practitioners, or both on the assumption that the relative importance of given variables and their influences on rehabilitation outcome is known. In reality, many candidates who might be ready and able to improve are denied services. Some would argue that all aphasic persons are candidates for a trial period of treatment to determine their candidacy for further treatment and that trial periods should be provided at different points in the recovery course. Experience suggests that the factors that prevail at one point do not necessarily obtain at another.

The extent to which the person with aphasia should determine their own rehabilitation regimens is an unresolved issue. Should speech therapy be provided to a patient who does not want it but whose family desperately wants him to undergo therapy? Should a severely impaired aphasic patient be included in family decision-making even if he clearly has little comprehension of the discussion at hand? Obviously, in the ideal situation, the patient's right to have as much control as possible over his or her life would be respected and encouraged. One way to facilitate patients' self-determination is to allow them to take over the goal-setting process gradually as they improve. To what degree is this possible, however, if the patient is severely impaired?

One of the most difficult dilemmas in aphasia rehabilitation is the setting of goals, as there are often marked discrepancies in the expectations of patient, family, speech pathologist, physician, and society. How long treatment should be provided is another difficult decision, especially as current studies point toward language and affective changes occurring over an extended period (Borenstein et al., 1987a, b). Should linguistic, functional, *and* quality of life goals dictate the criteria for the termination of intervention? If so, whether patients have come to terms with their limitations becomes an important factor.

There are several additional aspects to the problem. Should therapy goals relate specifically to linguistic improvement or to general adjustment? Is the patient to return to the community and to work? Should the goals relate to a presumed potential level of improvement? Who should set the goals: the patient, the family, the speech pathologist, the physician? Whose standards and values should direct the continuing of care? Where should rehabilitation medicine properly end and educational, community, and social agency care begin? Is the termination of speech therapy for the aphasic patient sometimes the equivalent of abandonment in the rehabilitation context? At what point during rehabilitation does a patient "fail" a trial period? What about the phenomenon of a "plateau"? How is it defined? Does it stand for a temporary period of "status quo," or does it indeed represent the end of a dynamic period of improvement and the beginning of the "chronic" stage?

CONCLUSION

This chapter has attempted to articulate a philosophy of aphasia rehabilitation in contrast to an "approach." This point of view considers that the most pressing needs of patients and their families are those related to aphasia as a chronic disability and its psychosocial impact, which depends on a patient's stage of recovery. Appropriate and effective management must address these aspects of the consequences of aphasia if it is to be meaningful and responsible.

REFERENCES

Albert, M.A., and Helm-Estabrooks, N. (1988). Diagnosis and treatment of aphasia. Part II. *J.A.M.A.*, **259**, 1205–1210.

Baretz, R., and Stephenson, G. (1976). Unrealistic patient. *N.Y. State J. Med.*, **76**, 54–57.

Bates, E. (1976). *Language in context.* Orlando: Acdemic Press.

Benson, D.F. (1979). *Aphasia, Alexia and Agraphia.* New York: Churchill Livingstone.

Benson, D.F. (1980). Psychiatric problems in aphasia. In: M.T. Sarno and O. Hook, eds., *Aphasia: Assessment and Treatment,* pp. 192–201. Stockholm: Almquist & Wiksell.

Benton, A.L. and Joynt, R.J. (1960). Early descriptions of aphasia. *Arch. Neurol.,* **3,** 109–126.

Blumstein, S., and Zurif, E. (1988). Special issue in honour of Harold Goodglass. *Aphasiology,* **2,** 3–4.

Borenstein, P., Linell, S., and Warborg, P. (1987a). An innovative therapeutic program for aphasia patients and their relatives. *Scand. J. Rehabil. Med.,* **19,** 51–56.

Borenstein, P., Wahrborg, P., Linell, S., Hedberg, E., Asking, M., and Ahlsen, E. (1987b). Education in "Folk High School" for younger aphasic people. *Aphasiology,* **1,** 263–266.

Broadbent, D. (1879). A case of peculiar affection of speech [with commentary]. *Brain,* **1,** 484–503.

Broca, P. (1885). Du siege de la faculte du langage articule. *Bull. Soc. Anthropol.,* **6,** 377–399.

Brooks, N.E., ed. (1984). *Closed Head Injury: Psychological, Social and Family Consequences.* Oxford: Oxford University Press.

Brumfitt, S., and Clarke, P. (1980). An application of psychotherapeutic techniques to the management of aphasia. Presented at Summer Conference, Aphasia Therapy, Cardiff, England.

Brust, R.J., Shafer, S., Richter, R., and Brown, B. (1976). Aphasia in acute stroke. *Stroke,* **7,** 167–174.

Caplan, A.L., Callahan, D., and Haas, J. (1987). *Ethical and Policy Issues in Rehabilitation Medicine. A Hastings Center Report* (special supplement). Briarcliff Manor, NY: Hastings Center.

Chapey, R., ed. (1986). *Language Intervention Strategies in Adult Aphasia,* 2nd ed. Baltimore: Williams & Wilkins.

Code, C., and Muller, D.J. (1983). *Aphasia Therapy.* London: Edward Arnold.

Coelho, C.A., and Duffy, R.J. (1987). The relationship of the acquisition of manual signs to severity of aphasia: a training study. *Brain Lang.,* **31,** 328–345.

Critchley, M. (1952). Articulatory deficits in aphasia. *J. Laryngol. Otol.,* **66,** 1–17.

Critchley, M. (1970). *Aphasiology and Other Aspects of Language.* London: Edward Arnold.

Darley, F. (1970). Language rehabilitation: presentation 8. In: A. Benton, ed. *Behavioral Change in Cerebrovascular Disease.* New York: Harper.

Darley, F. (1972). The efficacy of language rehabilitation in aphasia. *Journal of Speech and Hearing Disorders,* **37,** 3–21.

Darley, F. (1975). Treatment of acquired aphasia. *Adv. Neurol.,* **7,** 111–145.

Davis, G.A. (1983). *A Survey of Adult Aphasia.* Englewood Cliffs, NJ: Prentice-Hall.

Davis, G.A., and Wilcox, M.J. (1981). Incorporating parameters of natural conversation in aphasia treatment. In: R. Chapey, ed. *Language Intervention Strategies in Adult Aphasia.* Baltimore: Williams & Wilkins.

Davis, G.A., and Wilcox, M.J. (1985). *Adult Aphasia Rehabilitation: Applied Pragmatics.* San Diego: College Hill Press.

Derman, S., and Manaster, A. (1967). Family counseling with relatives of aphasic patients at Schwartz Rehabilitation Hosptial. *J. Am. Speech Hear. Assoc.,* **9,** 175–177.

Donnelley, S. (1988). Rehabilitation and evolving selves. Presented at the Rehabilitation Institute of Chicago Conference: Ethics in Rehabilitation Medicine: Issues and Dilemmas, Chicago.

Eisenson, J. (1973). *Adult Aphasia: Assessment and Treatment.* Englewood Cliffs, NJ: Prentice-Hall.

Eisenson, J. (1986). In: R. Chapey, ed. *Language Intervention Strategies in Adult Aphasia,* 2nd ed. Baltimore: Williams & Wilkins.

Espmark, S. (1973). Stroke before 50: a followup study of vocational and psychological adjustment. *Scand. J. Rehabil. Med.* [*Suppl. 2*].

Friedman, M. (1961). On the nature of regression. *Arch. Gen. Psychiatry,* **5,** 60–64.

Gardner, H., Zurif, E., Berry, T., and Baker, E. (1976). Visual communication in aphasia. *Neuropsychologia,* **14,** 275.

Garrett, J., and Levine, E., eds. (1973). *Psychological Practices with the Physically Disabled.* New York: Columbia University Press.

Glass, A., Gazzaniga, M., and Premack, D. (1975). Artificial language training in aphasia. *Neuropsychologia,* **2,** 95–103.

Glosser, G., Wiener, M., and Kaplan, E. (1986). Communicative gestures in aphasia. *Brain Lang.,* **27,** 345–359.

Glosser, G., Wiener, M., and Kaplan, E. (1988). Variations in aphasic language behaviors. *J. Speech Hear. Disord.,* **53,** 115–124.

Goldscheider, A. (1902). *Handbuck der physikalischer therapie,* Vol. 2, part 2, Leipzig.

Goldstein, K. (1948). *Language and Language Disturbances.* Orlando: Grune & Stratton.

Goodglass, H. (1985). Aphasiology in the United States. *Int. J. Neurosci.,* **25,** 307–311. (Cited: *Amnestic aphasia and agraphia,* 1879.)

Goodglass, H. (1987). In: M. Meier, A. Benton, and L. Diller. (eds.) *Neuropsychological Rehabilitation.* New York: Guilford Press.

Goodglass, H., and Kaplan, E. (1972). *Assessment of Aphasia and Related disorders.* Philadelphia: Lea & Febiger.

Granger, C., and Gresham, G. (1984). *Functional Assessment in Rehabilitation Medicine.* Baltimore: Williams & Wilkins.

Green, E. (1969). Phonological and grammatical aspects of jargon in an aphasic patient: a case study. *Lang. Speech,* **12,** 103–118.

Guitzmann, H. (1894). *Des kindes sprache und sprachfehler.* Leipzig.

Haas, J. (1988). Admission to rehabilitation centers: selection of patients. *Arch. Phys. Med. Rehabil.,* **69,** 329–332.

Haas, J., Caplan, A.L., and Callahan, D.J. (1988). *Case Studies in Ethics and Rehabilitation.* Briarcliff Manor, NY: Hastings Center.

Halper, A., and Burns, M. (1988). *Speech/Language Treatment of the Aphasias: An Integrated Clinical Approach.* Rockville, MD: Aspen Publishers.

Hartman, J., and Landau, W. (1987). Comparison of formal language therapy with supporting counseling for aphasia due to acute vascular accident. *Arch. Neurol.,* **44,** 646–649.

Head, H. (1926). *Aphasia and Kindred Disorders of Speech.* New York: Hafner Publishing (reprinted 1963).

Holland, A.L. (1977). *Estimators of aphasic Patients' Communicative Performance in Daily Life: Final Report.* Washington, D.C.: National Institute of Health, NINCDS.

Holland, A.L. (1980). *Communicative Abilities in Daily Living: Manual.* Baltimore: University Park Press.

Holland, A.L. (1982). Observing functional communication of aphasic adults. *J. Speech Hear. Disord.,* **47,** 50–56.

Holland, A.L. (1984). *Language disorders in Adults: Recent Advances.* San Diego: College-Hill Press.

Hooper, C.R., and Dunkle, R.E. (1984). *The Older Aphasic Person: Strategies in Treatment and Diagnosis.* Rockville, MD: Aspen Systems Corp.

Horenstein, S. (1970). Presentation 17. In: A.L. Benton ed. *Behavioral Changes in Cerebrovascular Disease,* pp. 171–194. New York: Harper & Row.

Hun, T. (1847). A case of amnesia. *Am. J. Insanity,* **7,** 358.

Hupet, M., Seron, X. and Frederix, M. (1986). Aphasics' sensitivity to contextual appropriateness conditions for pragmatic indicators. *Brain Lang.,* **28,** 126–140.

Jakobson, R. (1968). *Child Language, Aphasia and Phonological Universals.* The Hague: Mouton.

Johannsen-Horback, H., Ceyla, B., Mager, V., Schempp, B., and Wallesch, C.W. (1985). Treatment of chronic global aphasia with a nonverbal communication system. *Brain Lang.,* **24,** 74–82.

Kenin, M., and Swisher, L. (1972). A study of patterns of recovery in aphasia. *Cortex,* **8,** 56–68.

Kertesz, A. (1979). *Aphasia and Associated Disorders: Taxonomy, Localization and Recovery.* New York: Grune & Stratton.

Kinsella, G.F., and Duffy, F.D. (1979). Psychosocial readjustment in the spouses of aphasic patients. *Scand. J. Rehabil. Med.,* **7,** 129–132.

Kubler-Ross, E. (1969). *On Death and Dying.* New York: Macmillan.

Lenneberg, E. (1967). *Biological Foundations of Language. New York: Wiley.*

Lesser, R. (1978). *Linguistic Investigations of Aphasia.* London: Edward Arnold.

Lindemann, E. (1944). Symptomatology and management of acute grief. *Am. J. Psychiatry,* **101,** 141–149.

Licht, S. (1975). Brief history of stroke and its rehabilitation. In: S. Licht, ed., *Stroke and Its Rehabilitation,* pp. 1–27. Baltimore: Waverly Press.

Linnell, S., and Steg, G. (1980). Family treatment in aphasia—experience from a patient association. In: M.T. Sarno and O. Hook, eds., *Aphasia: Assessment and Treatment.* Stockholm: Almquist & Wiksell.

Lomas, J., and Kertesz, A. (1978). Patterns of spontaneous recovery in aphasic groups: a study of adult stroke patients. *Brain Lang.,* **5,** 388–401.

Lubinski, R. (1986). Environmental language intervention. In: R. Chapey, ed., *Language Intervention Strategies in Adult Aphasia,* 2nd ed. Baltimore: Williams & Wilkins.

Ludlow, C. (1977). Recovery from aphasia: a foundation for treatment. In: M. Sullivan and M. Krommers, eds., *Rationale for Adult Aphasia Therapy.* Omaha: University of Nebraska Medical Center.

Luria, A.R. (1948). *Rehabilitation of Brain Functioning After War Traumas.* Moscow: Academy of Sciences Press.

Luria, A.R. (1970). *Traumatic Aphasia.* The Hague: Mouton.

Malone, R. (1969). Expressed attitudes of families of aphasics. *J. Speech Hear. Disord.,* **34,** 146–150.

Marks, M., Taylor, M.L., and Rusk, H. (1957). Rehabilitation of the aphasic patient: a survey of three years experience in a rehabilitation setting. *Neurology,* **7,** 837–843.

Martin, A.D. (1986). An examination of Wepman's thought-centered therapy. In: R. Chapey, ed., *Language Intervention Strategies in Adult Aphasia,* 2nd ed. Baltimore: Williams & Wilkins.

Mettler, C.C. (1947). *History of Medicine.* Philadelphia: Blakiston.

Mills, C.K. (1880). *Medical Bulletin.* (Cited in Mills, 1904.)

Mills, C.K. (1904). Treatment of aphasia by training. *J.A.M.A.,* **43,** 1940–1949.

National Aphasia Association. (1988). NAA questionnaire response summary. Unpublished report. New York: National Aphasia Association.

National Institute of Neurological & Communicative Disorders and Stroke. (1979). *Aphasia: Hope Through Research.* Washington, D.C.: U.S. Department of Health, Education and Welfare.

Osgood, C.E., and Miron, M.S., eds. (1963). *Approaches to the Study of Aphasia.* Urbana: University of Illinois Press.

Pittner, M.S., and Houston, B.K. (1980). Response to stress, coping strategies and the type A behavior pattern. *J. Pers. Soc. Psychol.,* **39,** 147–157.

Prins, R., Snow, C., and Wagenaar, E. (1978). Recovery from aphasia: spontaneous speech versus language comprehension. *Brain Lang.*, **6,** 192–211.

Prutting, C., and Kirchner, D. (1983). Applied pragmatics. In: T. Gallagher and C. Prutting, eds., *Pragmatic Assessment and Intervention Issues in Language,* pp. 29–64. San Diego: College-Hill Press.

Reinvang, I. (1969). Functional language in aphasia. *Scand. J. Rehabil. Med.,* **1,** 112–116.

Reinvang, I., and Engvol, E. (1980). Language recovery in aphasia from 3–6 months after stroke. In: M.T. Sarno and O. Hook, eds., *Aphasia: Assessment and Treatment.* Stockholm: Almquist & Wiksell.

Robinson, R.G., and Szetala, B. (1981). Mood change following left hemispheric brain injury. *Ann. Neurol.* **9,** 447.

Rollin, W. (1984). Family therapy and the adult aphasic. In: J. Eisenson, ed., *Adult Aphasia.* Englewood Cliffs, N.J.: Prentice Hall. 252–80

Sands, E., Sarno, M.T., and Shankweiler, D. (1969). Long-term assessment of language function in aphasia due to stroke. *Arch. Phys. Med. Rehabil.,* **50,** 203–207.

Sarno, M.T. (1969). *The Functional Communication Profile: Manual of Directions.* New York: New York University Medical Center, Institute of Rehabilitation Medicine.

Sarno, M.T. (1980). Analyzing aphasic behavior. Aphasia rehabilitation. Review of research in aphasia: recovery and rehabilitation. In: M.T. Sarno and O. Hook, eds., *Aphasia: Assessment and Treatment,* pp. 15–76. Stockholm: Almquist & Wiksell.

Sarno, M.T. (1981). Recovery and rehabilitation in aphasia. In: M.T. Sarno, ed., *Acquired Aphasia,* pp. 485–529. Orlando: Academic Press.

Sarno, M.T. (1984). Functional measurement in verbal impairment secondary to brain damage. In: C. Granger and G. Gresham, eds., *Functional Assessment in Rehabilitation Medicine,* pp. 210–222. Baltimore: Williams & Wilkins.

Sarno, M.T. (1986). *The Silent Minority: The Patient with Aphasia.* Fifth Annual James C. Hemphill Lecture. Chicago: Rehabilitation Institute of Chicago.

Sarno, M.T. (1988). The case of Mr. M: the selection and treatment of aphasic patients. In: *Case Studies in Ethics and Rehabilitation,* pp. 24–28. Briarcliff Manor, N.Y.: Hastings Center.

Sarno, M.T., and Hook, O. (1980). *Aphasia: Assessment and Treatment.* Stockholm: Almquist & Wiksell.

Sarno, M.T., and Levita, E. (1979). Recovery in treated aphasia in the first year post-stroke. *Stroke,* **10,** 663–670.

Sarno, M.T., and Levita, E. (1981). Some observations on the nature and recovery in global aphasia after stroke. *Brain Lang.,* **13,** 1–12.

Sarno, J.E., and Sarno, M.T. (1981). *A Guide for Patients and Their Families,* revised, 2nd ed. New York: McGraw-Hill.

Sarno, J.E., Sarno, M.T., and Levita, E. (1971). Evaluating language improvement after completed stroke. *Arch. Phys. Med. Rehabil.,* **52,** 73–78.

Schuell, H., Jenkins, J., and Jimenez-Pabon, E. (1964). *Aphasia in Adults.* New York: Harper & Row.

Singer, H., and Low, A. (1933). The brain in a case of motor aphasia in which improvement occurred with training. *Arch. Neurol. Psychiatry,* **29,** 162–165.

Starkstein, S., and Tanner D. (1980). Loss and grief: implications for the speech-language pathologist and audiologist. *ASHA,* **22,** 916–928.

Taylor Sarno, M. (1965). A measurement of functional communication in aphasia. *Arch. Phys. Med. Rehabil.,* **46,** 101–107.

Turnblom, M.L., and Myers, J.S. (1952). A group discussion program with families of aphasic patients. *J. Speech Hear. Disord.,* **17,** 393–396.

Ullman, M. (1962). *Behavioral Changes in Patients Following Strokes.* Springfield: Charles C. Thomas.

Vignolo, L. (1964). Evolution of aphasia and language rehabilitation: a retrospective exploratory study. *Cortex,* **1,** 344–367.

Wahrborg, P. (1988). Behavioral Changes and Therapeutic Intervention in Aphasics and Their Relatives Following Stroke. Unpublished doctoral dissertation, University of Goteborg, Goteborg, Sweden.

Wahrborg, P., and Borenstein, P. (1986). Behavioral changes in aphasic patients and their relatives following stroke—a review of the literature. Presented at the 2nd International Aphasia Rehabilitation Congress, Goteborg, Sweden.

Weigl, E., and Bierwisch, M. (1970). Neuropsychology and linguistics: topics of common research. *Foundations of Lang.,* **6,** 1–18.

Weinrich, M.P. (1987). Computerized visual communication (C-VIC) therapy. Presented at the Academy of Aphasia, Phoenix, Arizona.

Wepman, J.M. (1951). *Recovery from Aphasia.* New York: Ronald Press.

Wepman, J.M. (1972). Aphasia therapy: a new look. *J. Speech Hear. Disord.,* **37,** 203.

Wepman, J.M. (1976). Aphasia: language without thought or thought without language. *ASHA,* **18,** 131–136.

Wepman, J.M., and Morency, A. (1963). Filmstrips as an adjunct to language therapy for aphasia. *J. Speech Hear. Disord.,* **28,** 191.

Williams, S.E., and Canter, J. (1982). The influence of situational content on naming performance in aphasia syndromes. *Brain Lang.,* **17,** 92–106.

Wint, G. (1967). *The Third Killer: Meditations on a Stroke.* New York: Abelard-Schuman.

Yarnell, P., Monroe, P., and Sobel, L. (1976). Aphasia outcome in stroke: a clinical neuroradiological correlation. *Stroke,* **7,** 514–522.

17

Rehabilitation of Cognitive and Neuropsychological Deficit Following Stroke

DAVID E. TUPPER

Each year stroke leaves more than 250,000 Americans, many of them elderly, handicapped with permanent disability (National Institute of Neurological and Communicative Disorders and Stroke [NINCDS], 1983a, b). Cognitive deficits contribute dually to the problems of rehabilitation of stroke patients. These deficits are themselves a primary treatment focus of rehabilitation and are related to the extent of the recovery of sensory and motor impairments often associated with stroke (Kinsella and Ford, 1980; Meier et al., 1982). Many of the approximately two million people in the United States currently disabled by stroke require rehabilitation to make significant progress toward more independent living (NINCDS, 1979).

Many therapists in the past believed that neuropsychological deficits following stroke were resistant to rehabilitation. In recent years, however, a more optimistic view of recovery and response to treatment has emerged (Newcombe, 1985; Williams and Long, 1987). This optimism is due in part to the increased quality of treatment research, in part to pressures from third party payors regarding treatment efficacy, and in part to unbridled enthusiasm without empiric backing. Whatever the cause of this optimism, a clinician is still too often left with a variety of largely unvalidated strategies, procedures, and theoretical frameworks from which to choose.

In this chapter is described a comprehensive approach to the rehabilitation of cognitive and neuropsychological deficits that emphasizes the practical and functional aspects of impairment following stroke. The need for a comprehensive approach to the management of stroke is outlined, the outcome of rehabilitation efforts for various cognitive and functional disturbances is reviewed, and past comprehensive approaches are surveyed to develop an appreciation of the practical needs of stroke patients. The chapter focuses on nonlinguistic cognitive and neuropsychological disturbances, as the problem of language impairment is considered elsewhere (see Chapter 16).

NEED FOR COMPREHENSIVE REHABILITATION

Frequent neurobehavioral sequelae of stroke include speech and language disturbances, visuoperceptual difficulties, memory and learning deficits, emotional disorders, disorders of other aspects of higher cognitive function, and the resultant adaptive functioning difficulties of daily life (Benton, 1970). All of these difficulties, whether in an acute or a more chronic stage, create significant handicaps for the individual (Kotila et al., 1984). Without further recovery, these deficits can lead to lifelong disability unless some adjustments or interventions are made (Bach-y-Rita and Balliet, 1987).

The daunting multiplicity of behavioral effects of strokes requires that interventions be carefully conceived and thoroughly studied. However, with few exceptions (e.g., Franz, 1923; Diller and Weinberg, 1977; Gordon and Diller, 1983), past rehabilitative efforts of common cognitive and neuropsychological consequences of stroke have not been well researched or well described for practicing clinicians. In contrast, the rehabilitation of physical and motor deficits has a long and well described history (Sharpless, 1982; Dombovy and Bach-y-Rita, 1988), as does the rehabilitation of language deficits, although the latter efforts have been controversial (Howard and Hatfield, 1987).

The varied behavioral effects of stroke require a comprehensive framework on which to base cognitive interventions and plan appropriate treatments. Too often past research and treatment efforts in rehabilitation have focused narrowly on a single type of behavioral deficit following stroke and have evaluated the patient in too few settings. At times past efforts have ignored the intact competence of the patient, failed to address his or her overall adaptive abilities, and overlooked the social implications of the patient's deficit. A comprehensive model of the consequences of disease and appropriate interventions form the framework for the discussion of cognitive rehabilitation in the rest of this chapter. This model distinguishes among neuropsychological impairments, functional disabilities, and related handicaps following stroke. These distinctions reflect the core concepts of a comprehensive and flexible view of rehabilitation.

MODEL OF NEUROPSYCHOLOGICAL CONSEQUENCES OF STROKE

In 1980 the World Health Organization adopted a categorization of the functional consequences of disease, including stroke, that can be applied to the process of intervention (World Health Organization, 1980; Fuhrer, 1987). The following review of the framework is based on the writings of Frey (1984). This model considers the consequences of illness in terms of impairments, disabilities, and handicaps.

Impairment

An impairment is a loss or alteration in psychological, physiologic, or anatomic structure or function. In the case of stroke, the basic physiologic/anatomic alteration in cerebral function is attributable to loss of blood supply causing parenchymal damage. Stroke-related neuropsychological impairments are alterations in basic neural processes consequent to cerebral pathology, e.g., hemiplegia, aphasia, neglect, and agnosia. Traditional neuropsychological concerns, such as determining the location (e.g., focal versus nonfocal, cortical versus subcortical or brain stem), severity, and onset of the stroke, are important at this level (Brown et al., 1986). The underlying impairments are often a priority for treatment during the acute or subacute phases of intervention and rely on medical or surgical intervention in the hopes of influencing recovery of function (Novack et al., 1984). Treatment is often curative in focus, and the alleviation of the deficit is the major goal. The few preventive strategies that have been suggested with regard to the neuropsychological impairments following stroke deal primarily with alterations of the person's premorbid life style or the prevention of secondary medical complications from the cerebrovascular or cardiac accident itself (Kurtzke, 1985).

Functional Disabilities

Lasting impairment creates, on another level, a functional disability for the affected individual. A disability, then, is a restriction or lack of ability to perform an activity in the manner or within the range considered normal for a human. Disability results from impairment, although not all impairments create disabilities. For example, at the impairment level an alteration of the corticospinal tract unilaterally may lead to a hemiparesis, whereas at the disability level it creates difficulties in ambulation (the integrated activity or task) to varying degrees depending on the severity of the injury. Treatment directed at the levels of impairment and disability differ. Thus in this example a physical therapist may assist with range-of-motion and strengthening exercises to the patient but may also provide assistive devices and ambulation practice to improve functional ambulation.

Intervention at the level of a person's functional disabilities is generally considered to be the typical domain of rehabilitation, and the concern is usually individual improvement in a functional area. Such traditional disciplines as occupational, physical, and speech and language therapy and physiatry often function as a team at this level of intervention. A great deal of work has gone into the understanding and treatment of difficulties in "activities of daily living" (ADL) (e.g., Carter et al., 1988).

Cognitive and neuropsychological disabilities, however, are more difficult to conceptualize at this level; they pervade many aspects of an individual's functioning, requiring special expertise and intervention strategies that cut across disciplines. Examples of cognitive disabilities include, but are not limited to, communicative difficulties (e.g., understanding or expressing oneself in social situations, reading or writing difficulties), learning and memory problems (e.g., forgetting to turn off the stove, not remembering someone's name), disabilities due to visuoperceptual impairments (e.g., visual scanning problems that affect one's ability to do grocery shopping), and emotional disabilities such as uncontrolled or labile expression of emotional dis-tress. The interaction of cognitive disabilities with the components of everyday life tasks has only recently become a matter for neuropsychological investigation during assessment or treatment (Hart and Hayden, 1986). Nagele's (1985) review provided an interesting methodology for cognitive inference-making in daily tasks. Other common daily tasks affected by cognitive impairments and disabilities include driving and wheelchair maneuvering.

Deficit reduction is not the only or best method of treatment of cognitive disabilities. Treatment aimed at the impairment level may not be effective in certain areas of function. Rather, direct functional retraining at the level of integrated tasks (disabilities), taking into consideration the person's impairments, may also be a productive treatment approach (Giles and Clark-Wilson, 1988); this issue is discussed further later. In some cases, rehabilitation strategies attempt to alter the context in which the person's deficits are displayed (e.g., advising an individual to avoid circumstances in which his or her disability would normally be demonstrated). However, the traditional context for rehabilitation has been intervention at the level of disabilities by functional retraining or practice.

Handicap

Stroke-related handicaps occur as the result of impairments or disabilities. A handicap is a disadvantage for an individual that limits or prevents the fulfillment of a role normal for that individual. A handicap has social implications that are not implied by the concepts of impairment or disability. Although the appropriate intervention for a handicap is traditionally defined as a change in society through legislation or education, more practical intervention for handicaps occur at the individual level with attempts to alter the real-life circumstances of stroke victims. Not all disabilities lead to corresponding handicaps. Handicap is traditionally viewed as an interaction between the environment and a disabled person. Vocational, social, personal, educational, and community-based handicaps have all been experienced by stroke patients (Tobis, 1976; Fowler, 1981). The intervention of handicaps is complicated by a number of issues, the most important of which may be the age of the patient. Elderly patients, who are often the victims of stroke (Roth, 1988), have different life circumstances than young patients, and the handicaps they display may be both more subtle and more devastating. Vocational and educational handicaps may be significant when considering the cognitive potential and rehabilitation needs for young stroke patients but less so for older patients. On the other hand, personal (e.g., not being able to vist the grandchildren) handicaps may be more significant in the elderly patient and may be prime targets for appropriate intervention (Feibel and Springer, 1982).

A truly comprehensive intervention approach to the management of stroke-related difficulties deals with the neurologic, behavioral, and social levels of this model to varying degrees, depending on the area of dysfunction and the individual's particular life circumstances. Goals for rehabilitation need to be selected and prioritized appropriately (Livneh, 1988). Cognitive and neuropsychological impairments, because they are so pervasive and long-lasting, require special attention in the intervention hierarchy.

REHABILITATION OUTCOME OF NEUROPSYCHOLOGICAL IMPAIRMENTS

General Principles

The efficacy of stroke rehabilitation has only relatively recently been investigated in terms of outcome or the quality of the intervention process as a whole (Dombovy et al., 1986; Granger et al., 1988, 1989). Generally, stroke rehabilitation has been shown to be effective in increasing independent function but has a negligible effect on the pure neurologic deficit, which typically improves spontaneously during the course of rehabilitation and natural recovery (Lind, 1982; Bach-y-Rita et al., 1988). Usually early implementation of comprehensive rehabilitation programs results in better outcome, especially with moderately disabled survivors (Johnston and Keith, 1983; Reding and McDowell, 1987). Recovery is rarely complete, however, even after extensive rehabilitation; and most stroke patients require continued long-term support for residual impairments, disabilities, and handicaps. In fact, only about 10% of the stroke survivors in the Framingham Study (Goldberg, 1987) had no discernible functional disability as a result of the stroke.

Cognitive rehabilitation, a term that emerged during the mid-1970s to 1980s, attempts to reduce or circumvent cognitive disruptions in order to decrease the effects of these deficits on an individual's functional skills (Gouvier et al., 1986). Cognitive interventions have been applied in the past (e.g., Goldstein, 1942), but the evolution of specific interest in the remediation of cognitive or information-processing deficiencies is a relatively recent development. Neuropsychological rehabilitation, a more encompassing term, reflects an area of practice within clinical neuropsychology that deals with the cognitive, psychosocial, and other consequences of brain injury (Prigatano, 1986; Alfano and Finlayson, 1987).

Few outcome studies of cognitive or neuropsychological rehabilitation have been performed. Therefore the empiric foundation for cognitive remediation is tenuous. The remainder of this section provides a general discussion of the effectiveness of cognitive rehabilitation and an exposition of some of the principles of rehabilitation within the context of a comprehensive approach to stroke rehabilitation. It is followed by a review of the outcome of rehabilitation of specific neurobehavioral consequences of stroke.

Neuropsychological rehabilitation, as most other rehabilitation specialties, is often oriented toward the alleviation of impairments and disabilities. Typically, an assumption is made that the alteration or reorganization of cognitive processes can yield a productive outcome at the level of handicap (Williams, 1987). It should be noted, however, that a great deal of controversy surrounds the efficacy of both specific cognitive interventions and neuropsychological rehabilitation as a whole (Butler and Namerow, 1988). This chapter reviews previous research and current opinion in this area. Mechanisms of recovery and rehabilitation are discussed later in the chapter (see also Chapter 14).

Moehle and colleagues (1987) reviewed the theories utilized in the development and application of cognitive rehabilitation. Despite a lack of clearly validated models, these authors described five primary models currently in use that guide treatment programming. These models include (1) the functional system approach suggested by Luria and his colleagues (Luria and Tzvetkova, 1968; Tsvetkova, 1988); (2) developmental models (e.g., Craine, 1982); (3) learning theory models, or the application of behavioral psychology techniques in cognitive rehabilitation; (4) process training models (Sohlberg and Mateer, 1989); and (5) pragmatic or functionally applied models, which are not necessarily theory-based. These models are not reviewed further except to identify common neuropsychological principles during rehabilitation. The reader is referred to the original sources for greater detail or to several reviews of methodologic considerations in the application of these models (Gordon, 1987; Harter, 1987).

Craine (1982) has outlined examples of treatment principles for cognitive rehabilitation. The following guidelines are representative of the principles developed by others: (1) Recovery following cortical damage is possible; (2) the cerebral cortex is an open, malleable system; (3) cortical learning comes from repeated activity, which can then become organized into a functional system; (4) activities of retraining must recapitulate cognitive development; (5) stimulation through multiple modalities supplement each other in learning; (6) the primary objective is to develop the processes underlying learning; (7) training should be deficit-specific; and (8) consistent and systematic feedback is needed. In addition, investigators from specific perspectives have added other principles. For example, Sohlberg and Mateer (1989), in a process-specific approach, provided six more guidelines: (9) A theoretically motivated model defines each cognitive process area; (10) therapy tasks are administered repetitively for overlearning to take place; (11) goals and objectives are hierarchically organized; (12) remediation involves data-based and directed treatment; (13) the use of generalization probes provides measurement of treatment success; and (14) ultimate measures of success must be improvements in level of vocational ability and independent living. These principles and guidelines, which were derived from a variety of models, require further empiric support. Nevertheless, as noted by Wepman (1951), the practical treatment of cognitive and neuropsychological problems requires a broad, comprehensive, flexible approach that recognizes both theory in treatment and the adjustment needs of the patient. In this way, the process of reeducation or rehabilitation can be truly facilitative for the patient, and the multifaceted needs of the patient can be recognized for further research and clinical practice.

Except for individual case reports and group studies oriented toward specific deficits, there have been few comprehensive outcome studies of cognitive or neuropsychological rehabilitation in stroke. One possible exception is the work of Diller, Gordon and colleagues at New York University Medical Center, which approximates a comprehensive approach. Carter and coworkers (1983), in a controlled study with acute stroke patients, demonstrated that several specific thinking skills can be improved as the result of a regular cognitive retraining program that incorporates paper and pencil tasks, simple cuing procedures, positive reinforcement, and immediate feedback. Outcome studies of neuropsychological rehabilitation in other populations, such as those with traumatic head injury, however, show both general and specific changes in cognitive processes following cognitive rehabilitation (Prigatano, 1986, 1988; Diller, 1988). It is thus necessary to review the evidence documenting improved rehabilitation outcomes following specific neuropsychological impairments.

Specific Disorders

Visuoperceptual Disturbances

The most widely investigated area in the cognitive rehabilitation of stroke is that of visuoperceptual disturbances or visual information-processing disorders. Common difficulties include left-sided neglect, visual field cuts, hemiinattention, and, more rarely, cortical blindness and visual agnosia. These deficits tend to be associated with damage to the right cerebral hemisphere (Hier et al., 1983; Hier, 1986), although this chapter focuses on the function impaired and not the hemisphere involved. The rehabilitation of visuoperceptual disturbances have been reviewed elsewhere (Diller and Weinberg, 1977; Gordon and Diller, 1983; Gianutsos and Matheson, 1987; Gouvier and Warner, 1987), and accumulating evidence suggests that these disturbances are among the impairments most amenable to treatment.

There have been several studies on the recovery of visuoperceptual deficits in stroke patients as an indicator of spontaneous improvement (Wade et al., 1988). It appears that visuoperceptual dysfunction is particularly prevalent during the first few months of recovery (Eriksson et al., 1988). Although steady improvement of the gross manifestations occurs (Egelko et al., 1989), these deficits remain at discharge from the hospital and contribute to difficulties in home-based activities.

The most organized remediation of visuoperceptual deficits has been described and executed by the New York University (NYU) group (Gordon et al., 1985), who have published extensively and have made some of their training methods and data available for others (Gordon et al., 1984, 1986). Visual scanning training has been the most commonly used treatment approach for perceptual remediation, particularly for visual neglect. Scanning training attempts to train the patient to attend to and survey the whole stimulus field, particularly the left side, before or while making a response. Various stimuli have been used to facilitate this process, including lightboards ("scanning machines"), money placed throughout the field, and letter cancellation tasks (see example in Figure 17–1).

Weinberg et al. (1977) compared a group of patients who had undergone 1 month of scanning training to a group that had received only standard rehabilitation. Notable improvements were seen on not only letter cancellation-type tasks but also on other dependent measures, such as the Wide Range Achievement Test and general cognitive tasks. Patients with severe neglect showed the most improvement with training, although patients with mild neglect also showed some improvement. Not all remediation attempts have been successful (Diller and Weinberg, 1986). Gordon and Diller (1983) reviewed the findings in their series of visuoperceptual rehabilitation studies. These authors have found that deficits in visual scanning vary widely among patients and typically form the basis for the visual-processing disorders in right hemisphere injury cases on neuropsychological tests and in day-to-day behavior. Gordon and Diller have also concluded that competence in processing of visual information is layered, such that patients must acquire gross scanning skills before learning to locate words on a line. Furthermore, gains made in perceptual training were independent of the degree of initial processing impairment as well as of the locus and extent of brain damage. Finally, it was concluded that certain principles of training scanning could be developed from the program (e.g., anchoring a left-side stimulus, pacing of responses, use of feedback).

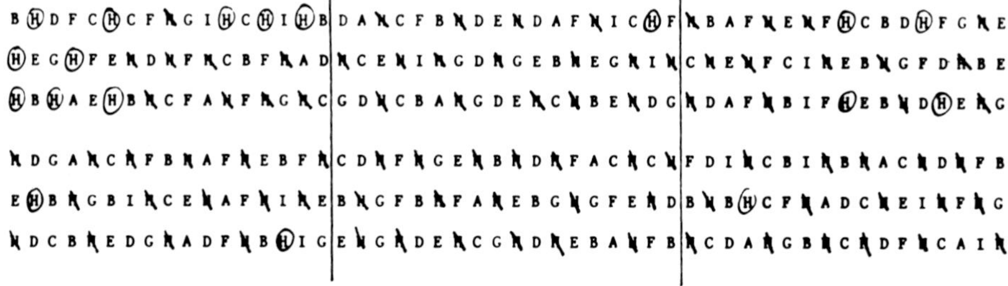

(a) time: 75 seconds
18 errors
6/1/81

(b) time: 85 seconds
0 errors
7/9/81

Figure 17–1 Improvement in a letter cancellation task following perceptual retraining. (A) Pretesting, (B) Post-test, approximately 5 weeks later. (Reproduced with permission from Gordon and Diller, 1983.)

Young and colleagues (1983) studied scanning training with the addition of training on a block design task. The study included three groups of subjects who underwent 1 hour of occupational therapy (OT) per day; OT plus cancellation and scanning training; or block design, cancellation, and lightboard scanning training only. All groups underwent twenty 1-hour treatment sessions. Dependent measures included WAIS Performance subtests, letter cancellation, WRAT, copying addresses, and counting faces tasks. The results indicated that the two groups with scanning training performed better than the OT-only group, but that the third group showed the best performance, implying that specific intensive scanning training yielded the best results. However, the impact of the training may have been limited to only a narrow range of behaviors (the dependent measures). OT itself, when oriented appropriately toward perceptual deficits, may achieve significant changes in visuoperceptual function (Neistadt, 1988). Further work is needed to assess generalization in this type of study.

Many sets of materials and treatment manuals have been developed to serve as practice materials for patients with perceptual deficits (Anderson and Miller, 1984; Burns et al., 1985; Siev et al., 1986). The theoretical basis of many of these methods are not known (Raymond, 1987; Hecht et al., 1988). Computer programs have also been developed that address visuoperceptual difficulties (Long, 1987). Whatever the actual perceptual training that takes place, the issue of the generalization of the training, or the "breadth" of the training (Egelko et al., 1986), needs to be considered. In the terminology of this chapter, it means that once the effect of the impairment is reduced it should have clear positive (and measurable) effects on the patient's disabilities and, ultimately, handicaps.

Webster et al. (1984) examined the generalization of lightboard scanning training to wheelchair navigation in a study designed to assess clinically significant effects of a treatment program on disabilities. With a multiple baseline, small N design they were able to show that lightboard scanning and letter cancellation improved dramatically for all subjects but that navigation abilities showed variable improvement across subjects. The subjects showed fewer direct collisions following scanning training, a finding which was maintained after 1 year of follow-up.

Gordon and Diller (1983) described the disabilities associated with visual information-processing disorders following right hemisphere injury. It can serve as a catalog of the various manifestations of impairment and may provide examples through which the generalization of remediation effects can be investigated.

Memory and Learning Difficulties

Memory disorders are frequent consequences of stroke, but efforts toward rehabilitation have infrequently been described. Memory is obviously a pervasive and complex skill, and one that is difficult to remediate. The history of memory improvement in normal subjects is long, but many questions about its effectiveness in that population remain unanswered.

Various forms of memory impairment may occur with stroke (Luria, 1976). Many of the amnesias following stroke are material-specific deficits related to unilateral hemispheric injury. More global memory disorders are seen with brain stem strokes, bilateral posterior cerebral artery infarctions, anoxic events, or rupture of an anterior communicating artery aneurysm. Disorientation due to amnesia is a frequent acute consequence of stroke. Certainly, memory and learning disorders are important to the patient's life and to the rehabilitation process, as new learning, mastery, and carryover are expected parts of most cognitive rehabilitation efforts (Wade et al., 1986; Caplan et al., 1988).

A discussion of the remediation of memory must recognize the complexity of not only current theories of memory function and amnesia but also the variety of treatment strategies that have been described. Memory retaining approaches have included retention, recall, internal and external mnemonic strategies, and physical treatments (Little, 1987; Wilson, 1987). Figure 17–2 illustrates the theoretical organization and practical examples of each of these strategies. As with perceptual retraining, repetition or repeated practice is a key element in the expected effectiveness of most strategies. Most of the published research in memory remediation is on

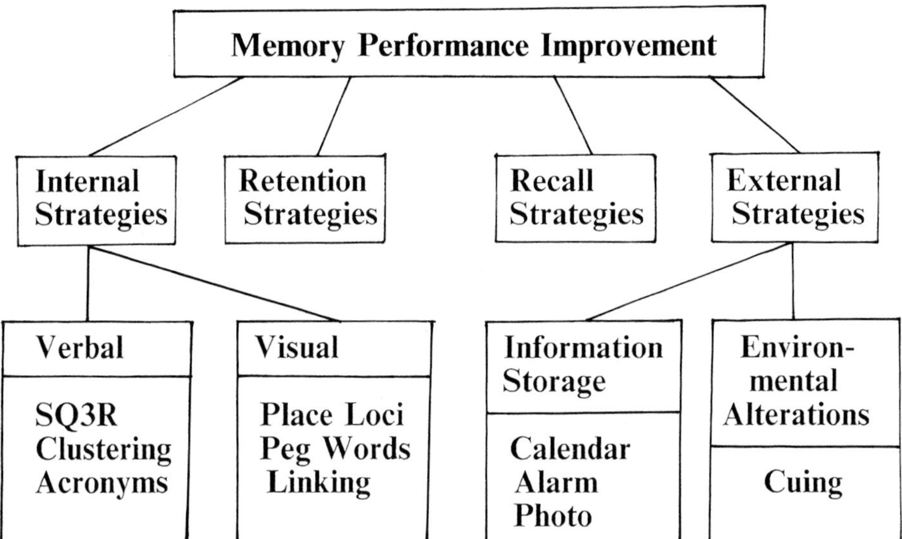

Figure 17–2 Memory retraining strategies. (Reproduced with permission from Little, 1987.)

head-injured patients, who often show markedly different patterns of impairment. To this author's knowledge, there are few studies of memory retraining exclusively with groups of stroke patients. Research with other populations has used visual imagery strategies, semantic elaboration, and provision of encoding and retrieval cues as internally mediated strategies for the patient. In addition, external memory aids have included the use of notebooks, reality orientation schedules, home computers, and wristwatches with signal alarms (Gouvier et al., 1986; Sohlberg and Mateer, 1989). Based on negative experiences with these methods as well as a critical review of the literature, Schacter and Glisky (1986) recommended the use of well focused, domain-specific attempts at memory remediation. As Mateer and Sohlberg (1988) pointed out, the minimal gains from some memory treatment methods may indicate that they lack sufficient ecologic validity to affect memory function in everyday life. Mateer and Sohlberg therefore recommended a greater focus on treatment of the memory process itself as well as the functional application of the memory process.

In a group study of stroke patients, Towle and colleagues (1986) investigated memory rehabilitation using computer-presented games. Eleven stroke patients with memory impairment were utilized. The patients spent 40 minutes a day on the computerized memory games during a 6-week treatment course. Seven of the patients showed some improvement (one standard deviation or more) on at least one memory outcome measure, but few group changes were seen. The authors concluded that specific memory skills can be learned as a result of memory retraining, but these skills generalize poorly to untrained memory tasks, as noted in other populations. Further group work is needed to evaluate the effectiveness of memory retraining, particularly as this study did not include a control group.

Wilson (1982) reported one of the few cases of memory retraining in a stroke patient. The case was a 51-year-old patient with confusion and severe memory difficulties. A computed tomography (CT) scan demonstrated softening in the territory of both posterior cerebral arteries, with better-defined atrophy on the left side, suggesting a more long-standing lesion. The patient recovered well physically and showed an intellectual level in the very superior range and few other cognitive difficulties, except for a severe and incapacitating memory disorder for both verbal and nonverbal material. The patient did not know his age or the year, and he had difficulty remembering his way around the rehabilitation center and his house.

He was offered a 6-week treatment program targeting four specific memory-related problems. The specific problems treated were (1) remembering the daily timetable, (2) remembering people's names, (3) remembering a shopping list, and (4) remembering short routes. A multiple baseline design was used to assess progress. Following baseline assessment, he was given strategies to deal with each problem on which he worked 4 days a week. Overall, the patient was able to achieve 100% success on two of the targeted problems. Although he did not show clear success on the other problems, he did show some improvement and was generally better on verbal than on nonverbal tasks. He was also able to remember a great deal of the information at a 3-month follow-up, but it was apparent that he did not fully incorporate use of the strategies into his daily life.

Based on the few available studies, it appears that some general conclusions and recommendations can be made. Memory dysfunction, like many other neuropsychological impairments, is complex and difficult to improve in a functional way without a great deal of concerted rehabilitation effort directed at its generalization to everyday life. It appears that the "abstract" strategies tried in other populations may not be clearly effective in the stroke population. It may be more effective to remediate memory problems by attempting to alter the patients' functioning in real life tasks directly through a behavioral approach and by altering the patients' needs in their lives to rely on their memory (Wilson, 1987), i.e., by intervention at the level of the resulting handicap.

Disorders of Higher Cognitive Functioning: Thinking Skills, Abstract Thought, Awareness

General intellectual deficiencies are infrequent in stroke victims unless the insult has been widespread and has caused more diffuse brain injury. Nonetheless, some aspects of higher order cognition have been noted to be impaired in a more global way, such as the capacity for abstract thought or the person's own awareness of his or her disabilities. In particular, Lehmann et al. (1975) stated that patients who have combined intellectual *and* perceptual deficits are less likely to gain during the rehabilitation process and are more likely to be institutionalized after discharge. Intellectual deficits are likely to affect progress in other areas and may create significant disabilities and handicaps. Thus disorders of higher cognitive function are a logical target for remediation, especially in a comprehensive program.

Carter et al. (1983) assessed whether a cognitive skills remediation program could help acute stroke patients regain important thinking skills. Patients in a community hospital were pretested and randomly assigned to either a treatment or a control group. The treatment group underwent 3 weeks of cognitive skill retraining, emphasizing higher order thinking skills. The control group underwent conventional therapies only. The treated patients had skill improvement scores that were significantly better than those for control patients. The authors stated that cognitive skill retraining was effective in stroke patients, and that it should be started early in the rehabilitation process, even during the acute phase. Unfortunately, there was insufficient psychometric data concerning the patients' intellectual status, although the study did suggest that general intellectual changes can be made.

A more frequent consequence of stroke that has been described is a lack, or altered awareness, of deficits (Cutting, 1978). Babinski in 1914 (quoted in McGlynn and Schacter, 1989) first reported a lack of awareness of a hemiplegia in two stroke patients with left hemiplegia. Babinski used the term anosognosia to describe this lack of awareness or recognition of the disease. Although the patients did not initially show intellectual deficits, some generalized mental deterioration was later observed. Weinstein and Kahn (1955) suggested that anosognosia was related to intellectual deterioration, although that conclusion is still open to question (McGlynn and Schacter, 1989). Certainly, there are cases where lack of awareness of deficit is clearly due to altered higher cognitive function. This author has seen several cases of severe lack of awareness of deficits correlated with reduced mental capacity in stroke patients, particularly after rupture and repair of an anterior communicating artery aneurysm.

There may be several reasons for the lack of studies aimed at improving stroke patients' awareness of deficits. The most obvious reason is that these difficulties are more common in the most severely impaired patients during the acute phases of recovery. These patients either recover quickly or remain severely disabled, requiring a great deal of support. Another reason is that this deficit is difficult to treat because it is not a simple cognitive dysfunction, and its improvement may depend on the improvement of other, more fundamental cognitive dysfunctions, such as a perceptual deficit (McGlynn and Schacter, 1989). This area is certainly one that needs investigation.

Emotional Disorders: Lability, Depression, Anxiety, Catastrophic Reactions

Depression and other emotional problems are often either primary or secondary sequelae of brain injury, including stroke (see Chapter 8). For example, the current literature suggests that approximately 30 to 60% of the stroke survivors in the United States are depressed (Ruckdeschel-Hibbard et al., 1987). Since the 1950s there has been increasing interest in the proposition that damage to the cerebral hemispheres can lead to primary emotional disturbances as well as cognitive difficulties. A growing body of research has described the affective disturbances associated with damage to each hemisphere (Ruckdeschel-Hibbard et al., 1986; see also Chapter 8). In general, indifference and denial of deficit are associated with right brain injuries; and anxiety and catastrophic reactions have been associated with left brain injuries (Starkstein and Robinson, 1988). In addition, right brain injured patients have difficulty recognizing faces, discriminating facial expressions, and choosing the appropriate emotions for a situation. Emotional disorders are a frequent consequence or reaction to stroke and require appropriate treatment within a comprehensive rehabilitation program.

Several writers have recommended a psychotherapeutic approach to the treatment of stroke-based emotional disorders (Gordon and Diller, 1983; Ruckdeschel-Hibbard et al., 1987). Medications have also been suggested, at least in a subgroup of stroke patients, but review of that work is outside the scope of this chapter. Diagnosis of depression or other emotional disorders is usually the first step toward treatment. Clear diagnosis is not always easy, as the patient often has cognitive problems that may mask the depression or precipitate the increased anxiety reaction. Many left hemisphere stroke patients, for instance, have major catastrophic reactions to their communication difficulties. Aphasia therapy with a concurrent psychotherapeutic approach may be productive in such a case (Wepman, 1951). Ruckdeschel-Hibbard et al. (1987) suggested that for the diagnosis of depression in stroke patients somatic symptoms should not be heavily weighed because somatic complaints are not particularly useful discriminators of the presence or severity of depression in stroke or other medically ill populations. In addition, the resistance to psychological evaluation common in the elderly should be kept in mind. Furthermore, existing assessment instruments (e.g., the Beck Depression Inventory) may be too cognitively complex for the stroke patient and may need to be modified to make the responses less demanding.

A second step in appropriate neuropsychological treatment is to determine whether the depression is transitory or reactionary, or if it is a chronic affective response. The type of intervention, as in other patient groups, varies according to the chronicity of the disorder. Premorbid reactions to illness may be particularly important to understand in this context.

In terms of actual treatment, most clinicians recommend a cognitively based psychotherapeutic approach to many brain-injured patients (Prigatano, 1986; Ruckdeschel-Hibbard et al., 1987). Such an approach deals with both the cognitive distortions of the patient and the altered emotional reactions. Although a full review of the principles of cognitive therapy is outside the scope of this chapter, several key points, borrowed from Ruckdeschel-Hibbard et al. (1987), are presented.

Opportunities should be provided within therapy sessions for modeling and overlearning, as well as mastery, of tasks prior to their attempts in everyday life. In this way, the chances of successful accomplishment and integration of the skill are increased. Emphasis is placed on the patient's assets and residual abilities. Finally, the focus of cognitive therapy is the identification and reality testing of cognitive distortions that serve to maintain the patient's altered mood. Therefore a close therapeutic relationship between the patient and family members helps the patient avoid feeling threatened by the process and thus enhances the likelihood of generalization.

Adaptive Functioning Difficulties

The loss of independent function is one of the greatest handicaps following stroke. The disabilities inolved are generally more integrated skills than those described to this point, and the cognitive skills underlying these integrated functions are not fully known. The major adaptive areas addressed thus far have included ADLs (particularly self-care and wheelchair transfers) and mobility, including wheelchair navigation and automobile driving. Neuropsychological impairments underlying these functions appear to be visuoperceptual deficits (Diller and Weinberg, 1970), apraxia (see Miller, 1986, regarding its management), attentional disorders, memory difficulties (Wade et al., 1986), and the patient's personality characteristics.

A study investigating remediation of the cognitive skills thought to underlie ADLs was performed by Carter et al. (1988). ADL scores were collected on acute patients who did or did not undergo cognitive skills remediation. Patients that received the training demonstrated significantly better personal hygiene, bathing, and toilet activity improvement scores. Additional analyses investigated the progress of 21 stroke patients given OT intervention that included training in both ADLs and cognitive skills. Results indicated that ADLs and cognitive skills performance increased significantly for these patients. Furthermore, improvement in cognitive skills was found to be positively related to improvement in performance of ADLs. Although these two analyses are preliminary and without an appropriate control group, they do show the potential for improved functional activities in acute stroke patients. A similar study of functional changes in more chronic patients would be useful.

Wheelchair transfer training was investigated in a case study (Stanton et al., 1983) of a 44-year-old woman who had failed to master safe transfers. Following a task analysis of safe transfers, she was given step-by-step instructions for each step as well as a sheet for self-monitoring her transfer behavior. As these steps were mastered and the training trials faded, the steps were reduced from 26 discrete steps to 13 larger steps. Intense repetition improved the patient's performance, so that 6 weeks after the program was implemented she was able to complete safe transfers and was discharged home. This study demonstrated that using a patient's verbal strengths as well as a careful task analysis can improve a behavior that is important to future discharge disposition.

Research regarding wheelchair navigation was touched on previously. Studies by Gouvier and colleagues (1984) and Webster et al. (1989) have demonstrated the successful treatment of perceptual deficits (hemispatial neglect) affecting wheelchair navigation around an obstacle course following right hemispheric stroke. In both of these studies, subtle residual problems in performance remained, leading the authors to recommend comprehensive, practical treatment of these navigational difficulties.

Driving an automobile is a complex task affected frequently by brain injury. Given the frequency of perceptual deficits following stroke and the elderly nature of the stroke population, it is surprising that there is not a greater database concerning its requisite skills and remediation. Sivak et al. (1984) attempted to demonstrate that remediation of perceptual/cognitive deficits would correlate with improved driving ability. Eight subjects (mixed diagnoses but mostly stroke) were given 8 to 10 hours of paper-and-pencil perceptual retraining (cancellation, pathfinding, pattern visualization, visual line tracing, pattern matching, and design construction and analysis tasks). The training was preceded and followed by repeated evaluations of perceptual ability and in-traffic driving performance. Results indicated that perceptual skills improved following the training, and that the training was associated with improved driving performance. Although subjects showed varying degrees of perceptual skill change, the degree of driving performance improvement was directly related to the degree of improvement of perceptual skills. Sivak et al. (1984) have therefore shown a strong relation between the remediation of a particular neuropsychological deficit and a real-life disability affecting independent mobility.

PROCESS OF REHABILITATION

Despite the progress in deficit reduction, many of the processes of neurologic recovery and rehabilitation remain a mystery. Nevertheless, some of the important concerns have been identified and several of the more salient contemporary intervention issues are dealt with here.

Neuropsychological Mechanisms

Neuropsychology and rehabilitation have a brief and still evolving relation in terms of understanding recovery of function (Beauvois and Derouesné, 1982; Miller, 1984). Two major theories regarding improvement in behavior due to recovery and remediation of function have been proposed (Rothi and Horner, 1983). The first theory—restitution of function—assumes that behavioral improvement results from the increasing integrity of the injured brain. This spontaneous recovery comes about through the physiologic changes due to diaschisis, decreased inhibitory influences on neurons, axonal regeneration, collateral sprouting, and denervation supersensitivity, as well as the decreased edema present at the site. These processes are most likely operative during the acute phases of recovery, and experimental evidence suggests that spontaneous changes in function secondary to these physiologic gains are seen from the first few weeks up to 6 months after injury (Rothi and Horner, 1983). Stimulation-based treatment methods are generally recommended during this time frame.

As more chronic physiologic changes are possible during the late phases of recovery (6 months or more later) (Geschwind, 1974), substitution of function has long been recognized as the most viable recovery mechanism (Luria and Tzvetkova, 1968). Several versions of this theory describe the "takeover" or circumvention of deficits by other cerebral regions to be the mechanism involved. This functional reorganization as a recovery model may be the result of dynamic processes, such as intra- or interhemispheric substitution, where higher cortical functions are improved owing to the cooperative interaction of different brain regions. Clearly, more variability, due to differences in the individual (Meier et al., 1987) and the environment, is seen here.

These two general theories of recovery of function provide, in a complementary way, a rationale for neuropsychological rehabilitation. Because further research support is needed to link these theories with intervention methodologies, they offer a direction for well designed rehabilitation efforts.

Maintenance and Generalization of Treatment Effects

Cognitive and neuropsychological rehabilitation, perhaps more than any other rehabilitation discipline, requires a concerted attempt to demonstrate maintenance and generalization of treatment effects. Therefore several suggestions regarding transfer of treatment effects to real-life behaviors are made here.

Gordon (1987) has described three levels of generalization from neuropsychological treatment to functional behaviors. At level I, rehabilitation should demonstrate that the result of training persists from one training session to the next as well as on alternate forms of the training materials. It is a demonstration of the maintenance of treatment gains. Level II improvement is noted on psychometric tests that are (1) similar to and (2) different from the task demands that are being trained. In cognitive psychology terminology, it is a demonstration of the near transfer of treatment effects. At level III, the emphasis is on the transfer (or generalization) of what has been learned from training to functioning as it occurs in day-to-day living. As Gordon (1987) noted, it is "the sine qua non for judging the effectiveness of an intervention program" (p. 125). In the terminology used in this chapter, it means that a rehabilitative outcome must be demonstrated not only at the level of deficit reduction but at the level of reduction of disability or handicap.

A developing technology is emerging in other rehabilitative spheres that provides strategies useful in training for maintenance and generalization, rather than just using a "train and hope" strategy for generalization. Application of these strategies to neuropsychological populations is a relatively new endeavor. Stokes and Osnes (1988) reviewed the various tactics and principles developed and applied in other areas. A major point is that generalization is not an all-or-none phenomenon, and that it needs to be appropriately programmed in advance. Heller (1979) also reminded professionals that an effective way to manage and program generalization is through altering the social environment of the patient. By using family members and relatives as reinforcers and supporters of treatment interventions, generalization can more often occur in the patient's natural environment. Use of family members also facilitates the maintenance of treatment gains.

Functional and Vocational Retraining

Ultimately, a neuropsychological rehabilitation effort needs to focus on improving functional and adaptive behaviors. Treatment programs designed to maintain a patient's progress (Marsh, 1984) must encourage appropriate performance of the functional behaviors attained previously. Often an emphasis on more practical behaviors fosters a patient's motivation to make further change.

Prigatano (1986) has noted, in a head injury population, how a focus on vocational programming can serve a useful function in increasing adaptive behaviors and in making the person a productive member of society. Work is the most evident handicap that can be altered in stroke patients. Diller (1970) has discussed vocational rehabilitation concerns in the stroke population. Wehman and Moon (1988) also discussed issues related to the vocational rehabilitation of stroke with an emphasis particularly on supported employment alternatives.

Coping with Chronic Neurologic Disorder

The personal struggles of individuals recovering from stroke have been well described (Moss, 1972; Sacks, 1985; Humphreys and Riddoch, 1987; Fishman, 1988). Interestingly, many of these cases have been rare disorders following stroke; and many of the routine, everyday difficulties in living with a chronic neuropsychological condition have not been fruitfully described. The neuropsychologist treating a stroke patient within a comprehensive framework must be cognizant of the many psychological and adjustment needs of these patients. Long-term counseling for both the patient and the family should be a frequent recommendation.

NEEDS FOR FUTURE RESEARCH AND PRACTICE

Neuropsychologically oriented rehabilitation of the stroke victim must go beyond a deficit reduction perspective and move to a position where it provides information regarding treatment strategies so that practical functional changes can be achieved. This chapter has advocated an approach emphasizing intervention at several levels of deficit so that rehabilitation neuropsychologists and other professionals can maintain a clear effort toward the multiple changes needed to increase the independent function of individuals after stroke. There is a strong need for more empiric studies of the effectiveness of specific neuropsychological interventions, as well as assessments of their effects on the patient's outcome environment. Continued creativity, as well as empiricism in future efforts, will pay off in increased hope for the person with neurobehavioral deficit following stroke.

REFERENCES

Alfano, D.P., and Finlayson, M.A.J. (1987). Clinical neuropsychology in rehabilitation. *Clin. Neuropsychol.*, **1,** 105–123.

Anderson, K., and Miller, P.C. (1984). *Recovery from Right Hemisphere Brain Damage* [5 workbooks]. Tigard, OR: C.C. Publications.

Bach-y-Rita, P., and Balliet, R. (1987). Recovery from stroke. In: P.W. Duncan and M.B. Badke, eds., *Motor Deficits Following Stroke,* pp. 79–107. Chicago: Year Book.

Bach-y-Rita, P., Lazarus, J.C., Boyeson, M.G., Balliet, R., and Myers, T.A. (1988). Neural aspects of motor function as a basis of early and post-acute rehabilitation. In: J.A. DeLisa, D.M. Currie, B.M. Gans, P.F. Gatens Jr., J.A. Leonard Jr., and M.C. McPhee, eds., *Rehabilitation Medicine,* pp. 175–195. Philadelphia: Lippincott.

Beauvois, M.F., and Derouesné, J. (1982). Recherche en neuropsychologie et education: quels rapports? In: X. Seron and C. Laterre, eds., *Rééduquer le Cerveau? Logopédie, Psychologie, Neurologie,* pp. 163–189. Brussels: Pierre Mardaga.

Benton, A.L., ed. (1970). *Behavioral Change in Cerebrovascular Disease.* New York: Harper & Row.

Brown, G.G., Baird, A.D., and Shatz, M.W. (1986). The effects of cerebrovascular disease and its treatment on higher cortical functioning. In: I. Grant and K.M. Adams, eds., *Neuropsychological Assessment in Neuropsychiatric Disorders,* pp. 384–414. New York: Oxford University Press.

Burns, M.S., Halper, A.S., and Mogil, S.I., eds. (1985). *Clinical Management of Right Hemisphere Dysfunction.* Rockville, MD: Aspen.

Butler, R.W., and Namerow, N.S. (1988). Cognitive retraining in brain injury rehabilitation: a critical review. *J. Neurol. Rehabil.*, **2,** 97–101.

Caplan, B., Cushman, L. Fink, W., and Reidy, K. (1988). Carryover in rehabilitation: neuropsychological data. *Arch. Phys. Med. Rehabil.*, **69,** 758–759.

Carter, L.T., Howard, B.E., and O'Neil, W.A. (1983). Effectiveness of cognitive skill remediation in acute stroke patients. *Am. J. Occup. Ther.*, **37,** 320–326.

Carter, L.T., Oliveira, J.O., Duponte, J., and Lynch, S.V. (1988). The relationship of cognitive skills performance to activities of daily living in stroke patients. *Am. J. Occup. Ther.*, **42,** 449–455.

Craine, J. (1982). Principles of cognitive rehabilitation. In: L. Trexler, ed., *Cognitive Rehabilitation: Conceptualization and Intervention,* pp. 83–98. New York: Plenum Press.

Cutting, J. (1978). Study of anosognosia. *J. Neurol. Neurosurg. Psychiatry,* **41,** 548–555.

Diller, L. (1970). Psychomotor and vocational rehabilitation: presentation 11. In: A.L. Benton, ed., *Behavioral Change in Cerebrovascular Disease,* pp. 81–105. New York: Harper & Row.

Diller, L. (1988). Rehabilitation in traumatic brain injury: observations on the current US scene. In: A.L. Christensen and B. Uzzell, eds., *Neuropsychological Rehabilitation,* pp. 53–68. Boston: Kluwer Academic Publishers.

Diller, L., and Weinberg, J. (1970). Evidence for accident-prone behavior in hemiplegic patients. *Arch. Phys. Med. Rehabil.,* **51,** 358–363.

Diller, L., and Weinberg, J. (1977). Hemi-inattention in rehabilitation: the evolution of a rational remediation program. In: E.A. Weinstein and R.P. Friedland, eds., *Hemi-inattention and Hemisphere Specialization,* pp. 63–82. New York: Raven Press.

Diller, L., and Weinberg, J. (1986). Learning from failures in perceptual cognitive retraining in stroke. In: B.P. Uzzell and Y. Gross, eds., *Clinical Neuropsychology of Intervention,* pp. 283–293. Boston: Martinus Nijhoff.

Dombovy, M.L., and Bach-y-Rita, P. (1988). Clinical observations on recovery from stroke. In: S.G. Waxman, ed., *Functional Recovery in Neurological Disease,* pp. 265–276. New York: Raven Press.

Dombovy, M.L., Sandok, B.A., and Basford, J.R. (1986). Rehabilitation for stroke: a review. *Stroke,* **17,** 363–369.

Egelko, S., Ruckdeschel-Hibbard, M., Gordon, W.A., and Riley, E. (1986). Cognitive treatment of RBD patients: depth vs breadth approach. *Arch. Phys. Med. Rehabil.,* **67,** 675.

Egelko, S., Simon, D., Riley, E., Gordon, W., Ruckdeschel-Hibbard, M., and Diller, L. (1989). First year after stroke: tracking cognitive and affective deficits. *Arch. Phys. Med. Rehabil.,* **70,** 297–302.

Eriksson, S., Bernspang, B., and Fugl-Meyer, A.R. (1988). Perceptual and motor impairment within 2 weeks after a stroke: a multifactorial statistical approach. *Occup. Ther. J. Res.,* **8**(2), 114–125.

Feibel, J.H., and Springer, C.J. (1982). Depression and failure to resume social activities after stroke. *Arch. Phys. Med. Rehabil.,* **63,** 276–278.

Fishman, S. (1988). *A Bomb in the Brain.* New York: Charles Scribner.

Fowler, R.S., Jr. (1981). Stroke and cerebral trauma: psychosocial and vocational aspects. In: W.C. Stolov and M.R. Clowers, eds., *Handbook of Severe Disability,* pp. 127–135. Washington, D.C.: U.S. Department of Education, Rehabilitation Services Administration.

Franz, S.I. (1923). *Nervous and Mental Re-education.* New York: Macmillan.

Frey, W.D. (1984). Functional assessment in the '80s: a conceptual enigma, a technical challenge. In: A.S. Halpern and M.J. Fuhrer, eds., *Functional Assessment in Rehabilitation,* pp. 11–43. Baltimore: Paul H. Brookes Publishing.

Fuhrer, M.J. (1987). Overview of outcome analysis in rehabilitation. In: M.J. Fuhrer, ed., *Rehabilitation Outcomes: Analysis and Measurement,* pp. 1–15. Baltimore: Paul H. Brookes Publishing.

Geschwind, N. (1974). Late changes in the nervous system: an overview. In: D.G. Stein, J.J. Rosen, and N. Butters, eds., *Plasticity and Recovery of Function in the Central Nervous System,* pp. 467–508. Orlando: Academic Press.

Gianutsos, R., and Matheson, P. (1987). The rehabilitation of visual perceptual disorders attributable to brain injury. In: M.J. Meier, A.L. Benton, and L. Diller, eds., *Neuropsychological Rehabilitation,* pp. 202–241. New York: Guilford Press.

Giles, G.M., and Clark-Wilson, J. (1988). Functional skills training in severe brain injury. In: I. Fussey and G.M. Giles, eds., *Rehabilitation of the Severely Brain-Injured Adult: A Practical Approach,* pp. 69–101. London: Croom Helm.

Goldberg, G. (1987). Principles of rehabilitation of the elderly stroke patient. In: R.F. Dunkle and J.W. Schmidley, eds., *Stroke in the Elderly: New Issues in Diagnosis, Treatment, and Rehabilitation,* pp. 103–143. New York: Springer Publishing.

Goldstein, K. (1942). *Aftereffects of Brain Injuries in War.* Orlando: Grune and Stratton.

Gordon, W.A. (1987). Methodological considerations in cognitive remediation. In: M.J. Meier,

A.L. Benton, and L. Diller, eds., *Neuropsychological Rehabilitation*, pp. 111–131. New York: Guilford Press.

Gordon, W.A., and Diller, L. (1983). Stroke: coping with a cognitive deficit. In: T.G. Burish and L.A. Bradley, eds., *Coping with Chronic Disease: Research and Applications*, pp. 113–135. Orlando: Academic Press.

Gordon, W.A., Ruckdeschel-Hibbard, M., Egelko, S., Diller, L., Simmens, S., Langer, K., Sarno, M., Orazem, J., and Weinberg, J. (1984). *Evaluation of the Deficits Associated with Right Brain Damage: Normative Data on the Institute of Rehabilitation Medicine Test Battery.* New York: Institute of Rehabilitation Medicine, N.Y.U. Medical Center.

Gordon, W., Hibbard, M., Egelko, S., Diller, L., Shaver, M., Lieberman, A., and Ragnarsson, K. (1985). Perceptual remediation in patients with right brain damage: a comprehensive program. *Arch. Phys. Med. Rehabil.*, **66,** 353–359.

Gordon, W.A., Ruckdeschel-Hibbard, M., Egelko, S., Weinberg, J., Diller, L., Shaver, M.S., and Piasetsky, E. (1986). *Techniques for the Treatment of Visual Neglect and Spatial Inattention in Right Brain Damaged Individuals.* New York: Rusk Institute of Rehabilitation Medicine, N.Y.U. Medical Center.

Gouvier, W.D., and Warner, M.S. (1987). Treatment of visual imperception and related disorders. In: J.M. Williams and C.J. Long, eds., *The Rehabilitation of Cognitive Disabilities*, pp. 109–122. New York: Plenum Press.

Gouvier, W.D., Cottam, G., Webster, J.S., Beissel, G.F., and Wofford, J. (1984). Behavioral interventions with stroke patients for improving wheelchair navigation. *Int. J. Clin. Neuropsychol.*, **6,** 186–190.

Gouvier, W.D., Webster, J.S., and Blanton, P.D. (1986). Cognitive retraining with brain-damaged patients. In: D. Wedding, A.M. Horton Jr., and J. Webster, eds., *The Neuropsychology Handbook: Behavioral and Clinical Perspectives*, pp. 278–324. New York: Springer Publishing.

Granger, C.V., Hamilton, B.B., and Gresham, G.E. (1988). The stroke rehabilitation outcome study. Part I. General description. *Arch. Phys. Med. Rehabil.*, **69,** 506–509.

Granger, C.V., Hamilton, B.B., Gresham, G.E., and Kramer, A.A. (1989). The stroke rehabilitation outcome study. Part II. Relative merits of the total Barthel index score and four-item subscore in predicting patient outcomes. *Arch. Phys. Med. Rehabil.*, **70,** 100–103.

Hart, T., and Hayden, M.E. (1986). The ecological validity of neuropsychological assessment and remediation. In: B.P. Uzzell and Y. Gross, eds., *Clinical Neuropsychology of Intervention*, pp. 21–50. Boston: Martinus Nijhoff.

Harter, G.W. (1987). Methodological issues in cognitive retraining research. In: J.M. Williams and C.J. Long, eds., *The Rehabilitation of Cognitive Disabilities*, pp. 95–107. New York: Plenum Press.

Hecht, J.S., Plummer, T., Fryer, B., and Meyer, R. (1988). Cognitively directed rehabilitation: use of left brain learning strengths to facilitate transfer in right brain stroke. *Arch. Phys. Med. Rehabil.*, **69,** 718 (abstract).

Heller, K. (1979). The effects of social support: prevention and treatment implications. In: A.P. Goldstein and F.H. Kanfer, eds., *Maximizing Treatment Gains: Transfer Enhancement in Psychotherapy*, pp. 353–382. Orlando: Academic Press.

Hier, D.B. (1986). Recovery from behavioral deficits after stroke. In: P.E. Kaplan and L.J. Cerullo, eds., *Stroke Rehabilitation.* Boston: Butterworths, pp. 147–157.

Hier, D.B., Mondlock, J., and Caplan, C.R. (1983). Recovery of behavioral abnormalities after right hemisphere stroke. *Neurology*, **33,** 345–350.

Howard, D., and Hatfield, F.M. (1987). *Aphasia Therapy: Historical and Contemporary Issues.* Hillsdale, NJ: Lawrence Erlbaum Associates.

Humphreys, G.W., and Riddoch, M.J. (1987). *To See But Not To See: A Case Study of Visual Agnosia.* Hillsdale, NJ: Lawrence Erlbaum Associates.

Johnston, M.V., and Keith, R.A. (1983). Cost-benefits of medical rehabilitation: review and critique. *Arch. Phys. Med. Rehabil.,* **64,** 147–154.

Kinsella, G., and Ford, B. (1980). Acute recovery patterns in stroke patients: neuropsychological factors. *Med. J. Aust.,* **2,** 663–666.

Kotila, M., Waltimo, O., Niemi, M.L., Laaksonen, R., and Lempinen, M. (1984). The profile of recovery from stroke and factors influencing outcome. *Stroke,* **15,** 1039–1044.

Kurtzke, J.F. (1985). Epidemiology of cerebrovascular disease. In: F.H. McDowell and L.R. Caplan, eds., *Cerebrovascular Survey Report 1985,* pp. 1–34. Washington, D.C.: National Institute of Neurological and Communicative Disorders and Stroke.

Lehmann, J.F., Delateur, B.J., Fowler, R.S., Warren, C.J., Arnold, R., Schenlzer, G., Hurka, R., Whitmore, J.J., Masock, A.J., and Chambers, K.H. (1975). Stroke rehabilitation: outcome and prediction. *Arch. Phys. Med. Rehabil.,* **56,** 383–389.

Lind, K. (1982). Synthesis of studies on stroke rehabilitation. *J. Chronic Dis.,* **35,** 133–149.

Little, M.M. (1987). The remediation of everyday memory deficits. In: J.M. Williams and C.J. Long, eds., *The Rehabilitation of Cognitive Disabilities,* pp. 123–138. New York: Plenum Press.

Livneh, H. (1988). Rehabilitation goals: their hierarchical and multifaceted nature. *J. Appl. Rehabil. Counseling,* **19**(3), 12–18.

Long, C.J. (1987). The current status of computer-assisted cognitive rehabilitation. In: J.M. Williams and C.J. Long, eds., *The Rehabilitation of Cognitive Disabilities,* pp. 79–93. New York: Plenum Press.

Luria, A.R. (1976). *The Neuropsychology of Memory.* Washington, D.C.: V.H. Winston.

Luria, A.R., and Tzvetkova, L.S. (1968). The re-education of brain-damaged patients and its psychopedagogical application. In: J. Hellmuth, ed., *Learning Disorders,* Vol. 3, pp. 139–154. Seattle: Special Child Publications.

Marsh, M. (1984). A day rehabilitation stroke program. *Arch. Phys. Med. Rehabil.,* **65,** 320–323.

Mateer, C.A., and Sohlberg, M.M. (1988). A paradigm shift in memory rehabilitation. In: H.A. Whitaker, ed., *Neuropsychological Studies of Nonfocal Brain Damage,* pp. 202–225. New York: Springer-Verlag.

McGlynn, S.M., and Schacter, D.L. (1989). Unawareness of deficits in neuropsychological syndromes. *J. Clin. Exp. Neuropsychol.,* **11,** 143–205.

Meier, M.J., Ettinger, M.G., and Arthur, L. (1982). Recovery of neuropsychological functioning after cerebrovascular infarction. In: R.N. Malatesha and L.C. Hartlage, eds., *Neuropsychology and Cognition,* Vol. 2, pp. 552–564. Boston: Martinus Nijhoff.

Meier, M.J., Strauman, S., and Thompson, W.G. (1987). Individual differences in neuropsychological recovery: an overview. In: M.J. Meier, A.L. Benton, and L. Diller, eds., *Neuropsychological Rehabilitation,* pp. 71–110. New York: Guilford Press.

Miller, E. (1984). *Recovery and Management of Neuropsychological Impairments.* New York: Wiley.

Miller, N. (1986). *Dyspraxia and Its Management.* Rockville, MD: Aspen Publishers.

Moehle, K.A., Rasmussen, J.L., and Fitzhugh-Bell, K.B. (1987). Neuropsychological theories and cognitive rehabilitation. In: J.M. Williams and C.J. Long, eds., *The Rehabilitation of Cognitive Disabilities,* pp. 57–76. New York: Plenum Press.

Moss, C. (1972). *Recovery with Aphasia: The Aftermath of My Stroke.* Urbana: University of Illinois Press.

Nagele, D.A. (1985). Neuropsychological inferences from a tooth brushing task: a model for understanding deficits and making interventions. *Arch. Phys. Med. Rehabil.,* **66,** 558.

National Institute of Neurological and Communicative Disorders and Stroke. (1979). *Report of the Panel on Stroke, Trauma, Regeneration, and Neoplasms.* N.I.H. Publ. No. 79-1915. Washington, D.C.: U.S. Department of Health, Education, and Welfare.

National Institue of Neurological and Communicative Disorders and Stroke. (1983a). *National Survey of Stroke.* Bethesda: U.S. Department of Health and Human Services.

National Institute of Neurological and Communicative Disorders and Stroke. (1983b). *Stroke: Hope Through Research.* N.I.H. Publ. No. 83-2222. Bethesda: National Institutes of Health.

Neistadt, M.E. (1988). Occupational therapy for adults with perceptual deficits. *Am. J. Occup. Ther.,* **42,** 434–440.

Newcombe, F. (1985). Rehabilitation in clinical neurology: neuropsychological aspects. In: J.A.M. Frederiks, ed., *Handbook of Clinical Neurology, Vol. 2(46): Neurobehavioral Disorders,* pp. 609–642. New York: Elsevier.

Novack, T.A., Satterfield, W.T., Lyons, K., Kolski, G., Hackmeyer, L., and Connor, M. (1984). Stroke onset and rehabilitation: time lag as a factor in treatment outcome. *Arch. Phys. Med. Rehabil.,* **65,** 316–319.

Prigatano, G.P. (1986). *Neuropsychological Rehabilitation After Brain Injury.* Baltimore: Johns Hopkins University Press.

Prigatano, G.P. (1988). Rehabilitation interventions after traumatic brain injury. *BNI Q.,* **4**(2), 30–37.

Raymond, M.J. (1987). Neuropsychological investigation in right hemisphere stroke: a rehabilitation case study. Presented at the Seventh Annual Meeting of the National Academy of Neuropsychologists, Chicago.

Reding, M.J., and McDowell, F. (1987). Stroke rehabilitation. *Neurol. Clin.,* **5,** 601–630.

Roth, E.J. (1988). The elderly stroke patient: principles and practices of rehabilitation management. *Topics Geriatr. Rehabil.,* **3**(4), 27–61.

Rothi, L.J., and Horner, J. (1983). Restitution and substitution: two theories of recovery with application to neurobehavioral treatment. *J. Clin. Neuropsychol.,* **5,** 73–82.

Ruckdeschel-Hibbard, M., Gordon, W.A., and Diller, L. (1986). Affective disturbances associated with brain damage. In: S. Filskov and T.J. Boll, eds., *Handbook of Clinical Neuropsychology,* Vol. 2, pp. 305–337. New York: Wiley.

Ruckdeschel-Hibbard, M., Gordon, W.A., Egelko, S., and Langer, K. (1987). Issues in the diagnosis and cognitive therapy of depression in brain-damaged individuals. In: A. Freeman and V.B. Greenwood, eds., *Cognitive Therapy: Applications in Psychiatric and Medical Settings,* pp. 183–198. New York: Human Sciences Press.

Sacks, O. (1985). *The Man Who Mistook His Wife for a Hat.* New York: Summit Books.

Schacter, D.L., and Glisky, E.L. (1986). Memory remediation: restoration, alleviation, and the acquisition of domain-specific knowledge. In: B.P. Uzzell and Y. Gross, eds., *Clinical Neuropsychology of Intervention,* pp. 257–282. Boston: Martinus Nijhoff.

Sharpless, J.W. (1982). *Mossman's A Problem-Oriented Approach to Stroke Rehabilitation,* 2nd ed. Springfield, IL: Charles C. Thomas.

Siev, E., Freishtat, B., and Zoltan, B. (1986). *Perceptual and Cognitive Dysfunction in the Adult Stroke Patient: A Manual for Evaluation and Treatment,* rev. ed. Thorofare, NJ: Slack.

Sivak, M., Hill, C.S., Henson, D.L., Butler, B.P., Silber, S.M., and Olson, P.L. (1984). Improved driving performance following perceptual training in persons with brain damage. *Arch. Phys. Med. Rehabil.,* **65,** 163–167.

Sohlberg, M.M., and Mateer, C.A. (1989). *Introduction to Cognitive Rehabilitation: Theory and Practice.* New York: Guilford Press.

Stanton, K.M., Pepping, M., Brockway, J.A., Bliss, L., Frankel, D., and Waggener, S. (1983). Wheelchair transfer training for right cerebral dysfunctions: an interdisciplinary approach. *Arch. Phys. Med. Rehabil.,* **64,** 276–280.

Starkstein, S.E., and Robinson, R.G. (1988). Lateralized emotional response following stroke. In: M. Kinsbourne, ed., *Cerebral Hemisphere Function in Depression,* pp. 23–47. Washington, D.C.: American Psychiatric Press.

Stokes, T.F., and Osnes, P.G. (1988). The developing applied technology of generalization and maintenance. In: R.H. Horner, G. Dunlap, and R.L. Koegel, eds., *Generalization and Maintenance: Life-style Changes in Applied Settings,* pp. 5–19. Baltimore: Paul H. Brookes Publishing.

Tobis, J.S. (1976). Re-evaluating the management of the stroke patient. In: A.A. Buerger and J.S. Tobis, eds., *Neurophysiologic Aspects of Rehabilitation Medicine,* pp. 319–330. Springfield, IL: Charles C Thomas.

Towle, D., Edmans, J.A., and Lincoln, N.B. (1986). Use of computer-presented games with memory-impaired stroke patients. *Clin. Rehabil.,* **2,** 303–307.

Tsvetkova, L.S. (1988). Theory and practice in rehabilitation. In: P.M. Deutsch and K.B. Fralish, eds., *Innovations in Head Injury Rehabilitation,* pp. 52-1–52-26. New York: Matthew Bender.

Wade, D.T., Parker, V., and Hewer, R.L. (1986). Memory disturbance after stroke: frequency and associated losses. *Int. Rehabil. Med.,* **8,** 60–64.

Wade, D.T., Wood, V.A., and Hewer, R.L. (1988). Recovery of cognitive function soon after stroke: a study of visual neglect, attention span and verbal recall. *J. Neurol. Neurosurg. Psychiatry,* **51,** 10–13.

Webster, J., Jones, S., Blanton, P., Gross, R., Beissel, G., and Wofford, J. (1984). Visual scanning training with stroke patients. *Behav. Ther.,* **15,** 129–143.

Webster, J.S., Cottam, G.,Gouvier, W.D., Blanton, P., Beissel, G.F., and Wofford, J. (1989). Wheelchair obstacle course performance in right cerebral vascular accident victims. *J. Clin. Exp. Neuropsychol.,* **11,** 295–310.

Wehman, P., and Moon, M.S., eds. (1988). *Vocational Rehabilitation and Supported Employment.* Baltimore: Paul H. Brookes.

Weinberg, J., Diller, L., Gordon, W., Gerstman, L., Lieberman, A., Lakin, P., Hodges, G., and Ezrachi, O. (1977). Visual scanning training effect on reading-related tasks in acquired right brain damage. *Arch. Phys. Med. Rehabil.,* **58,** 479–486.

Weinstein, E.A., and Kahn, R.L. (1955). *Denial of Illness: Symbolic and Physiological Aspects.* Springfield, IL: Charles C Thomas.

Wepman, J.M. (1951). *Recovery from Aphasia.* New York: Ronald Press.

Williams, J.M. (1987). The role of cognitive retraining in comprehensive rehabilitation. In: J.M. Williams and C.J. Long, eds., *The Rehabilitation of Cognitive Disabilities,* pp. 43–55. New York: Plenum Press.

Williams, J.M., and Long, C.J., eds. (1987). *The Rehabilitation of Cognitive Disabilities.* New York: Plenum Press.

Wilson, B. (1982). Success and failure in memory training following a cerebral vascular accident. *Cortex,* **18,** 581–594.

Wilson, B.A. (1987). *Rehabilitation of Memory.* New York: Guilford Press.

World Health Organization (1980). *International Classification of Impairments, Disabilities, and Handicaps.* Geneva: WHO.

Young, G.C., Collins, D., and Wren, M. (1983). Effect of pairing scanning training with block design training in the remediation of perceptual problems in left hemiplegics. *J. Clin. Neuropsychol.,* **3,** 201–212.

Index